W0017822

Herbs and Roots

Herbs *and* Roots

A History of Chinese Doctors
in the American Medical Marketplace

TAMARA VENIT SHELTON

Yale UNIVERSITY PRESS/NEW HAVEN & LONDON

Published with assistance from the foundation established in memory of Henry Weldon Barnes of the Class of 1882, Yale College.

Copyright © 2019 by Tamara Venit-Shelton.
All rights reserved.
This book may not be reproduced, in whole or in part, including illustrations, in any form (beyond that copying permitted by Sections 107 and 108 of the U.S. Copyright Law and except by reviewers for the public press), without written permission from the publishers.

Yale University Press books may be purchased in quantity for educational, business, or promotional use. For information, please e-mail sales.press@yale.edu (U.S. office) or sales@yaleup.co.uk (U.K. office).

Set in Minion type by Newgen North America, Austin, Texas.
Printed in the United States of America.

Library of Congress Control Number: 2019937531
ISBN 978-0-300-24361-1 (hardcover : alk. paper)

A catalogue record for this book is available from the British Library.

This paper meets the requirements of ANSI/NISO Z39.48-1992 (Permanence of Paper).
10 9 8 7 6 5 4 3 2 1

In memory of Anne Cramnik Venit (1909–2012)
and Rose May Fong (1918–2017)

Contents

Preface

Herbs and Roots: A History of Chinese Doctors in the American Medical Marketplace chronicles approximately two hundred years of traditional Chinese medicine in the United States, from the transoceanic trade of its *materia medica* in the late eighteenth century to its rediscovery and the flourishing of acupuncture in the late twentieth century. It is the first book to situate herbalism, acupuncture, and other ancient Chinese therapies squarely within the narrative of American medicine. *Herbs and Roots* is not a work of advocacy or medical science. Therefore, it does not take a position for or against the therapeutic efficacy of traditional Chinese medicine. The book's principal concern is the social history of the individuals and institutions that shaped the spread of ancient healing traditions in a new place. While people of many national origins, races, and ethnicities practiced Chinese therapies in the United States, this book focuses on practitioners of Chinese descent and the unique relationship that they had with American law and politics, particularly early experiments in exclusion and changing diplomatic relations between the United States and China. It also considers the interplay between traditional Chinese medicine and Western-style scientific medicine. Practitioners of these different medical knowledge systems professionalized, competed, and collaborated over the course of the nineteenth and twentieth centuries. The story that this book recounts will appeal equally to readers curious about the experiences of Chinese immigrants in the United States and to readers interested in the social history of American medicine.

Acknowledgments

I started researching Chinese herbalists while on the faculty at Reed College, where one of my students, Jillian Jackson, introduced me to Ing Hay and Kam Wah Chung in John Day, Oregon. Her interest in the state's preservation of the historic apothecary led me toward years of work that became this book. Beth Howlett, a faculty member and administrator at the Oregon College of Oriental Medicine, graciously shared the resources of her research group, which translates the prescriptions written by "Doc Hay." At Reed, I benefited from the mentorship and encouragement of my colleague Jacqueline Dirks, and with her help I became the recipient of a fellowship at the Oregon Historical Society that allowed me to conduct preliminary research. I thank the editor of its journal, Eliza Canty-Jones, for her early support and enthusiasm.

I am enormously grateful to Gilbert Hom, a dogged researcher with a genuine passion for the history of Chinese herbalists in the United States. His guidance and generosity gave shape to the core of this book. My thanks also go to archivists at the Huntington Library, Wing Luke Museum, Ethnic Studies Library at the University of California at Berkeley, Stanford Medical School Library, the University of California at San Francisco Archives, and the Chinese Historical Society of Southern California, with special acknowledgment to Eugene Moy.

I also extend my gratitude to my San Francisco Chinatown relatives—especially Corinne Fong Venit, Priscilla Leong Genis, Laurie Chang Kum, and Ron Lee—who connected me with the descendants of Chinese American herbalists.

Several individuals shared their personal and family histories with me: Morton Barke, Pedro Chan, Anna Cho-Wong, Anna Don, Calvin Fong, and Jane Leung Larson. Victoria Maizes and Andrew Weil of the Center for Integrative Medicine at the University of Arizona talked me through the evolving place of integrative medicine in contemporary medical education. My special gratitude goes to Ka-Kit Hui of the Center for East-West Medicine at UCLA for extending to me so much of his time.

This project could not have come to fruition without the financial support of several foundations and research libraries. This research was assisted by a Frederick Burkhardt Residential Fellowship for Recently Tenured Scholars from the American Council of Learned Societies. My sincere thanks go as well to the Huntington Library and the College of Physicians of Philadelphia. At Claremont McKenna College, funds from the Dean of Faculty, the Gould Center for the Humanities, and the Center for Innovation and Entrepreneurship have enabled me to complete this scholarship.

Student research assistants at Claremont McKenna have helped me comb through newspapers and compile bibliographies in English and Chinese. To Evelyn Linyue Chen, Yi Luo, Frances MacKercher, and Yizhou (Jack) Tao, I extend my fond appreciation.

Numerous friends and colleagues have shared comments on early drafts, sent me obscure citations for Chinese herbalists, and reassured me that I was writing something that might one day have an audience. Matthew Klingle was wonderfully and energetically helpful from this project's start to its finish. His perspective and advice on the field of environmental health and the publishing process have been invaluable to me. My gratitude also goes to Shana Bernstein, Matthew Morse Booker, Connie Chiang, and Colin Fisher as well as my Claremont McKenna history department colleagues, especially Glen Cooper, Lily Geismer, and Heather Ferguson, who all provided concrete feedback as my manuscript took shape over the years. My former graduate advisers, Richard

White and Gordon Chang, probably thought they got rid of me when I finished my Ph.D. more than a decade ago, but I have continued to rely on their insightful questions and guidance anyway.

I also thank the many colleagues who enabled me to test out ideas (however half-baked) at conferences, writing workshops, and invited talks, including Linda Barnes, Sharla Fett, Mark Fiege, Lori Flores, Jane Hong, Moon-Ho Jung, Beth Lew-Williams, Christof Mauch, Catherine McNeur, Natalia Mehlman-Petrzela, Char Miller, Gregg Mittman, Nancy Tomes, Rachel St. John, Louis Warren, and Mei Zhan. I extend particular gratitude to William Deverell, Steven Hindle, and the twenty-five long-term fellows in residence at the Huntington Library in the 2017–2018 academic year. The community and collegiality I experienced while in residence with the USC-Huntington Institute for California and the West were intellectually invigorating and inspiring. Alan Kraut gave the manuscript a final read and offered substantive and helpful comments before it made its final journey to the publisher.

My most heartfelt thanks go to Cameron Shelton, the best partner I could ask for in this crazy juggling act, and to our beloved children—Evelyn, Damian, and Elliott—the three rings of our family circus.

My grandmother Rose May Fong introduced me to traditional Chinese medicine long before I had any academic interest in the subject. To treat a common cold, she steeped some herbs in hot water, which I drank and promptly threw up. "That's how you know it's working," she said with a casual but nonetheless authoritative shrug. I dedicate this book to her memory and to that of my other grandmother, Anne Cramnik Venit. They inspired my love of history.

Note on Terminology

When discussing the nineteenth century and first half of the twentieth century, I use the terms "regular medicine" or "Western-style scientific medicine" to refer to therapeutic principles and practices that emerged from the study of anatomy and principles of empiricism and universalism popularized in eighteenth- and nineteenth-century Europe and transmitted to the United States. In the American context, "regular medicine" or "scientific medicine" became the system most frequently and widely sanctioned by medical professional associations of doctors and public health institutions, state licensing boards, and major medical schools. I use "irregular medicine" as a catchall for medical knowledge systems that existed at the margins or outside of the "regular" community. I prefer "regular" and "irregular" to "orthodox" and "unorthodox" or "allopathic" and "alternative" because of the etymological link between "regular" and "regulation" and its close connection to "standardization." Since the end of the eighteenth century, Western-style medical scientists have been leaders and foot soldiers in movements to regulate and standardize medical practices in the United States.

"Regular" and "irregular" are admittedly problematic and ahistorical terms. What distinguished regular from irregular medicine was dynamic, contingent, and not always apparent to patients. Yet such terms become impossible to avoid. I have tried to indicate in the text where there was slippage between these categories. During and after World War II, regular medicine more systematically incorporated the life sciences into clinical practice, giving the terms "biomedicine" or "biomedical science" meaning for that era. The last chapters of the book, concerning the post–World War II period, therefore use "biomedicine" where appropriate.

Note on Transliterations

I have transliterated Chinese words into pinyin Romanization except in the case of individuals or businesses most commonly known by names based in other systems of Romanization. In the case of place names like Peking/Beijing or Canton/Guangzhou/Guangdong, I have used the transliteration that would have been most common for the period under discussion, with the alternative Romanization in parentheses.

In the Chinese custom, family names precede given names, but European American patients often called doctors by their given name. Thus, Tom Foo Yuen was known as "Foo"; his cousin Tom Leung advertised as "T. Leung"; and Ing Hay went by "Doc Hay." In many instances, Chinese doctors worked under pseudonyms that were more easily pronounced by their American patients or recognizably similar to famous doctors' names. In this book, I principally identify Chinese doctors by the names they used with their non-Chinese patients and in their English- and Spanish-language advertisements, and wherever possible, I mention other names they assumed.

Chinese names present a unique challenge in the context of American immigration history. Immigration restrictions often prioritized entry of blood relations. To circumvent the law, Chinese in the United States adopted "paper sons and daughters," fictive relations who changed their surnames to avoid detection. Although immigration records and other sources sometimes include the multiple aliases taken on by Chinese immigrants, it is not always possible to determine the true names of Chinese doctors through these many layers of identity.

Herbs and Roots

Introduction

Curiosity no longer bothered Moy Yuk. In the fall of 1885, when a visiting reporter from the *Arizona Sentinel* appeared at his doorstep, Moy simply smiled and readied himself to answer the usual litany of questions.[1] Peddling Chinese medicine in Chicago, Moy had grown accustomed to receiving travelogue writers and gawking tourists alongside health-seekers at his apothecary. Wherever there were Chinese immigrants, there were Chinese herbalists, and Moy counted himself among the few who tended to the health of Chicago's Chinatown residents, a community underserved by American physicians and hospitals, to say the least. In Chicago, the Chinese population was small—about seven hundred people, mostly men who had built railroads to the eastern terminus and never left.[2] Back in China, doctors like Moy would have apprenticed in a family shop specializing in one proprietary remedy, but in the United States, they had to become general practitioners. They brought books with them to learn how to compound medicine for all manner of ailments, to set broken bones, and—in some cases—to deliver babies and provide abortions. When their neighbors, friends, and relatives succumbed to their sufferings, doctors like Moy signed their death certificates even though they knew that a combination of professional territorialism and

1

pervasive nativism would lead the State Board of Health to reject the opinion of a "Chinaman."[3]

Not all the work Moy did for his community was strictly medical. A Chinese herbalist might also serve as Chinatown's postmaster, banker, translator, labor broker, and defender. Legally and extralegally, doctors like Moy made it possible for the Chinese to endure and survive in America. In the 1880s, anti-Chinese violence was as rampant in Chicago as it was in other parts of the country. Impoverished and overcrowded, Chinatowns attracted vice industries, and the police raided Chinese homes and businesses that may or may not have been opium dens or brothels. Meanwhile, the nascent field of bacteriology gave public health officials scientific cover to quarantine, expel, and otherwise control Chinese bodies. By the 1880s, an anti-Chinese working-class movement that began in California had spread east to Chicago. Local trades unions passed resolutions against the employment of any Chinese laborers in 1882, the same year that the U.S. Congress restricted Chinese immigration with the passage of the nation's first law targeting Chinese laborers entering the country.[4]

In this historical moment, the touristic appeal of the Chinatown apothecary may seem incongruous, but it was not. In the logic of anti-Chinese racism, forces of repulsion and attraction were closely paired. The *Arizona Sentinel* reporter who stumbled across the threshold of Moy Yuk's Chicago apothecary in the fall of 1885 aimed to feed the lurid fascination of his readers back home. For the Chinese herbalist, prying eyes and probing inquiries would have been relatively tolerable when compared to the many hardships and dangers of being Chinese in America in the 1880s. To his visitor, Moy patiently explained the differences between Chinese and "American" medicine. Both schools had their strengths, Moy conceded; Chinese doctors were superior diagnosticians while American doctors were better surgeons. Moy emphasized that Chinese and American physicians were all "scientists," not quacks, and he criticized American physicians for their "arrogant assertions that nothing was to be learned from the sages of the Orient." In this way, Moy defended his community and his professional integrity. At the same time, however, he gamely played the part of the "Oriental sage" for his Arizona visitor. He spun tales of miraculous Chinese remedies made of pulverized pearls and known only to students of the "unbroken teachings of thousands of years past."[5] Moy's time in America had taught him how to fulfill American fantasies of Chinese healing arts as decadent, ancient, and irrevocably other. In the United States, Chinese doctors were servants equally to the realities of immigrant life and the expectations of the Orientalist imagination.

This book is about men and women like Moy Yuk. Chinese medicine has a long history in the United States, dating back to America's colonial period and extending up to the present. Well before mass emigration from China to the United States began, Chinese *materia medica* crossed the oceans, in both directions: Chinese medicinal teas and herbs came West while Appalachian ginseng went East. In the early nineteenth century, medical missionaries to China assimilated Chinese herbalism into their practices and published reports that circulated among American readers. Beginning in the 1850s, Chinese immigrants came to the United States in significant numbers and transplanted their health practices, sometimes quite literally by propagating medicinal plants in their adopted home. Chinese doctors established businesses that catered to both Chinese and non-Chinese patients. They marketed their services in English-, Spanish-, and Chinese-language newspapers distributed in urban and rural areas across the United States. Although acupuncture is the modality most commonly associated with Chinese medicine in today's medical marketplace, up until the 1970s Chinese healers in the United States typically specialized in diagnosis by pulse (or pulsology) and prescriptions derived from mineral, zoological, and botanical (or herbal) sources. This book chronicles roughly two hundred years of Chinese medicine as a system of knowledge, therapies, and *materia medica* brought to the United States and transformed by immigrants, doctors, and patients as well as missionaries, scientists, and merchants. Over time, Chinese medicine—along with other medical knowledge systems deemed "irregular," "alternative," or "unorthodox"—both facilitated and undermined the consolidation of medical authority among formally trained, Western-style medical scientists.[6]

Throughout this book, I use the term "traditional Chinese medicine" or "classical Chinese medicine" as an umbrella for a wide array of therapies, some dating back thousands of years and ranging from herbalism to acupuncture, moxibustion (the burning of medicinal plants on or very close to the skin), cupping, faith healing, bone-setting and facial analysis, massage, dietary counsel, and exercise.[7] What we consider Chinese medicine finds its origins in many Asian cultures, religions, and philosophies. A rich scholarship on traditional medicine in China has laid the groundwork for this study of its dissemination to the United States. Historians and medical anthropologists have characterized Chinese healing traditions as tremendously heterogeneous and dynamic while insisting on a core set of principles that unify a system of medical knowledge.[8] The Han Dynasty (206 BCE–220 CE) was an important period of consolidation and canonization of the conceptual foundations of Chinese medicine.[9] By the third century BCE, theories of health and illness clustered around the central conception of the universe as balanced by the opposing, invisible forces of *yin* and *yang* (陰陽). Shamanic healers, believing the human body to be a microcosm of the universe, based their healing rituals on the doctrine of *yinyang*. By the first century BCE, a competing school of thought emerged that was organized by systems of correspondence. In this school, there were not two elements in balance but five: metal, wood, water, fire, and soil. References to earthly substances may make this doctrine (*wu-xing*, 五行) seem akin to Western traditions of "nature cures," but it should not be interpreted so simplistically. Like *yin* and *yang*, the five phases were largely invisible and abstract. Tsou Yen, the chronicler and perhaps creator of the five phases doctrine, used metal, wood, water, fire, and soil as symbols to represent those forces, but they did not have any direct relationship to their material counterparts. Historian Paul Unschuld has argued that "five phases" is a more appropriate translation of *wu-xing* because *xing* implies change and movement.[10] These core concepts— balance, correspondence, holism, and particularism—draw together the many modalities that have evolved and flourished, floundered and vanished in China and beyond.

While *Herbs and Roots* begins its story in the late eighteenth century and ends in the near present, its primary concern lies within the late nineteenth and early twentieth centuries—what historians often call the "long Progressive Era," a period when Chinese doctors became increasingly active in the American medical marketplace. These decades witnessed important changes in immigration law, scientific understandings of disease, and medical regulation. In 1882, Congress passed the first in a series of exclusion acts targeting immigrants from China, which caused a decline in the Chinese population in the United States over the subsequent decades. A shrinking stock of co-ethnic customers may have compelled some Chinese herbalists to cast a wider net for non-Chinese patients. Around the same time, a new science of disease transmission that located its source in microscopic organisms called germs gained traction among elite, formally trained physicians. The germ theory of disease worked in concert with nativism to embolden government officials targeting immigrant communities in the name of public health. Such efforts unfolded in the context of a broader campaign by members of the American Medical Association (AMA) to "regularize" medicine according to their professional standards. In collaboration with AMA physicians, state and local officials introduced public licensing exams that concentrated on medical science and pharmacology and imposed fines and jail sentences on doctors practicing without a license.

In the Progressive Era, practitioners of traditional Chinese medicine, as a racialized embodiment of irregular medicine, became a useful foil for regular physicians struggling to articulate the superiority of their practices. The popular association between Chinese doctors and Orientalist stereotypes of primitivism—cultivated in Chinatown travelogues and sensationalist journalism—provided American medical scientists with a vocabulary to describe their work as modern, scientific, and superior, and their competitors as ancient, unscientific, and therefore inferior. American Orientalist attitudes emerged out of the nineteenth-century history of trade, diplomacy, and conflict between the United States and its Asian neighbors around the Pacific Rim, especially China, and had much in common with an older, European-style of Orientalism, first developed in the Middle East. Orientalism constructed an image of the "Orient" populated by racially inferior people, possessed of a backwards and morally depraved culture, and destined to submit to the more powerful, racially fit, and morally upright "Occident." As an ideology, American Orientalism justified the supremacy of a "masculine, modern" America over a "feminine, primitive" Asia.[11] Such assumptions extended to the realm of Chinese medicine: if Chinese people were primitive, so was Chinese medical knowledge. Racist stereotypes and discriminatory policies made Chinese doctors the target for outside scrutiny, persecution, and contempt. The state refused them the right to sit for licensing exams and then arrested them for practicing without a license. Border control detained their family members, coworkers, and supplies, and denied them entry.

Yet criticism of Chinese medicine could constitute its allure, particularly for American patients skeptical of Western-style medical science. The Progressive Era might not have seemed like the most opportune time for Chinese herbalists to get into the American health care business, but the AMA monopoly on the medical marketplace was far from complete. Traditional Chinese medicine flourished in the spaces where regular medicine had not yet consolidated its control, and Chinese doctors did not always fight the racialized expectations imposed on them.[12] In fact, Chinese doctors often "self-Orientalized," using racist tropes to sell their services to non-Chinese patients. In their English-language advertisements, Chinese doctors pictured themselves amid images of dragons, pagodas, and scroll-toting Mandarin scholars, and they described their practice as ancient and mystical. What regular physicians labeled unscientific or backwards, Chinese physicians celebrated as closer to an essential, unchanging, and universally accessible nature than Western-style scientific medicine would ever be. That strategy enabled Chinese doctors to survive, and even thrive, in the American medical marketplace. Categories of social difference—in particular, the Orientalist assumption of Chinese racial inferiority—created hierarchies of medical knowledge in the American medical marketplace, but it did not do so in predictable ways. Western-style scientific medicine did not always come out on top.

Chinese doctors in the United States constituted a small, but significant cohort. In any given year, there were probably no more than two hundred practitioners of Chinese medicine working in the United States, but they assumed outsized importance within and outside their immigrant community.[13] Chinese doctors took up residence in nearly every state in the union (as well as Canada and Mexico), but unsurprisingly, they were more numerous in the places where Chinese immigrants concentrated, particularly in California and the West. To some

extent, place-specific circumstances shaped the professional possibilities for Chinese doctors. Local chapters of the AMA persecuted Chinese "quacks" with varying levels of vigor. Competition among herbalists was steeper in San Francisco and Los Angeles, where the Chinese
were more numerous, compared to other cities or rural areas. Yet there
were also similarities in medical cultures and institutions that cut across
regions. Through real and fictive kinship networks that spanned state
borders, Chinese doctors exchanged medical and cultural knowledge.
They confronted a common set of legal challenges concerning immigration restrictions and medical licensure, and they competed in a marketplace that medical scientists increasingly monopolized.

Some practitioners of Chinese medicine found extraordinary
success among a heterogeneous clientele; others failed and faded into
obscurity. The perception of therapeutic efficacy was certainly a factor
in the survival of Chinese medicine in the American medical marketplace and its growing popularity today. Patients would not have chosen
Chinese medicine if they did not experience relief from their ailments
or cures for their afflictions. Biographies of individual herbalists have
praised the efficacy (and perhaps superiority) of their treatments over
Western-style medical science. In a biography of Ing Hay, an herbalist
who practiced in John Day, Oregon, Jeffrey G. Barlow and Christine
Richardson assert that "Doc Hay" had a greater rate of success than did
other doctors in eastern Oregon.[14] Based on patient testimonials, letters,
and local lore, Barlow and Richardson portray Hay as almost preternat-
urally gifted.[15] While other authors have been less inclined to take tales
of miraculous cures at face value, they have similarly focused on glowing
patient testimonials to explain the widespread appeal of Chinese medicine outside of its ethnic community.[16]

This book does not focus on arguments about therapeutic efficacy.
First, there is a lack of useable historical evidence in this regard. Patient
testimonials exist in advertisements and lawsuits with expected biases.
Private correspondence between herbalists and their non-Chinese patients is scarce and inconclusive. Perhaps another historian will one
day discover a trove of patient diaries or letters that permits a robust
consideration of traditional Chinese medicine's effects on the American
consumer's body and consumer choice. At present, however, we have

only modern laboratory and clinical experiments to apply retrospectively to earlier generations of patient populations. As a historian, I am unqualified to assess medical science. For the purposes of this book, I pass no judgment on the merits of traditional Chinese therapies. Instead, *Herbs and Roots* analyzes the historical context that conditioned perceptions of traditional Chinese medicine. It focuses on cultures and politics that framed debates over therapeutic efficacy and perhaps made non-Chinese patients receptive to trying traditional Chinese medicine.

Historiography

As a social history of Chinese Americans and Chinese doctors in the United States, this book synthesizes and expands on a body of scholarship that has been primarily biographical. Among the hundreds of men and women who practiced traditional Chinese medicine in the United States, only a handful of men left behind more than a few fragmentary records. Two of them have been the subject of monographic biographies: Ing Hay of John Day, Oregon, and Yitang Chang (Yick Hong Chung) of Los Angeles, California.[17] In Boise, Idaho, C. K. Ah Fong—one of the few practitioners of Chinese medicine to receive a license from the state—similarly left behind a record of his business that has been the subject of several peer-reviewed essays.[18] Broader histories of nineteenth-century Chinese immigration to the United States sometimes include discussions of herbalists as a type of merchant and their responsibilities within the immigrant community.[19] *Herbs and Roots* draws together disparate biographies of individual herbalists and builds on them with the scraps and traces of others like them. Taking a wider perspective on Chinese doctors in the United States, the book offers a sense of the scale of their impact both within their community and on the American medical marketplace. It also aims to uncover the commonalities and variation among their lived experiences across regions.

To date, the scholarship on Chinese medicine in the United States has emphasized how Chinese medicine allowed its practitioners to resist assimilation by remaining financially, intellectually, and culturally connected to their homeland. In his biography of Yitang Chang and subsequent essays on Chinese herbalists, Haiming Liu repeatedly emphasizes

INTRODUCTION 9

the "resilience" of their medical traditions and their achievements as cultural ambassadors to American patient-consumers. According to Liu, the success of Chinese medicine in the American medical marketplace is evidence of the doctors' resistance "to being channeled into racially defined occupations such as laundries and restaurants."[20] Chinese immigrant doctors were undoubtedly courageous, creative, and entrepreneurial, and they won the respect and patronage of non-Chinese patients despite a hostile cultural and political climate, but their occupation was just as racially defined as that of Chinese launderers and restauranteurs. Biographies and histories that celebrate Chinese doctors' triumphs over adversity fail to acknowledge how Chinese doctors became complicit in the perpetuation of anti-Asian stereotypes. As members of the merchant class, herbalists played a role similar to the Tape family discussed in Mae M. Ngai's *The Lucky Ones: One Family and the Extraordinary Invention of Chinese America*. Like the Tapes, Chinese herbalists often helped Chinese immigrants navigate American institutions and customs, and like the Tapes, they acted as "culture brokers," whose liminality positioned them to profit from rampant anti-Chinese discrimination.[21]

Chinese doctors depended on the logic of American Orientalism to sell their services. *Herbs and Roots* draws on the historical scholarship on American Orientalism, which has largely considered its development through cultural artifacts and trade between the United States and China. John Kuo Wei Tchen and Mari Yoshihara have considered the long history of European American fascination with "Chinese things, ideas, and people" from the late eighteenth to the early twentieth centuries. While the American elite had a long history of collecting Chinese and Japanese objects and studying Eastern religions, the appeal of "Orientalia" became a more widespread cultural phenomenon by the end of the nineteenth century. Chinese and Japanese consumer goods were available to mass markets through mail-order catalogs and department stores. At the same time, World Fairs and traveling shows popularized "Oriental" arts, ideas, and religions. The contours of American Orientalism shifted with the changing relationship between the United States and China, and Tchen claims that by the end of the nineteenth century, "the fascination with Chinese goods and values had been eclipsed by attitudes of fear and loathing."[22] This was demonstrably untrue for

Chinese medicine, whose popularity ascended at the turn of the twentieth century.

Herbs and Roots draws on foundational work by Henry Yu, Karen J. Leong, Judy Tzu-Chun Wu, and Emma Teng as they have considered how Asian Americans contributed to the reimagining of "the Orient" in the early twentieth century. These historians have revealed the ways that Chinese in the United States appropriated Orientalist tropes to serve their own agendas in different spheres: academia, politics and commerce, and entertainment.[23] In many ways, the experiences of this generation foreshadowed those of their educated, affluent counterparts during the Cold War. By the mid-twentieth century, American Orientalism made Chinese civilizational deficiencies and Communist corruption discursively equivalent, but elite Chinese in the United States still found ways to turn racialist thinking to their advantage. As Ellen D. Wu, Madeline Yuan-yin Hsu, and Scott Kurashige have argued, American political and diplomatic imperatives depended on the invention of Asian Americans as a "model minority." Appearances of their social acceptance and upward social mobility served as evidence of the benevolence of American capitalism, but their assimilation could never be complete. They derived privileges and status as "model minorities" and "assimilating others" that simultaneously reinforced their permanent marginality within American society.[24] *Herbs and Roots* locates practitioners of traditional Chinese medicine in this history of elite Chinese interactions with the Asia of the American imagination. Herbalists were not simply defenders of their community and their heritage. Their livelihood depended on their capacity to embody and sustain American expectations of Oriental alterity.

As a history of American medicine, *Herbs and Roots* interrogates the social and cultural contexts in which Western-style scientific medicine gained meaning and asserted authority. In this way, it engages with scholarship on boundary conflicts between science and pseudoscience.[25] Historians interested in the social and cultural construction of medical authority in the modern era have written extensively about the sectarian wars between regular and irregular physicians. There is widespread consensus among historians that, over the course of the nineteenth century, scientific medicine developed instruments and theories that distinguished its practice from the alternatives. From the market perspective, however, that technological advantage only mattered where regular physicians could convince patient-consumers of the superiority of their theories and methods. The boundary between regular and irregular was inherently porous, unstable, and contingent. Regular and irregular physicians thus had to engage in an ongoing discursive rehearsal of difference. Popular media, academic journals, advertisements, and public reports mapped, remapped, and gave meaning to the boundaries between medical sects.[26] As Hans A. Baer has shown in *Biomedicine and Alternative Healing Systems in America*, Western-style scientific medicine consolidated and professionalized in the same era as homeopathy, Christian Science, hydropathy, osteopathy, and chiropractic medicine because these knowledge systems were mutually constitutive. Regular and irregular medical sects defined themselves in contradistinction, each asserting its authority in the spaces left absent by the others.[27] In *Nature Cures: The History of Alternative Medicine in America*, James C. Whorton argues that naturalism has been an important boundary marker. In their war against scientific medical hegemony, irregular physicians staked their claim to "nature" as the basis of their cultural authority.[28]

Herbs and Roots argues that, over more than two centuries, Chinese medical knowledge, *materia medica,* and practitioners helped give meaning to the assemblage of theories and practices that became characteristic of Western-style scientific medicine. Yet, histories of irregular medicine in the United States have largely ignored Chinese doctors in the American medical marketplace or have only acknowledged their contribution when discussing the American (re)discovery of acupuncture in the 1970s. Chinese herbalism only occupies two pages in Volney Steele's *Bleed, Blister, and Purge,* a history of "frontier" medicine. James Whorton situates the rising popularity of Chinese acupuncture within the holistic medicine movement in the 1970s but makes no mention of its practice in earlier periods. Likewise, Susan E. Cayleff's recent history of naturopathy solely references the post-1970s integration of Chinese herbalism and acupuncture into naturopath education.[29] Irregular medical traditions developed by non-Americans and shared with the United States via overseas immigration have not been similarly overlooked. For example, historians of medicine have treated homeopathy, created by

German physician Samuel Hahnemann and spread to the United States by German immigrants in the early nineteenth century, as a fixture in the early history of alternative medicine in America. Indeed, in his seminal work, *Homeopathy in America,* Martin Kaufman describes its history as the "history of every unorthodox sect" in the United States and gives scant attention to its origins abroad.[30] *Herbs and Roots* is thus an important corrective. The intersecting histories of traditional Chinese medicine and American scientific medicine in the Progressive Era United States demonstrate how regular and irregular physicians depended on one another to articulate their value propositions and authoritative claims in a pluralistic marketplace and society.

The history of public health is also an important context for this work. The success of Chinese doctors in the American medical marketplace depended not only on their appeal among American patients but also on their ability to overcome associations between Chinese spaces and bodies and epidemic disease. In the nineteenth century, the threat of contagion in urban spaces was constant, and periodic flare-ups of smallpox, plague, typhoid, cholera, yellow fever, and other infectious diseases created demand for centralized control. In the Progressive Era, public health bureaucracies—typically staffed by formally trained medical professionals—experimented with sanitation, quarantine, and other public health initiatives in immigrant urban enclaves. Densely populated and under-resourced, these communities suffered a disproportionate burden of environmental health hazards, and they rarely possessed the economic or political capital to resist such impositions. Alan M. Kraut's *Silent Travelers: Germs, Genes, and the "Immigrant Menace"* argues that by the turn of the twentieth century, Western-style scientific medicine became a "weapon" that Anglo-Saxon nativists deployed to "defend [their race] against the intrusion of those it regarded as an inferior breed."[31]

In the late nineteenth and early twentieth centuries, residents of San Francisco's Chinatown were particularly beleaguered by local, state, and federal efforts to enact a regime of physical regulation and containment. The conflation of "Oriental" difference with diseased bodies by public health bureaucracies has been the subject of numerous historical articles and monographs.[32] In *Contagious Divides: Epidemics and Race in San*

Francisco's Chinatown, Nayan Shah links the construction of white racial citizenship to anxieties about disease contagion. According to Shah, the science of public health at the turn of the twentieth century lent "legitimacy and plausibility" to the marginalization and exclusion of Chinese men and women from the American body politic.[33] Guenter B. Risse's *Plague, Fear, and Politics in San Francisco's Chinatown* offers a detailed portrait of the 1900 outbreak of bubonic plague in San Francisco to reveal how Chinatown merchants and diplomats preserved a degree of autonomy for their communities by manipulating internal discord among city, state, and federal officials. The politics of disease etiology and eradication extended beyond the mayor's office or the State Board of Health. It included Chinatown residents—particularly the elite—who participated in the process of defining their neighborhood as healthy or sickly according to Western-style scientific medical norms.[34]

Yet for Risse and Shah, Chinese doctors are ciphers. They appear only wherever they came into the view of local or state officials. In *Contagious Divides,* the main historical actors are white bureaucrats and physicians, not the Chinese men and women they policed. By comparison, Risse devotes more attention to Chinese diplomats and merchants, although not herbalists. *Herbs and Roots* explores how herbalists interacted with public health officials in both combative and collaborative ways but contextualizes that interaction in a longer and larger historical relationship between traditional Chinese and Western-style scientific medicine. Public health crises were just one moment of contact in that relationship. Non-Chinese patients' consumption of Chinese medicine ran counter to the officialized construction of Chinatowns as sites of filth and epidemic disease. The successes of Chinese medical entrepreneurs are evidence of the lack of consensus around the science of bacteriology and the effects of an enduring strain of anti-authoritarianism that has characterized American medical cultures.

The often subtle but meaningful shifts in the therapeutic practices of traditional Chinese medicine as it adapted to conditions in the United States have been the subject of prodigious scholarship by anthropologists including Paul D. Buell, Linda L. Barnes, and Mei Zhan, as well as archaeologists across the American West and British Columbia.[35] At the Oregon College of Oriental Medicine, Beth Howlett leads a translation team analyzing prescriptions written by Ing Hay in John Day, Oregon.[36] To this work, *Herbs and Roots* adds the perspective of environmental history. As a field, U.S. environmental history has typically been concerned with large-scale transformations of the nonhuman natural world by human activity. These dramatic alterations to the environment have led historians to ask important questions about the relationship between human society and nonhuman nature. The relationship has not been strictly material but rather has also been shaped by culture; environmental historians have studied the way that ideas about nature, especially those prompted by capitalist imperatives, have affected policies and practices.[37] More recently, there has been a historiographic turn toward contemplating human health as an important vector through which people, as individuals and as groups, interact with nature. In scholarship by Conevery Bolton Valencius, Gregg Mitman, Linda Nash, Nancy Langston and others, environmental historians have begun to understand the dialectical relationship between American landscapes and human health. Over time, societies have settled and shaped environments to promote wellness, and environments have responded, although not always in anticipated ways.[38]

As an environmental history of Chinese medicine in the United States, this book defines nature in three ways. First, nature was a material, trans-Pacific environment where practitioners procured, distributed, and consumed medicinal plants, animals, and minerals. At the same time, "Nature" helped draw the distinction between modern, scientific "regular" medicine and antimodern, unscientific "irregular" medicine, a process that reached a moment of crisis in the Progressive Era. Finally, *Herbs and Roots* considers the uses of nature as a reflection of the racialization of traditional health practices co-created by Chinese doctors and their American patient-consumers. Attention to the material and social meanings of nature points toward not only the physical environment in which Chinese immigrant herbalists made medicine but also the problematic discourse of "natural medicine" that emerged as a critique of scientific medicine in the nineteenth century. As James Whorton has argued in his book *Nature Cures,* in the United States the historically persistent coupling of irregular medicine—including traditional Chinese medicine—with the "natural," and scientific medicine with its opposite, has impeded conversation and collaboration between Western-style medical scientists and practitioners of other medical knowledge systems.[39]

Overview of Chapters

Chapter 1 begins with an examination of the transmission of Chinese medical knowledge and *materia medica* to the United States in the colonial period and early republic. Colonial Americans were, to varying degrees, familiar with Chinese medicine. Chinese *materia medica*—including ginseng, rhubarb, cassia (cardamom), and camphor—were vital to American international trade and integral to American habits of self-dosing. Colonial Americans were part of a larger European world with a longstanding fascination for all things Chinese. Early modern European observations of Chinese medicine circulated in the British colonies of North America as part of historical and philosophical texts. In the early nineteenth century, American and European medical professionals began to make their way to China as missionaries. They studied, reported, and sometimes adopted Chinese therapeutic practices and principles. Their reports primarily justified their intervention in China and upheld their claims to scientific authority, but they nonetheless became a major conduit through which Chinese medical knowledge first flowed to the United States. In the early nineteenth century, the trans-Pacific crossings of medical science and authority became entangled with the United States' imperial interests in China and an emergent American Orientalist imagination.

In the second and third chapters, I consider how Chinese doctors, who began immigrating to the United States in the 1850s, served Chinese and non-Chinese patients. Chinese doctors were present wherever Chinese men and women lived and worked, and in the late nineteenth and early twentieth centuries, they played a variety of roles within their community. They were, of course, medical practitioners and educators, training successive generations of their biological and adopted kin to attend to the health care needs of their community. Chinese doctors also typically assumed the responsibilities of grocer, labor broker, and translator. Chinatown apothecaries were not only drugstores but recreational and religious centers and post offices as well. As part of the merchant class, they often possessed moderate wealth and had the ability to extend individual loans and make charitable donations. After Chinese exclusion raised the barriers to entry for non-merchants, Chinese doctors coached their fellow immigrants on the new and complex requirements for getting into the United States. They sponsored applications and sheltered new arrivals in their homes. Some likely participated in the elaborate forgery and smuggling networks that permitted Chinese people to circumvent exclusion. Trans-Pacific networks of knowledge, supplies, and money supported Chinese American apothecaries, and chapter 2 traces connections observable in the United States, where Chinese doctors engaged with American institutions and regulations.[40]

Outside of their communities, Chinese doctors played a role more narrowly defined by Orientalist attitudes. Chapter 3 demonstrates how Chinese doctors regularly cared for non-Chinese patients, especially in the decades after exclusionary immigration policies diminished their co-ethnic clientele. To bridge the linguistic and cultural divide with non-Chinese patients, Chinese physicians implemented a variety of business strategies. For some Chinese doctors, American patients came to comprise the majority of their practice. The popularity of Chinese medicine, particularly among middle-class and affluent patient-consumers, ran counter to public health officials' campaigns to quarantine and control Chinatowns as sources of epidemic disease. Chinese doctors sometimes relocated their offices outside of Chinese neighborhoods to assuage concerns about contagion, but they more commonly stayed in ethnic enclaves, and their success was at least partly due to American patients' skepticism about the new science of public health. Moreover, this chapter argues that engaging a Chinese physician was, in many ways, a natural extension of the service economy in which Chinese labor was prevalent, particularly in the American West. In the late nineteenth century, consulting a Chinese physician for intimate, physical advice may have seemed akin to the other kinds of transactions non-Chinese customers had with Chinese service providers. As cooks, servants, restauranteurs, grocers, and launderers, Chinese people regularly entered into close bodily contact with non-Chinese customers.

Chapter 4 chronicles the rise of regular medicine and its implications for Chinese doctors at the turn of the twentieth century. As the meanings of Western-style medical science gradually consolidated, standardized licensing requirements formalized the distinction between regular and irregular medicine. Although many Chinese physicians presented degrees from Chinese medical colleges, their qualifications carried little weight among professional societies and state boards of health. Largely excluded from public licensing, Chinese medicine became part of an evolving category of medical knowledge systems labeled "irregular." When irregular physicians resisted regulation, Chinese physicians found themselves caught in the crossfire of a sectarian war. They were arrested and prosecuted for practicing without a license alongside naturopaths, abortionists, and other unorthodox practitioners. Regular physicians used Chinese medicine to explain the differences between irregular and regular medicine to the American public. As a target of persecution and as a rhetorical device, Chinese medicine helped define Western-style scientific medicine and legitimate the authority of regular doctors in the late nineteenth and early twentieth centuries.

The fifth chapter examines how Chinese doctors combated discriminatory licensing and other medically related policies in the early twentieth century. Chinese doctors defended their businesses through a number of public channels: in judicial and legislative proceedings, in newspaper interviews, and in printed advertisements. In the courtroom of public opinion and the actual courtroom, anti-Chinese racism denied them the protections their businesses needed, but it also presented an opportunity. They defended themselves by reappropriating and reversing the meanings of the Orientalist stereotypes used to justify discriminatory policies. Such defensive strategies offer a window onto the relations of power that shaped the lived experiences of Chinese immigrants and, more broadly, that affected matters of human health care in Progressive Era America.

Most histories and biographies of Chinese doctors in the United States vault over the decades between the 1930s and 1970s. Compared to the new legal regime of the Progressive Era and the frenzy over acupuncture in the 1970s, the challenges that Chinese doctors faced during the middle decades of the twentieth century seem, on the surface, un-remarkable, but as the sixth chapter reveals, the mid-twentieth century witnessed a profound reformulation of the roles that Chinese herbalists played within their communities. Like all small business owners, Chinese herbalists struggled during the Great Depression. Then, mid-century wars in Asia disrupted supply lines, making it difficult to restock apothecary drawers and shelves. World War II and the Cold War had other adverse effects on the Chinese American herb business. Wartime partnerships between the U.S. military and biomedical researchers ushered in a "golden age" of American medicine that diminished the competitiveness of irregular medicine in the medical marketplace. During the Cold War, the rivalry with the Soviet Union intensified American efforts to recruit scientists—including biomedical doctors—through new immigration policies and educational exchange programs. Refugees from China in the 1940s and American-born Chinese began to pursue careers in licensed medical professions rather than continue the practice of traditional Chinese medicine. While many Chinese herb companies in the United States shuttered their businesses in this period, this chapter details the strategies that the survivors deployed to get through these lean years.

Chapter 7 argues that conditions that precipitated the decline of Chinese medicine in the United States unexpectedly laid the foundations for its eventual renaissance. In the 1970s, a countercultural backlash to biomedical hegemony and warming relations between the United States and China helped popularize acupuncture among American patient-consumers. Demand for the therapy was met by a new supply of Chinese acupuncturists who had fled their war-torn country alongside Western-trained scientists. The seventh chapter concludes with a discussion of the state-by-state movement to license acupuncturists and practitioners of other traditional Chinese therapies, including herbalists. By the mid-1970s, legalization permitted Chinese medicine to move out of the hidden corners of the American medical marketplace, but its practitioners maintained an ambivalent relationship with Orientalism. Their medical authority remained in many ways tethered to their embodiment of Asian alterity.

An epilogue explores the still-unfolding history of traditional Chinese medicine in the United States after its rediscovery in the 1970s. In the last decades of the twentieth century, traditional Chinese modalities became part of an increasingly popular category of care, often called Complementary and Alternative or Integrative Medicine. The epilogue follows a new cohort of Chinese immigrant doctors, many of them beneficiaries of Cold War–era policies that prioritized entry among students and scientists. Formally trained in Western-style biomedicine but conversant with traditional healing practices, these doctors have dedicated their professional lives to explaining traditional therapies through the language, tools, and methodologies that have become most widely accepted by biomedical professionals. They have effectively "de-Orientalized" Chinese medicine. Largely because of their work, major American research institutes, medical colleges, and insurance companies have integrated Chinese therapies with their more conventional programs and offerings. The epilogue points toward an ongoing debate among scientists, practitioners, and patients over the place of traditional Chinese medicine in the American medical marketplace and considers the lessons of its long history for our time.

A Chinese Doctor

Long ago, in a Chicago Chinatown apothecary, Moy Yuk ended his interview with the *Arizona Sentinel* reporter by posing a question of his own. He was interested in growing his business to serve a non-Chinese clientele. Although his English was far from fluent, he could make himself understood, and he knew that other Chinese immigrants had turned a handsome profit selling traditional remedies to American patients. Moy asked the *Arizona Sentinel* reporter what he thought his chances of success might be. The reporter scoffed and "told him frankly that he thought the chances would be nil, although there might be some idiots discovered who would expend their money at the risk of their health." Moy kicked the insolent Arizonan out of his shop.[41]

But the herbalist may have known what the reporter did not; Americans avidly and regularly consumed Chinese remedies, and by

1885 they had been doing so for more than a century. The popularity of Chinese medicine among American patient-consumers befuddled its late nineteenth-century observers, who spilled no small amount of ink to ask how Chinese doctors attracted American patients. In a sense, this book is more spilled ink on the subject. A history of Chinese doctors in the United States recounts not only the experiences of Chinese immigrants and the unique challenges they faced but also the rarely acknowledged, often invisible work that Chinese medicine has done to create the diverse landscape of the American medical marketplace.

Herbs and Roots

I n April 1799, an advertisement ran in a Harrisburg, Pennsylvania, newspaper. A man identifying himself as "Chinese Doctor, Dr. John Howard" announced that he was receiving patients at his home on Second Street, across from "Mr. Stines's Tavern."[1] Howard claimed that he had come from Canton, China, and he promised to treat a range of ailments—from the merely uncomfortable to the mostly fatal—with "herbs and roots only." His advertisements appeared in the *Oracle of Dauphin and Harrisburgh Advertiser* throughout the spring and early summer of 1799 before he moved to a new location in nearby Carlisle and rented a room above George Weise's tavern on York Street. In the fall of 1800, he ran the same advertisement for his herbs and roots in Carlisle's *Weekly Gazette*.[2] At the turn of the nineteenth century, the Harrisburg area had no shortage of doctors. Laid out in 1785 on the east bank of the Susquehanna River, the trading depot that would eventually become the capital of Pennsylvania was a sickly place. In 1793, the same year that yellow fever famously devastated Philadelphia, more than a hundred miles away, the residents of Harrisburg suffered an unusually high death rate from uncertain causes.[3] Consequently, from its earliest days, Harrisburg was home to a number of professional healers, including John Howard, who may have been the first practitioner of Chinese medicine in the United States.

Advertisement for John
Howard in the *Oracle of
Dauphin and Harrisburgh
[Penn.] Advertiser,*
April 17, 1799. Courtesy
of NewsBank, Inc.

But who was John Howard, Chinese Doctor? Was he, in fact, Chinese? Chinese men and women did travel abroad and often at great distances in the early modern period. The Spanish conquest of the Philippines in 1571 opened a corridor of migration for thousands of Chinese to cross the Pacific and settle in Spanish-American colonies.[4] Chinese voyagers also went to Europe, India, and other parts of Asia as sailors, artisans, merchants, domestic servants, and religious students.[5] In Hawaii, the Chinese monopolized the sandalwood trade from the late eighteenth century. Yet comparatively few Chinese migrants went to the British colonies that would become the United States. Their presence on the Atlantic seaboard of North America went unrecorded until the 1810s. In 1817, British Protestant missionary Robert Morrison received a letter about a young Chinese man living in New York who claimed to have immigrated just prior to the War of 1812 as a domestic servant in the household of a Pennsylvania politician, James Milnor, and in 1818, Christian missionaries invited five Chinese men to attend their school in Cornwall, Connecticut.[6] John Howard, if he was Chinese, would have preceded those men's arrival in the United States by more than a decade. As a Chinese man, he might have adopted an American pseudonym that his English-speaking clientele could more easily pronounce. Alternatively, Howard may not have been Chinese by birth but could have spent significant time in China, perhaps among the foreign merchants or Protestant missionaries who took up seasonal residency in Canton, the only port open to European and American trade at that time.[7] There is no record of a "John Howard" in the 1800 census manuscript records for either Harrisburg or Carlisle. Federal census takers in that era did not include information about race beyond "negro" or "Indian" nor did they list national origin or occupation, which might have helped distinguish Howard from his neighbors. Census manuscripts from that era named only heads of household, but the advertisements for his business indicate that Howard was a renter. If he was Chinese, he may have been the free, nonwhite, non-Indian person enumerated as living in George "Wise's" home in Carlisle in 1800. Or he could have been one of the two free white males of majority age living under the same roof.[8]

Over a century later, the *Pennsylvania Medical Journal* remembered John Howard as a "charlatan," but there is no evidence that his contemporaries saw him as such.[9] A Connecticut newspaper celebrated his business in August 1800. The *Norwich Packet,* printed by Alexander and James Robertson, the Scottish loyalists and brothers who also published the *New York Chronicle,* declared, "Let the Patentees of Pills boast no longer when we inform them of the famous Chinese Doctor John Howard lately from Canton in China who has arrived in America." The *Norwich Packet* paraphrased Howard's advertisement, listing the many diseases and afflictions his roots and herbs promised to cure, and it praised his skill, calling him a "descendant of Galen and Hippocrates." The announcement ended with a little rhyme: "John's full of skill, from head to toe / And kills old death with one sage blow."[10]

To understand Howard's story and the long history of Chinese medicine in the United States, we need to pay equal attention to what the *Norwich Packet* emphasized and what it ignored. The announcement found nothing remarkable to say about Howard's nativity. Its failure to note such a detail might be evidence that he was not, in fact, Chinese. More importantly, the *Norwich Packet*'s untroubled coverage of Howard's Chinese "herbs and roots" reflected the fact that by 1800, Americans were, to varying degrees, already familiar with Chinese medicine.

Half a century before mass emigration from China to the United States began, Chinese herbal remedies had already become integral to American habits of self-dosing. Via British importers and domestic medicine guides, Chinese medicine freely voyaged to British North America in its colonial period and to the United States in its early national period. Americans learned about traditional Chinese medicine not only through the drugs they consumed but also through European and American merchants, missionaries, and medical scientists. Their observations were principally justifications for European and, eventually, American interventions in China, but nonetheless they became a major channel through which Chinese medical knowledge and goods flowed first to colonial North America and then to the United States. In those trans-Pacific crossings, new theories of scientific medicine became entangled with the United States' imperial interests in China and an emergent American Orientalist imagination.

Early European Encounters with Chinese Medicine

Early North America was, in many ways, an annex to a European world with a longstanding curiosity for all things Chinese, including its medicinal plants and therapeutic systems.[11] In 1253, the French king Louis IX dispatched a Franciscan friar named William of Rubruck to parlay with the Mongol leader Möngke Khan. Traveling in Karakorum (in modern-day central Mongolia), William paused to admire a Mongol or Chinese physician prescribing herbal remedies and practicing diagnosis by pulse. Later, he witnessed faith healing, which he failed to understand, and consumed a sickening excess of rhubarb tonic, which he confused with holy water.[12] The Franciscan scholar Roger Bacon later included William's observations in his 1292 *Opus majus,* and by these means, William's misunderstandings were passed down to later generations of

European naturalists, missionaries, and other travelers.[13] The potential for trade for Chinese *materia medica* sparked medieval European curiosity, and its travelers to Mongolia and China sent back reports of Chinese medicine. In the late thirteenth century, Marco Polo famously ventured into the Chinese empire, where he watched a physician perform an exorcism and then a healing by means of animal sacrifice.[14] The commercial motivations for Polo's journey meant that he also paid particular attention to local, marketable remedies such as crocodile bile and camphor.[15]

In the early modern period, European travelers to Asia continued to record their observations of Chinese medicine. Jesuit missionaries were among the first Europeans to establish a permanent presence in China. Drawn to the Far East by its millions of potential converts, representatives from various Catholic orders began to arrive in the late sixteenth century, but the Chinese emperor initially confined them to Macao. In this Portuguese-leased enclave, they waited for the emperor to extend official permission to proselytize on the mainland, which he did in the early seventeenth century.[16] For the Jesuits, documenting Chinese health practices became part of a strategy to acquire cultural knowledge that would assist missionaries in connecting with Chinese people, understanding their mentalities, and convincing them to convert to Catholicism. Jesuits wrote copious letters and reports on Chinese medicine and sent examples of Chinese medical texts back to their order as well as to European political and religious leaders. Because the missionaries were dismissive of Chinese religious traditions, and perhaps because their own early modern European culture was increasingly separating religion and science into separate spheres, their notes on Chinese health practices tended to exclude faith healing. Jesuits instead focused on herbalism, which may have seemed familiar to them given their own reliance on botanical and zoological drug therapies. In the mid-seventeenth century, Michael Boym, a Polish Jesuit missionary, translated Chinese herbal compendia to help describe the medical practices that he observed. His translations were incorporated into *China illustrata,* an anthology of missionary writing by the German Jesuit Athanasius Kircher. *China illustrata* informed much of early modern European knowledge of Chinese natural history. Boym and Kircher's

contemporary Jean-Baptiste du Halde, a French Jesuit, included transla-
tions of the *Bencao gangmu* (本草綱目), the famous sixteenth-century
Chinese pharmacopoeia, in his widely read and oft-quoted histories of
China.[17]

Jesuit missionaries traveled alongside traders, who were interested
in inventorying Chinese medical practices so that they might sell them
back home in Europe. The early fourteenth-century pharmacopoeia
compiled by the Florentine merchant Francesco Balducci Pegolotti included three medicinal plants of Chinese origin: rhubarb, camphor, and
galangal. In the sixteenth century, two Portuguese merchants in India,
García d'Orta and Cristóvão Acosta, each published a compendium of
Indian medicines that included several Chinese herbs, which they had
found in use in Goa. A Flemish botanist, Charles de l'Ecluse, translated
the compendia into Latin and illustrated them with images of the stock
available for purchase in Antwerp.[18]

European surgeons and physicians also made their way to Asia,
typically attending to the health of merchants, and they too gathered
and transmitted information on Chinese medicine. Beginning in the
late seventeenth century, surgeons posted in Batavia (present-day Ja-
karta) and Japan encountered Chinese medical practices while under
the employ of Dutch and British trading companies.[19] Although cultural and language barriers limited their ability to interpret what they
observed, their writings provided early modern European readers with
detailed accounts of Chinese theories of anatomy and herbalism.[20] Pulsology, acupuncture, and moxibustion also piqued their interest because those therapies spoke to a theory of circulation that was a major research concern for early modern European scientists. Physicians
with the Dutch East India Company—Jakob de Bondt and Willem
ten Rhijne—produced the first detailed accounts of acupuncture for
Western readers after observing it in practice in Japan in the late seventeenth century.[21] Around the same time, Andreas Cleyer, an officer with
the same company who happened to be a formally trained physician,
published a treatise on pulsology that included thirty plates illustrating
the physiological foundations for acupuncture.[22] The transmission of
knowledge of moxibustion from China to Europe followed a similar
timeline, carried via intellectual waystations in Java and Japan.[23]

Expanding European knowledge of Chinese *materia medica* depended on a partnership between traders and scientists. Images of exotic flowers, foliage, and nature scenes adorned Chinese embroidery, furniture, porcelain, and other manufactured goods, and they sparked the curiosity and admiration of European customers.[24] Sea captains or other officers sometimes ferried home a plant cutting or two, procured from the Canton nursery garden. If the plant managed to survive the long voyage, it could fetch a high price among collectors, but the nursery garden failed to offer the variety or comprehensiveness desired by naturalists.[25] In the late seventeenth century, the Qing imperial government permitted some formal exchange of botanical specimens, which allowed European scientists to expand their studies.[26] Those efforts intensified in the eighteenth and nineteenth centuries as European naturalists began to catalog Chinese plants as part of an Enlightenment project to comprehend all the earth's flora and fauna.

The "Canton System" limited what traders and naturalists could access firsthand. Set forth by the emperor in 1757, the system carefully

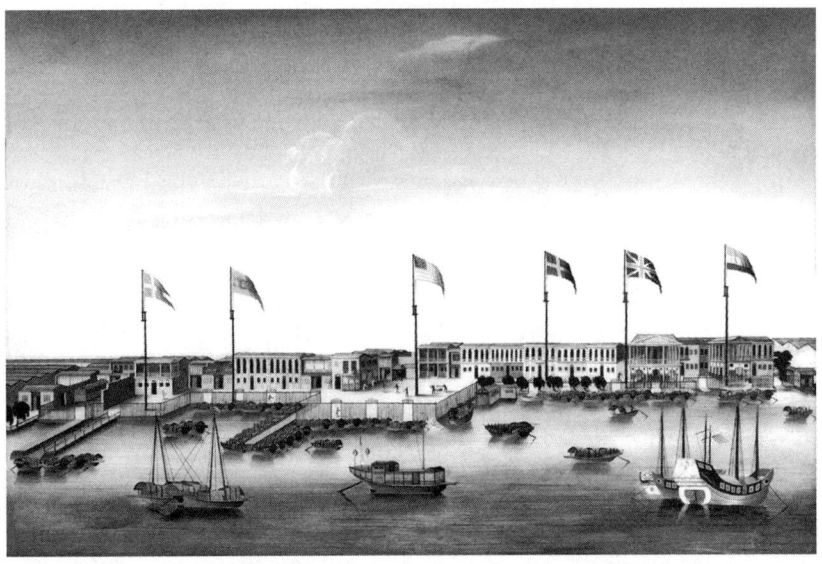

Canton Harbor and Factories with Foreign Flags,
ca. 1805. Wikimedia Commons.

managed the presence of European traders, subjecting them to an elaborate process of inspections and permitting before allowing them to disembark in the city of Canton. European traders were prohibited from entering China between the months of March and October and could not roam freely. They were almost entirely confined to the "foreign factories"—a walled residential district at the edge of the city of Canton. Their time in the country was highly supervised by Chinese merchants, interpreters, and compradors, who ensured the foreign traders' adherence to the emperor's "Eight Regulations," rules of comportment and prohibitions on women and weapons. The imperial government designed the Canton System to guarantee that the presence of foreigners in China was temporary and largely invisible.[27]

European visitors to China with an interest in its natural history thus had to rely on networks of Chinese intermediaries to help them gather specimens and information from beyond the walls. Customs officers were particularly good sources of information for naturalists as their work brought them into close contact not only with flora and fauna passing through Chinese ports but also with the traders and brokers who handled them. European naturalists encouraged customs officers to interview Chinese traders and brokers to ask for details about the goods and their origins. Occasionally, a customs officer might even confiscate a specimen for scientific study.[28]

The energy devoted to the study of China's flora and fauna extended to its *materia medica*. Robert Morrison, dispatched to China by the London Missionary Society in 1807, was instrumental in collecting Chinese medical texts and samples of its drugs.[29] Morrison was not a doctor, but he had a little basic medical training and worked closely with the surgeon to the British East India Company, John Livingstone, to establish a dispensary and clinic for the Chinese in Macao in the 1820s.[30] Eventually, Morrison's missionary duties took priority over his efforts to produce a comprehensive compendium of Chinese medicine. He abandoned the project, but other European visitors, including his former partner, Livingstone, took over his research.[31] Livingstone studied Chinese medical textbooks in hopes of discovering useful therapies and techniques for his own practice. He also worked closely with a Chinese physician at a Macanese charity clinic and cultivated a relationship with Cantonese herbalist Lee Seen-sang to learn more about commonly prescribed remedies. In 1819, Livingstone helped establish an Anglo-Chinese college in Malacca, where he hoped to employ a Chinese gardener skilled in cultivating medicinal plants.[32] Around the same time, Alexander Pearson, who famously introduced the smallpox vaccination to southern China, paid a Roman Catholic priest to interview Chinese doctors on treatments for paralysis. In the 1860s, Daniel Hanbury, a pharmacologist, endeavored to construct and analyze a Chinese pharmacopoeia from his London office. He relied on agents in China—including his brother Thomas, who worked as a merchant in Shanghai—to send him samples of Chinese drugs. His work, in conjunction with that of British botanist Henry Fletcher Hance, successfully identified a new species of rhizome used by the Chinese as a stimulant.[33]

Chinese Medicine in Early America

Information about Europe's medical discoveries in China flowed constantly across the ocean to North America.[34] In the era of the American Revolution, major political figures like Benjamin Franklin and Thomas Jefferson had copies of Jean-Baptiste du Halde's *General History of China* in their private libraries.[35] American scientists were intrigued by China's natural history and its possible contributions to the health and prosperity of their new nation. In 1771, the American Philosophical Society declared its intentions to study and implement Chinese horticultural and agricultural practices in the United States.[36] Formally trained American physicians often had strong ties with their colleagues in Europe. Many of them studied in European medical colleges, and American medical libraries collected European studies of Chinese herbalism, moxibustion, and acupuncture.[37] In 1825, Benjamin Franklin Bache, a physician and the grandson of the famous Philadelphian, reported in the *North American Medical and Surgical Journal* that a few American physicians employed acupuncture when treating inflammatory diseases, headaches, and other conditions with chronic pain.[38]

Nonelite Americans were most likely to encounter Chinese medicine via its *materia medica,* often imported through British merchants and stocked in local apothecaries or carried by itinerant drug peddlers.

Chinese herbalism's place in American lay medicine depended on what historian Roberta E. Bivins characterizes as "shared boundaries" in her study of early modern European, South Asian, and Chinese traditions. Bivins argues that the congruencies which existed among these diverse medical knowledge systems permitted "cross-cultural" exchanges of ideas and practices.[39] These congruencies made Chinese medicine legible to early American consumers as well.

In the late eighteenth and early nineteenth centuries, most ordinary Americans continued to believe in humoral theories of disease that equated good health with a balance of the body's humors: blood, phlegm, black bile, and yellow bile. Organs producing the humors were susceptible to seasonal changes, astrological conditions, and mental and physical actions, as well as the local environment and its potentially disease-carrying odors. A good healer attended to the patient's entire system, rather than a specific condition. Chinese doctors approached diagnosis in a similarly holistic way, an approach that had its roots in ancient traditions. The people of the Shang (1600–1046 BCE) and Zhou (1046–256 BCE) periods understood human bodies as embedded in families (living and dead), polities, and material environments. Sickness was a manifestation of a disruption in that system.[40] Central Chinese principles of *yinyang* and, perhaps more pointedly, *wu-xing,* or the five phases, resonated with European American theories of health and sickness as a disruption of counterbalancing forces within the body. Concepts of balance and holism brought the two knowledge systems into alignment and encouraged ordinary Americans to engage in cross-cultural medical sampling.

Practitioners of scientific medicine rejected theories of humors, but their profession was still in a nascent and largely inchoate state in the late eighteenth and early nineteenth centuries. The science of anatomy—popularized in Europe—was gaining traction among elite American doctors. In the early nineteenth century, many of them embraced French empiricism, with its emphasis on linking clinical observations to postmortem organ autopsies.[41] Not only did American medical scientists distinguish themselves as members of a privileged class, separated by a combination of affluence, race, and gender from other healers, but they also increasingly claimed that the relative importance of observed phenomena to theory differentiated their work from that of other knowledge systems. However, in the colonial period and early republic, their authority was far from certain. Although the first American colleges of scientific medicine organized in the last decades of the eighteenth century, and a handful of associated societies and journals soon followed, its practitioners continued to compete on relatively equal terms in a largely unregulated medical marketplace with faith healers, herbalists, and many other sects up until the late nineteenth century.[42]

Most health care at that time took place in the home, under the supervision of women or lay practitioners. Medical knowledge circulated informally through kinship networks or—for the literate—newspapers, almanacs, herbals, and recipe books.[43] Ordinary Americans were quite ecumenical in their approach to health care. Racial differences between healer and patient posed no barrier to the exchange of medical advice. Upon arrival in North America, European colonists often noted the good health of their Indian neighbors and attributed it to their knowledge of indigenous botanical remedies. In the nineteenth century, the *United States Pharmacopoeia* included 150 plants used medicinally by Native American communities.[44] "Indian doctors"—both real Native healers and non-Natives pretending to have learned from them—peddled herbs and nostrums up through the end of the nineteenth century.[45] African Americans were also important sources of healing knowledge in the early republic. Historian Sharla M. Fett has studied how enslaved African Americans, principally women, were critical to health care on American plantations in the antebellum period. In addition to nursing and midwifery, enslaved women prepared plant-based medicines and ritual objects and practiced healing traditions imported from Africa for both black and white patients.[46] Thus, early American patients would have been quite accustomed to consulting with nonwhite healers and sampling from non-European medical knowledge systems.

Perhaps most importantly for the adoption of Chinese *materia medica*, Americans of this era relied on plant-based medicine. In this respect, their medical tradition was no different from that of any premodern society. Families grew medicinal plants in their gardens, foraged for them in the wild, or purchased specimens from "root-and-herb doctors," men and women who dispensed raw, locally sourced botanical remedies. Prominent medical scientists of the colonial period and early republic including Cotton Mather and Benjamin Rush prescribed medicinal plants, and in the early nineteenth century the first irregular medical sects to professionalize—Thomsonians and its offshoot, the eclectics—promoted the exclusive use of botanical drugs. For Thomsonians, herbs were superior to mineral-based medicines because they grew toward the sun and were gentle and "life-giving," whereas minerals, lodged in the ground, were quite the opposite.[47] The well-to-do might purchase manufactured plant-based medicines, harvested in distant places and compounded into pills or powders in an apothecary. Drug sellers often imported such products from England and claimed to hold a "patent" from the king protecting their original list of ingredients.[48] Regardless of their origins, American drug preparations would have been identical to those of the Chinese. Plants with medicinal properties were dried for storage and then typically reconstituted in boiling water, vinegar, or alcohol. Ointments and poultices were also made by combining dried herbs with emollients, cornmeal, or other substrates.[49]

Remedies from far-flung, "exotic" places like those advertised by John Howard in Pennsylvania would have been right at home in the American apothecary or the peddler's cart. For centuries, European prospectors had scoured the globe for febrifuges, abortifacients, and other classes of drugs. Colonial America was a node in a well-established global network, importing and exporting medicinal plants. Its apothecaries customarily stocked medicinal plants from Africa, South America, and the Middle East.[50] Rhubarb, often used as a laxative, was among the most popular medicinal plants imported from China. Benjamin Franklin was a famous early adopter.[51] Chinese rhubarb competed on the market with the Turkish varietal, which was considered less flavorful but perhaps equally effective.[52] Along with rhubarb, cassia and camphor—while not exclusively grown in China—were often identified as the country's exports in American druggist catalogs and price lists.[53]

Seventeenth- and eighteenth-century books of domestic remedies often contained mention of more esoteric Chinese remedies. *The Family Physician, and the House Apothecary,* a guide published in England

and distributed in the American colonies in the late seventeenth century, included a description of the proper preparation for compound
powders made of "Oriental bezoar," sometimes called "Chinese snake
stones," which were in fact bovine gallstones believed to be an antidote
for poisons and toxins of all kinds. The guidebook notes that "Oriental"
bezoar was both more expensive and more effective than "Occidental"
bezoar.[54] Several decades later, in the 1740s, a French drug peddler who
went by the name Francis Torres sold "Chinese Stones" for twenty-five
shillings in colonial towns and cities up and down the Atlantic seaboard.
Although a Philadelphia skeptic dismissed the Frenchman's cure-all as
nothing more than burnt fragments of buckhorn, at the very least it
gestured toward familiarity with the real Chinese remedy.[55] In the early
nineteenth century, reports of a remarkable plant circulated in American newspapers from the mid-Atlantic to New England. The *Hias tea
Tomchon* was described as a "dirty yellow" root, which took the form
of a vegetable in the summer and a "worm" in the winter. Consuming
the root promised to restore energy. It is possible that the discovery was
Ophiocordyceps sinensis, the combination of a fungus and a caterpillar
native to the Tibetan plateau that is today sometimes called Himalayan
Viagra.[56]

By far China's most prevalent and successful medicinal export was
tea. Colonial Americans were, like all Britons, enthusiastic consumers
of Chinese tea, which Dutch traders had introduced to Western Europe
in the seventeenth century. While King Charles II popularized the consumption of tea in social settings, many European doctors touted its
preventative and curative functions. Some believed that tea energized
the body, enhanced the performance of major organs, and staved off
various illnesses.[57] There was, however, no consensus about tea's health
benefits, and some European and American physicians, startled by their
nations' escalating quantities of imported tea, began to warn against
overindulgence in the "Chinese drug."[58] Eighteenth- and nineteenth-
century discourses often closely linked physical wellbeing and moral
rectitude, and warnings about tea touched on both. In a publication
on health and longevity, esteemed Scottish scientist Sir John Sinclair
declared, "There can be no doubt, that tea is naturally a pernicious,
and if taken in any quantity, a poisonous plant. There is reason also to

suppose that the use of it has contributed to the weak bodies and ener-
vated minds of the Chinese."[59] Such language directly invoked Orientalist characterizations of China as an ancient and decaying civilization,
destined to submit to the vigor and youth of the West.

An 1810 advice book written in the voice of the imaginary "Farmer
Trueman" to his daughter, a serving girl, warned that "many destroy
their health" by consuming too much of a "Chinese drug called tea."
In this work, a racialized fear of contamination by the Chinese mingled
with concerns about maintaining class hierarchies as Farmer Trueman
expresses his disapproval for "servants [who] run mad about tea; they
spend a large portion of their wages in it, and squander too great a part
of their time."[60] The problems of an unsupervised underclass were common cause for conversation in the early nineteenth century. Industrialization in the northern states disrupted household economies and drew
individuals into a capitalist labor market. A growing wage-working class
exercised new freedoms not possible under an earlier system of apprenticeship. In this democratizing moment, old constraints on consumption and moderation fell away, and the ubiquity of the "Chinese drug"
could seem dangerous to the physical and moral health of the young
nation.

These early nineteenth-century exhortations to abstain from consuming Chinese medicine are a reminder of how precarious the fate of
the United States seemed. With the ink barely dried on the treaties end-
ing the wars with Britain (first in 1783 and then again in 1814), Americans were far from convinced that their republican experiment would
succeed. In such an environment, the critique of Chinese medicine was
not only shorthand for maintaining racial purity and social hierarchies
but also a means to prevent American dependence on foreign imports.
American physicians' concerns about tea sometimes mingled with pro-
tectionist sentiment. Anthony Florian Madinger Willich, a popular
author of domestic medicine manuals reprinted in the United States,
advised his readers, "A moderate use of tea may sometimes be of service to persons in a perfect state of health; yet for daily use, it cannot be
recommended." He urged his readers to abstain from Chinese tea: "It
would be a great proof of patriotic spirit in this country, if the use of this
exotic drug were either altogether abandoned, or, at least, supplied by

some indigenous plants of equal flavor and superior salubrity."[61] Willich's advice went unheeded. No domestically produced tea could compete with the Chinese import.

Over time, ordinary Americans learned to associate Chinese medicine with magical healing powers. In the Orientalist imagination, China was a mysterious, quasi-mystical land. From there, it was a short step to link Chinese products and knowledge to folklore and fantasies in which anything was possible, even the impossible. In the eighteenth century, the *Virginia Gazette,* a popular broadsheet published in Williamsburg, reprinted a satirical story from a London newspaper that described a five-thousand-year-old Chinese ointment possessed of miraculous regenerative capabilities. Within five days of application, an amputated limb would regrow as new.[62]

The association between Chinese medicine and the miracle cure was not always played for laughs. By the 1840s, patent medicine manufacturers used popular perceptions of Chinese otherworldliness to suggest the wondrous capabilities of their products. Historian James Harvey Young, who has published extensively on American medical quackery, has found several examples of mid-nineteenth-century nostrum companies that invented Chinese doctors or referenced China to sell their "miraculous" remedies, including Dr. Lin's Celestial Balm of China, Dr. Drake's Canton Chinese Hair Cream, and Carey's Chinese Catarrh Cure.[63] There were also "Oriental" or Chinese-branded toothpastes, including Bryan's Oriental Dentifrice ("a very superior article" according to its advertisement) and Joseph Burnett's "Oriental Tooth Wash" (which promised to preserve and beautify the gums).[64] Early Americans, who prided themselves on their long-lived citizenry, seem to have been particularly captivated by the Chinese reputation for longevity, and that myth inspired advertising copy for various drugs.[65] In the 1840s, *The General Family Directory,* a pamphlet on domestic medicine published in New York, ran full-page advertisements for Dr. Lin's Temperance Life Bitters and Chinese Blood Pills, which promised to purge the blood of alcohol and other toxicants. "Why do the Chinese live to such immense ages and still retain the powers of youth or middle age?" the advertisement queried. "Because they purify the blood."[66] An advertisement for hashish printed in Albany, New York's *Good Samaritan and Domestic*

Physician noted that all Asian civilizations, including the Chinese, relied on the universal remedy: "These were the most Beautiful, Happy, Healthy, Cheerful, and Long-lived Races of people that ever existed."[67]

Ginseng and Opium

The currents of trade also carried *materia medica* from American shores to China. By the end of the eighteenth century, Americans had become major producers and exporters of the popular Chinese remedy ginseng. The Chinese used *Panax ginseng* as a stimulant as well as a cure for a variety of illnesses. In 1717, Joseph-François Lafitau, a Jesuit missionary proselytizing to the Iroquois between Montreal and Ottawa, observed a plant with red berries growing in the forest near a house he was building. Lafitau thought the plant might be similar to Asian ginseng, which had been recently described by another French Jesuit, Pierre Jartoux, on his travels in Mongolia. Jartoux's 1711 report, "A Description of a Tartarian Plant Called Gin-seng, with an Account of Its Virtues," explained that ginseng flourished in a particular climate and soil type, both of which seemed, to Lafitau, much like Quebec's. Thus, Lafitau was actively on the lookout for ginseng as he went about his missionary work.[68] When he showed a cutting of a red-berried plant to an Iroquois woman at his mission, she was able to confirm its healing properties. The Iroquois also used ginseng for medicinal purposes, although not as prevalently as the Chinese. Lafitau then sent a specimen to Quebec City for scientific analysis, and reports of the discovery of *Panax quinquefolium,* a North American cousin to *Panax ginseng,* quickly made their way to Paris. By 1752, Canada's business exporting wild ginseng to China reached a half million francs per year.[69]

Ginseng hunters soon spread out to New England and Appalachia, and cities like Albany, New York, and Philadelphia became important entrepôts for the ginseng trade. French and British merchants leaned heavily on Indian labor to forage for the wild-growing root, a practice that alarmed New England religious leader Jonathan Edwards. In a 1752 letter to a fellow reverend, he wrote that the discovery of ginseng had "prejudiced the cause of religion among the Indians." With dismay, Edwards described how "Indians of all sorts, young and old" devoted an "abundance of time in wandering about the woods and sometimes to great distance, in the neglect of public worship, and of their husbandry," and went to Albany to trade the root for rum.[70] But Indians were not the only ones wandering about in the wilderness looking for ginseng. In 1752, a New York City newspaper noted that "great Numbers of the Five Nations and other Indians, as well as white People, are now out on the Search for it."[71] Fur traders, including the legendary Daniel Boone, often foraged for ginseng in the fall, a time usually spent scouting for the best winter trap sites.[72] The close scrutiny of the land necessary for laying traps was naturally compatible with spotting the easily overlooked plant. Several companies dedicated themselves to both trapping and ginseng hunting, including Lowe Fur and Herb and White Brothers' Fur and Ginseng Company among others.[73]

Prior to the Revolutionary War, all ginseng went to China through the British East India Company, whose merchants competed for the Chinese market with their French counterparts, but American independence freed the former colonists to sell ginseng directly to Chinese buyers. On February 22, 1784, the *Empress of China* sailed from New York, just behind a rival sloop called the *Harriet,* which sailed from Boston in 1783. Both vessels carried a range of American goods desired by the Chinese—silver and ginseng being the most valuable per ounce. The *Harriet's* five tons of ginseng never made it to Canton. The captain sought out a buyer for her cargo in the popular midway stopover port of Cape Town, South Africa. There, the British East India Company purchased the *Harriet's* entire cargo, and she returned to the United States in July 1784 laden with tea.[74] Meanwhile, the merchants backing the *Empress* readied their ship, packing it with thirty tons of ginseng among other commodities. To procure such a quantity of ginseng, a Philadelphia merchant had contracted with a local doctor, Robert Johnston, who scoured the frontier lands of Virginia and Pennsylvania for three months, then sent his haul via boat to New York, where clerks sorted it by quality and stored it in casks until the *Empress* was ready to set sail.[75]

Between 1783 and 1900, the United States shipped approximately 60 million pounds of wild-growing ginseng to Asia.[76] On top of that, Americans, who took the enormous demand in China as evidence

of its health benefits, consumed an unknown amount of the root
domestically.[77] The success of trade with China encouraged more collection of ginseng and expanded its geography as far west as Minnesota
and south to Georgia. Beginning in the last decades of the eighteenth
century, foragers could readily exchange "well-dried ginseng" for cash
or all manner of goods with local merchants.[78] John Jacob Astor, known
for his wide-ranging fur empire, made an additional fortune selling ginseng to China in 1786, with revenues of $55,000 in silver coin (or well
over $1 million in today's currency). Ordinary farmers found that sell-
ing a few wild-growing roots could become a means of securing a little
startup capital before their first harvest came in.[79] Articles recruiting
settlers to the western reaches of early America often mentioned the
availability of ginseng on the land. In 1759, advertisements for Crown-
Point, on the New York side of Lake Champlain, promised settlers
would find "the richest Lands in America" as evident by the abundance
of "Sugar Trees and Ginseng" to be found there.[80] Similarly, in 1787,
William Worth, a Virginia land speculator, reached out to the readers of
a Philadelphia newspaper to promote his tracts in Harrison and Ohio
Counties, where "the underwood abounds with plenty of spikenard,
spicey-wood, and ginseng."[81]

Ginseng merchants read about Chinese medicine to recognize
what properties made the root most valuable to their overseas buyers,
and this information tended to reinforce Orientalist understandings
of Chinese difference and inferiority.[82] In the late eighteenth and early
nineteenth centuries, texts that described how to process and store the
product for long-distance shipping might also detail how and why the
Chinese used ginseng, which helped inform American perceptions of
Chinese culture and customs. North American newspapers occasionally excerpted the parts of Jean-Baptiste du Halde's *A General History of
China* that concerned ginseng and its medicinal uses. Du Halde's interpretation of Chinese governance and culture mingled with advice that
the roots "largest, most uniform" and possessing the "fewest strings"
would likely fetch the highest prices. In his discussion of ginseng, du
Halde described the oppressive regime of the Mandarin emperor, who
compelled his Tartar (Turkic) soldiers to scour the countryside for ginseng: "These poor people suffer greatly," du Halde wrote, "for they carry

neither tents nor beds with them . . . They are obliged to sleep under a
tree, covering themselves with such branches or pieces of bark as they
can find."[83] The conscription of Tartar soldiers into ginseng hunting
may have mattered very little to American merchants, but it reinforced
an image of a despotic and distant Orient. Other accounts blended
practical information about ginseng with depictions of its consumers
that recalled Orientalist stereotypes of sexual depravity and irrationality.
William Cullen's 1789 *A Treatise of the* Materia Medica intimated that
the Chinese valued the root as a "powerful aphrodisiac," an unusual
claim for the remedy, which was more customarily attributed general
restorative powers.[84]

Eighteenth- and nineteenth-century compendia of American *materia medica* and native plants included entries on ginseng, and, noting
its high esteem among the Chinese, they often implied the presumed
inferiority of Chinese medical knowledge. In 1801, a medical dictionary
dismissed the medicinal benefits of ginseng: "The Chinese ascribe extraordinary virtues to the root of ginseng, and have no confidence in
any medicine unless in combination with it. In Europe, however, it is
very seldom employed."[85] An 1818 text on American medical botany
echoed the sentiment: "As far as Ginseng has been tried medicinally in
this country, and in Europe, its virtues do not appear, by any means,
to justify the high estimation of it by the Chinese."[86] John Bell, an early
eighteenth-century Scottish doctor who traveled in Asia, scoffed at the
Chinese affinity for ginseng: "If it really has any extraordinary virtues, I
never could discover them, after repeated experiments."[87] John Wilson,
a surgeon in the British Navy, claimed that the Chinese regarded ginseng with "admiration bordering on religious adoration."[88] To American readers, these scientific and popular texts conveyed an impression
of Chinese obsession with a root of dubious benefit.

While the price of ginseng fluctuated according to supply in the
early decades of America's China trade, there was nonetheless agreement among merchants that ginseng was a more profitable export than
opium.[89] That changed by the 1830s.[90] Opium is a milky substance produced by the seed capsule of *Papaver somniferum,* a kind of poppy. The
liquid contains various alkaloids—including morphine—with analgesic effects. Opium producers made small incisions into the opium poppy

seed capsule, collected the liquid, and dried it into bricks or balls. The use of medicinal-grade opium and its alkaloids was both ubiquitous and legal despite its well-known tendency to lead to addiction. Narcotic-grade opium required additional processing, which concentrated the drug and rendered it more potent.[91] American merchants did traffic in narcotic-grade opium, imported from Turkey, but not to the extent that their British rivals did. Prior to the outbreak of the First Opium War in 1839, the British imported thousands of chests of opium annually while the United States only brought in a few hundred. That number increased after the war's conclusion, when the "unequal treaties" gave European and American merchants greater latitude in China, but the United States remained a relatively unimportant player in the opium trade, accounting for not much more than 10 percent of the market.[92] American merchants who trafficked in opium narcotics to China did not seem to equate their trade with the medicinal-grade opium pre-scribed by Chinese and American doctors. Indeed, in the nineteenth century, opium with more than 9 percent morphia content, ostensibly used for medicine, could move into the United States duty-free.[93]

British and American Medical Missionaries

Medical missionary texts fed the imagination of American consumers of Chinese medicine. European doctors and nurses had been present in China as early as the sixteenth century, and some of them were ordained as friars or nuns.[94] Up until the nineteenth century, however, Western-style medicine offered little clear advantage over traditional Chinese medicine for Chinese patients. When smallpox struck southern China in the spring of 1805, a Portuguese subject imported the vaccine from Manila to Macao. Alexander Pearson, a surgeon with the British East India Company, trained Chinese doctors to vaccinate against the dis-ease with the financial support of local Chinese merchants. His succes-sor, Robert Livingstone, carried on the work after 1808 and spread the smallpox vaccination to nearby Jiangsu and Fujian. European doctors could also offer cataract surgeries that Chinese doctors did not. Between 1827 and 1832, the English surgeon Thomas Colledge operated an ophthalmic hospital in Macao, where he purportedly performed cataract surgery on between four and six thousand Chinese patients.[95] Around the same time, German Lutheran Karl Gutzlaff published an account of his forays into China, which the evangelical community widely read and reprinted. Gutzlaff traveled up the coast of China to Tientsin (Tianjin) and distributed religious tracts and rudimentary medical care. He reported that medicine gave him "the esteem and friendship of the whole clan or tribe of the Chinese, who never ceased to importune me to cure their natural or imaginary physical defects."[96] The success of Colledge and Gutzlaff inspired Protestant evangelists to incorporate health care into their efforts to spread the gospel of Jesus. In 1828, missionaries established dispensaries in Macao and Canton, where they gave out free medicine along with religious tracts, printed by Liang Afah, a Chinese convert to Christianity.[97]

Souring relations between Chinese officials and foreign guests in the 1830s forced Protestant missionaries to change tactics. After the British East India Company's monopoly on Chinese trade ended in 1833, the Crown appointed Lord William Napier as the first chief superintendent of relations between British traders and Chinese officials in 1834. Napier bristled at the restrictions of the Canton System and threatened to defy them with force of arms. In response, the chief magistrate of Nanhae suspended trade, placed Napier under house arrest, and fired on British ships in the Pearl River.[98] He also ordered the confiscation and destruction of all "evil and obscene books of the foreign barbarians."[99] The edict made it practically impossible for missionaries to print and distribute religious materials as openly as they had before. Chinese officials welcomed foreigners so long as they provided an essential service, and spreading the gospel of Jesus did not count as such. Thus, European and American missionary societies had to think of creative ways to make themselves essential in the eyes of Qing officials.

British and American churches began to envision full-fledged hospitals in which foreign doctors, ordained as Protestant missionaries, would simultaneously cure and convert. Behind the walls of missionary hospitals, beyond the prying eyes of Qing officials, ordinary Chinese people could attend church services, receive religious tracts, and seek out theological explanations, all while they waited for treatment.[100] Missionary societies well understood that doctors and patients forged intimate relationships, the necessary preconditions for conversion. In 1851, David Abeel, a missionary dispatched to China and Southeast Asia with the American Reformed Mission, testified to his sponsors that medical missionaries "have the best passport to the dwellings and the hearts of the heathen . . . Patients feel themselves under obligations and are disposed to comply with any methods which may be devised for their spiritual benefit." The native convert and printer of religious tracts Liang Afah concurred: "When I speak to my countrymen in the villages and suburbs about Jesus Christ, and His glorious gospel, they are careless, and utter expression of scorn; but in the hospital their hearts are soft, and they will listen to the gospel with serious attention."[101] Providing health care was not simply a means to circumvent Qing prohibitions. Medical missionaries believed in the compatibility of healing bodies and saving souls.

Medical missionaries also believed in the preeminence of Western-style medical science and its utter necessity to the Chinese people, but they worried about malpractice. The *Chinese Repository,* a journal on Chinese history and culture printed in Canton for Protestant missionaries, often included letters cautioning against sending ill-prepared physicians to administer to the Chinese.[102] In the 1830s, European and American missionary societies began to recruit men (and later women) formally trained as physicians who also happened to be ordained as ministers. In 1834, the American Board of Commissioners for Foreign Missions (ABCFM) sent its first medical missionary to China: thirty-year-old Peter Parker.[103]

To prepare himself for such a career, Parker pursued graduate degrees in medicine and theology at Yale University and finished both courses of study in three years. In 1834, the ABCFM ordained Parker as a missionary, and he set off for China that summer, accompanied by a seventeen-year-old Chinese convert, Ah Lun (or Ah Leang), who had been living for two years as a domestic servant in Middletown, Connecticut, with an American trader, Samuel Russell. Lun agreed to travel with Parker back to China and tutor him in the Chinese language on the way.[104] After brief stops in Canton and Macao, Parker continued his language studies in Singapore for nearly a year before making his way to Canton in the fall of 1835, where he took up residence at a makeshift hospital among the foreign factories, rented at five hundred dollars per year from a wealthy Chinese merchant named Howqua (or Wu Chong-yao).[105] Although the hospital intended to provide comprehensive health services, it was informally known as the Ophthalmic Hospital for its most popular service: cataract surgeries. Parker came to China with some expertise in ophthalmology, having written in the field and completed a rotation in a New York City eye hospital.[106] His skills were soon in high demand, and he wrote to the ABCFM that he had acquired three hundred patients within the first few weeks. By January 1836, Parker's first quarterly report to the ABCFM noted that number had increased to over nine hundred.[107]

The growing demand for Western-style medical care, especially cataract surgery, encouraged Parker to organize the Medical Missionary Society in Canton along with fellow doctor Thomas Colledge and missionaries David Abeel and Elijah Coleman Bridgman, the founder of the ABCFM station in Canton.[108] They began to formulate the idea for the association in a circular they distributed in 1836, but its members did not meet until 1838. The Medical Missionary Society of Canton aimed to provide mutual assistance for medical missionaries working in China, language instruction, recruitment of qualified medical missionaries in Britain and the United States, and management of all necessary funds. With thirty-four members in its inaugural year, the society flourished. By 1887, it had sponsored 150 medical missionaries, both British and American, whose ranks included 27 women. The society eventually began to train Chinese students in Western-style medicine and helped secure a place for that therapeutic system in modern Chinese medicine.[109]

The society's foundational documents portrayed its members as entering a kind of vacuum of medical knowledge. In their address before the first meeting, Parker, Colledge, and Bridgman described the Chinese medical arts as beset by superstition and falsehoods: "An amusing and ridiculous compound of astrological dogmas and dissertations on the influence of the elements like the 'Ethers and Elements' of Heraclitus, takes the place of the well-established principles of physiology and chemistry now received in the West."[110] Parker and his colleagues ridiculed the core doctrines of traditional Chinese medicine and proclaimed the "obligation upon enlightened nations" like their own to impart "the incalculable benefits received from the application of chemistry and natural and inductive philosophy to the subject of health."[111] They expressed their confidence that the Chinese were receptive to such missionary work and reprinted an article Colledge had earlier published in the *Chinese Repository:* "The Chinese have always shown themselves more sensible to what affects their temporal or personal interests, than to any efforts which have been made to improve their moral and intellectual condition. This must necessarily be the case with a people whose more refined and exalted mental powers are but partially developed."[112] By these means, society members rehearsed an old Orientalist trope: the Chinese were like children, capable of recognizing and seeking to fulfill their basic human needs but developmentally incapable of any higher order reasoning. A physician caring for the Chinese body might coax his patient not only toward better health but also toward the path to greater enlightenment and Christianity.

Parker and his colleagues believed they were on a civilizing mission that physicians were uniquely equipped to fulfill. Prior to his departure for China in 1834, Parker had gained familiarity with its history and culture from the *Encyclopaedia Americana,* which described Chinese people as "slavish" and intellectually stultified.[113] Edward Vose Gulick, Parker's principal biographer, noted that Parker frequently described China as a "moral wilderness."[114] Parker's journals from his early days in China expressed his low estimation of Chinese culture and his optimism that Western-style medical science could make such necessary and sweeping change: "The time is coming when [China's] people will be delivered from their burdens of perpetual disease . . . when, under the rule of Jesus, China will be wonderfully different from the China of today."[115] For his part, Colledge also saw himself as serving a "benighted race," equally in need of Western-trained physicians and Christian evangelists.[116] Elijah Bridgman's opinion was more floridly stated in his memoirs: "Darkness covers the land, and gross darkness the people. Idolatry, superstition, fraud, falsehood, cruelty, and oppression everywhere predominate, and iniquity, like a mighty flood, is extending far and wide its desolations."[117]

Other European and American physicians traveling through China validated medical missionary work and applauded its civilizing efforts. In 1846, John Wilson, a doctor with the British Navy, published his observations of medical missionaries: "In their frequent, and from its very nature, familiar intercourse with the afflicted . . . [they have] potent means of touching the heart and turning feelings of gratitude into instruments by which they may act powerfully on the dark mind." In terms that recalled the linked traditions of the European Enlightenment and Orientalism, Wilson expressed his confidence that medical missionary work would "assail the strongholds of bigotry and conceited ignorance" among the Chinese, and, in time, "undermine these antiquated structures that they may ere long annihilate them, rearing in their room institutions of light and liberty."[118] In contrast to Western-style medical science, Wilson described Chinese medicine as "a chaos of unfounded conceits, contradictory notions, and pompous phrases."[119] He diagnosed their problem as civilizational: "The system of the West has long made way for more truthful systems, while that of the East remains in all its force and gives no sign of alteration or decay . . . [The Chinese] appear to have fallen into a petrified fixedness, which nothing but the most powerful external agents can move."[120] The presumption of the Orient as ancient and static gave definition and supremacy to the dynamism of European science.

Yet, while medical missionaries and their supporters projected an image of China as a great void of knowledge, they had to confront the reality that its indigenous medical traditions were both deeply entrenched and highly respected by potential Chinese patients and converts. Short articles on ancient Chinese medical texts or theories printed by the *Chinese Repository* suggested that missionaries paid close attention to Chinese healing practices.[121] Such knowledge not only armed medical missionaries with better knowledge of their patients' mentalities, but it also served as a rhetorical defense of their presence in China for their supporters back home. British Protestant missionary Robert Morrison included several entries on Chinese medical terms and phrases in part 3 of his English-Chinese dictionary, published in 1822. He briefly described the *yinyang* doctrine and referred his reader to a more extensive discussion of it in the *Indo-Chinese Gleaner* of January 1821.[122] In the dictionary entry on "physician," he outlined a typical Chinese physician's approach to pulse diagnosis. Translating "physician" as "the writer of prescriptions," Morrison described their work: "Physicians should observe, listen to, enquire of, and feel the pulse of the patients."[123] The entry on "pulse" alluded to the system of correspondences underpinning its diagnostic significance: "The right or *yew* pulse has a relation (they say) to *fe, pe, ming,* the lungs, the stomach, and the *ming* region; and the left to *sin, kan, hin,* the heart, liver, and kidneys."[124] The brevity of dictionary writing gave Morrison little room to opine, but perhaps the parenthetical comment "they say" speaks to some skepticism on his part.

In the early nineteenth century, when the status of regular medicine remained uncertain in the American medical marketplace, medical missionaries looked to Chinese medicine as a powerful, negative example and justification for their own scientific authority. William Lockhart, a British medical missionary sponsored by the London Missionary Society, observed and wrote about Chinese medicine during his twenty-five-year career in China. His memoirs, published in 1861, detailed the Chinese use of various "native remedies" and devoted the better part of a chapter to explaining the "state of medical science in China," with particular attention to research and education. Lockhart framed his discussion of Chinese healing practices in ways that highlighted the supposed backwardness and depravity of Chinese civilization. He appended a section on "native remedies" to an extensive recounting of grisly murders and suicides.[125]

His account of Chinese medical science in a later chapter drew an explicit comparison between Western-style science and what he perceived to be its absence in China: "In Europe," he wrote, "much talent and energy have been spent in ascertaining the true principles of medicine and in improving its practice; and in consequence, the advance in every department of medical science has been both remarkable and rapid." Lockhart, not surprisingly, found no such advances in the "heathen lands" of China: "Though a great, populous, and civilized country, with a people largely educated, medicine has not yet been studied to any purpose."[126] He sketched the basic contours of the five phases (*wu-xing*) and their corresponding elements for his reader but left out their larger philosophical or practical meanings, either through ignorance or an unwillingness to learn. Of pulsology, Lockhart was openly dismissive: "The pulse helps [the doctor] much in arriving at his conclusions. To this great attention is paid, and its indications are divided into almost endless variety, which are for the most part fanciful."[127] By demeaning Chinese medicine, Lockhart elevated his own scientific and moral authority.

Lockhart's memoirs also included a long excerpt from a report submitted by his colleague Benjamin Hobson, who managed the London Missionary Society's Shanghai Hospital in 1858. Like Lockhart, Hobson began by comparing Chinese medicine unfavorably to the Western medical tradition: "Medical science in China is at a low ebb. It does not equal the state of the medical art in the time of Hippocrates and Celsus. The knowledge of anatomy and surgery in ancient Greece and Rome was much superior to anything now in India and China."[128] Hobson went on to disparage the Chinese theory of anatomy. He characterized the Chinese understanding of the circulatory system as both "preposterously confused and erroneous," and Chinese anatomical drawings as replete with "glaring errors." Hobson's report conveyed no attempt to make sense of the philosophy underpinning what he had observed. He evaluated Chinese medical knowledge and found it irredeemable: "In this condition of things," he asserted, "it seemed very desirable to attempt to introduce the well-established principles and facts of western medical science."[129] A medical missionary's memoirs served a dual purpose: they were both a justification for the European American civilizing project in China and an argument for the supremacy of Western-style medical science.

What remained invisible to the readers of such memoirs was the extent to which medical missionaries and foreign doctors working in China had absorbed certain elements of Chinese traditional medicine, particularly herbalism, into their practices. By the 1850s, missionary hospitals regularly stocked Chinese *materia medica* in their pharmacies.[130] Peter Parker and his fellow founders of the Medical Missionary Society encouraged their colleagues to learn the Chinese language so that they might research and gain insight into the unique elements of the Chinese

pharmacopoeia: "We may therefore look for a great many valuable ad-
ditions to our dispensatories."[131] Benjamin Hobson may have sneered
at Chinese theories of anatomy, but he boasted of his success treating
leprosy with chaulmoogra oil, produced by a tree native to South Asia
and long used in traditional Chinese medicine to cure various skin disorders.[132] Hobson's colleague William Lockhart also wrote dismissively
about *yinyang* doctrine and the system of correspondences, but he
praised Chinese drug therapies: "Though their theory of medicine is
imperfect, yet they have learned the use and properties of many medicines; they have seen the propriety of various forms of diet . . . Finding certain plans of treatment successful, they adapt their action to the
disease empirically. Though ever in the dark as to their principles of
treatment, they are by these means frequently successful."[133] C. Toogood
Downing, a medical officer on a British merchant ship, similarly conceded that "however deplorable the state of the *science* of medicine may
be at the present time in China, it cannot be denied that the native practitioners have yet much more success than might be expected from their
small stock of knowledge. The experience of thousands of years must
have brought forth something of general utility."[134]

Several medical missionaries sought out assistance and instruction
from practitioners of Chinese medicine. In Canton, Downing befriended
a local apothecary, whom he called his "professional brother" and consulted regularly.[135] George Tradescant Lay, a British naturalist and vice
president of the Medical Missionary Society, collaborated with a Chinese physician and made house calls with him when Lay worked as a
missionary for the British and Foreign Bible Society in southern China
from 1836 to 1839. Lay aimed not only to convert his partner's patients
but also to learn Chinese methods of diagnosis and prescription.[136]

The British victory in the first Opium War in 1842 allowed medical
missionary activity in China to accelerate and expand. In 1844, the United
States signed its own treaty with China at Wangxia, with Bridgman and
Parker serving as translators for the American emissary. The missionaries may have been instrumental in drafting an article that guaranteed
Americans the right to build hospitals along with other necessary buildings in treaty ports.[137] In the decades thereafter, medical missionaries
continued to observe, interpret, and even practice Chinese medicine.

Conclusion

Long before there were Chinese doctors in the United States, there was Chinese medicine. American druggists sold tea, rhubarb, cassia, camphor, and occasionally something more esoteric like Chinese snakestones or *Hias tea Tomchon,* the "dirty root." American physicians experimented with acupuncture and moxibustion while ginseng hunters, seeking to understand what properties made the root most valuable to their buyers, developed incomplete and incorrect impressions of Chinese medical traditions. In between the lines of letters, reports, and memoirs meant to justify the imposition of Western medical and religious norms, medical missionaries—like traders and naturalists—provided an important conduit for information moving across the Pacific to the United States. Chinese healing practices that medical missionaries dismissed as unscientific, superstitious, or "fanciful" found their way to elite and ordinary Americans in the colonial period and early republic. Knowledge of Chinese medicine thus came to early America refracted through a lens distorted by greed, overseas imperialism, and Orientalism. This corrupted perspective created the cultural environment that Chinese doctors would encounter when they began immigrating to the United States in the mid-nineteenth century.

T • W • O

Transplanted

L i Po Tai was buried with jade bracelets around his wrists and gold rings on his fingers. But first, a grand funeral procession escorted him from his apothecary in San Francisco's Chinatown to his grave. Guards carrying umbrellas shielded Li's coffin from a spring rain in March 1893. An American hearse, pulled by black horses, led a parade of mourners, representing a veritable who's who of Chinese America: the Chinese consul-general marched alongside the presidents of the Six Companies (the most prominent district organizations in Chinatown) and members of the Li family, including two grandchildren, dressed in the Chinese funereal color of white. A handful of Li's European American friends and patients joined the procession. From Li's shop at the corner of Washington Square to Stockton Street, Broadway, and Grant Avenue, and finally on to Market Street, his coffin toured San Francisco to the sound of cymbals and a medley of American- and Chinese-inspired band music. In keeping with Chinese traditions, there were offerings and a ritual sacrifice as well as money distributed in packets tied with red thread. Finally, Li's coffin was sealed and buried until such a time as his family might send his remains home to China to rest forever with their ancestors.[1]

Li had come to the United States in the early 1850s around the age of thirty-four from his birthplace in Canton Province. By some reports, he had worked in Shuntak (Shunde) County as a barber, likely acquiring skills ranging from personal grooming to dental surgery and bloodletting. In his first years in California, Li kept a shop selling general merchandise, including medicinal herbs, and dispensed medical advice as a side business, but he quickly recognized the potential gains from specialization. He went on to amass his fortune and his fame working exclusively as a doctor.[2] Diagnosing illnesses and selling medicines made him one of the wealthiest men, not just in Chinatown but in all of San Francisco. At his peak, he saw between 150 and 300 patients each day, both Chinese and non-Chinese, charging the latter $10 for a week's medications along with a $2 interpreter's fee.[3] Newspapers estimated his revenues at varying amounts: $6,000 per month, $15,000 per month, or more.[4] By the end of his life, Li was a local celebrity, with an estate totaling $50,000, including personal property, cash, and two properties: the site of his first store on Dupont Street and a second one on Washington Square.[5]

Li Po Tai's success attracted the scrutiny of tourists, journalists, and other voyeurs, who made him the object of their Orientalist desires and fears. Two newspapers—the *San Francisco Chronicle* and the *San Francisco Call*—covered his funeral in detail, and an obituary appeared in the *Los Angeles Times*. The article in the *Call* luxuriated in the ceremony's exoticism and opulence. It described the occasion as a demonstration of "rich, barbaric mourning," The *Chronicle* declared, "Should an Eastern visitor have suddenly landed yesterday at the corner of Washington Street and Brenham Place . . . he would have declared that he was in the most uncivilized portion of the Chinese empire."[6] Yet long before Li's opulent funeral became a public display of strange and splendid "Oriental" culture, his shop on Washington Square had been a popular destination for European American tourists seeking an immersive experience in the most exotic aspects of Chinatown.

The death and life of Li Po Tai open a window onto how Chinese doctors bridged their immigrant enclaves and the world beyond in the late nineteenth-century United States. The curiosity that Chinese medicine inspired among non-Chinese made its practitioners highly visible to outsiders. Tourists who frequented their shops and newspaper reporters who detailed their lives and deaths perpetuated images

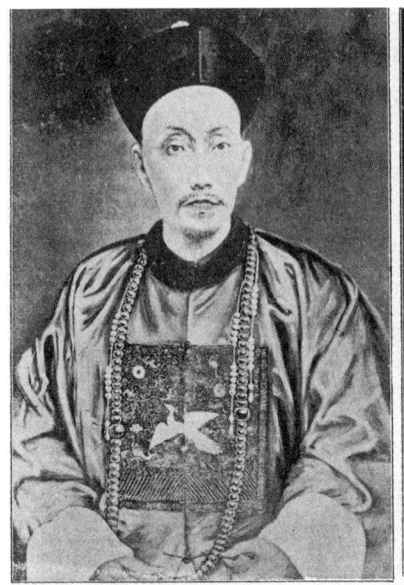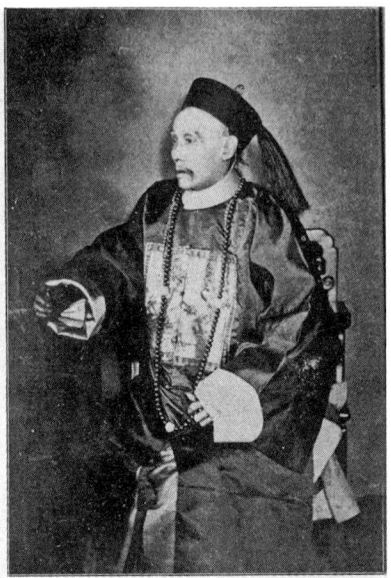

LI PO TAI
When 50 Years Old

LI PO TAI
When 75 Years Old

The above are portraits of Dr. Li Po Tai, the celebrated Chinese
Physician, who practiced his profession among the white residents of
San Francisco for nearly half a century. Among the people whom he
cured of difficult and dangerous disorders were Senator Leland
Stanford and Governor Mark Hopkins, who were for many years
among his warmest friends. People sought his advice from all the
great cities of the United States, and the average attendance at
his office was three hundred patients daily for a long time. He
made a fortune and a record of which any physician in any
country might well be proud.

Li Po Tai depicted at age fifty (left) and age seventy-five. From Foo and Wing
Herb Company, *The Science of Oriental Medicine: A Concise Discussion of
Its Principles and Methods, Biographical Sketches of Its Leading Practitioners,
and Its Treatment of Various Prevalent Diseases, Useful Information on Matters of Diet, Exercise, and Hygiene* (Los Angeles: G. Rice and Sons, 1897), 3.

of Chinese immigrants as eternally foreign and inassimilable. Willingly and unwillingly, Chinese doctors became an embodiment of Oriental exoticism. But outsiders typically failed to notice the diverse functions that herbalists fulfilled within their communities.

Li and other physicians like him were medical practitioners and educators, training successive generations of their biological and adopted kin to attend to the health care needs of their communities, but Chinatown apothecaries were not only drugstores. Decades before American pharmacies diversified their retail offerings beyond compounded drugs to surgical supplies, hygiene and cosmetic products, convenience food, candies, and other sundries, Chinese apothecaries provided imported foods and other goods to their immigrant customers.[7] They also served their communities in ways that American pharmacies never did. Chinese immigrants congregated in Chinese apothecaries to play cards, worship at shrines, and send mail. They were as likely to purchase medicine from Chinese doctors as they were to buy groceries or borrow money. As part of the merchant class, Chinese doctors could act as labor brokers or translators. Many of them were literate in Chinese and English, and as such, they were uniquely positioned to resist the prejudices that confined and oppressed their immigrant community, particularly after Chinese exclusion raised the barriers to immigration. As this chapter details, Chinese doctors sustained the literal and figurative health of American Chinatowns.

Chinatown Tourism and the Chinese Apothecary

When immigration from China to the United States began in earnest in the mid-nineteenth century, Chinese men and women tended to gather in neighborhoods or encampments labeled Chinatowns. First and foremost, Chinatowns were homes and businesses, but they also attracted the curiosity of non-Chinese visitors. Tourists who went to Chinatown, whether independently or with a hired guide, carried expectations conditioned by American Orientalism. The potential to glimpse a so-called Chinese underworld held the most appeal for tourists because it embodied what they associated with the foreign culture: exoticism, decadence, and depravity. Chinatown tourists delighted in encounters with gamblers and gangsters ("high binders"), opium "fiends," women with bound feet, or prostitutes. As historian Barbara Berglund writes of San Francisco's Chinese neighborhood, "Chinatown's appeal combined a number of overlapping impulses—the desire to see the exotic; the pull of an encounter with a different culture; the draw of slumming; and the attraction of experiencing, from a safe distance or with a police guide, racially charged urban dangers."[8] Tourism to Chinatowns spawned its own subgenre of travel literature, published in short guides, newspaper articles, or books, all of which reinforced the script of Chinese racial otherness. Theaters, restaurants, and temples attracted visitors, and retailers catered to Chinatown tourists seeking exotic goods from "the Orient," including medicines.[9]

The Chinese apothecary, with its picturesque jumble of jars and pots, became a regular feature of the Chinatown travelogue and a stop on the Chinatown tour. As chapter 1 details, Chinese medicine—particularly its *materia medica*—had long been part of American medical culture and practice, but very few nineteenth-century Americans would ever actually travel to China. A visit to a Chinatown apothecary was an immersive encounter with an Oriental fantasy. Given the number of Chinese doctors who opened their doors to non-Chinese voyeurs in the late nineteenth and early twentieth centuries, it seems likely that they had a hand in attracting such traffic to their shops. Perhaps they even orchestrated encounters with the most exotic aspects of their practice.[10] In a 1900 advertisement for their Los Angeles herb company, Tom Foo Yuen and Li Wing extended an invitation to "the invalid tourist" to soak up the salubrious southern California climate while they patronized their shop on South Olive Street.[11] In the 1930s, Oakland herbalist Fong Wan served on the tourist committee of the city Chamber of Commerce and, with his business partners, operated a cluster of businesses that catered to non-Chinese visitors including a hotel and two restaurants offering American and Chinese cuisine.[12]

One of the earliest traveler's accounts of an American Chinatown apothecary appeared in the *New York Daily Times* in 1854. Accompanied by a Chinese translator, Gustavus L. Simmons described his visit to an herb shop in Sacramento. Upon arrival, he noted that the storefront was "in no wise dissimilar to those of other occupations," except that it

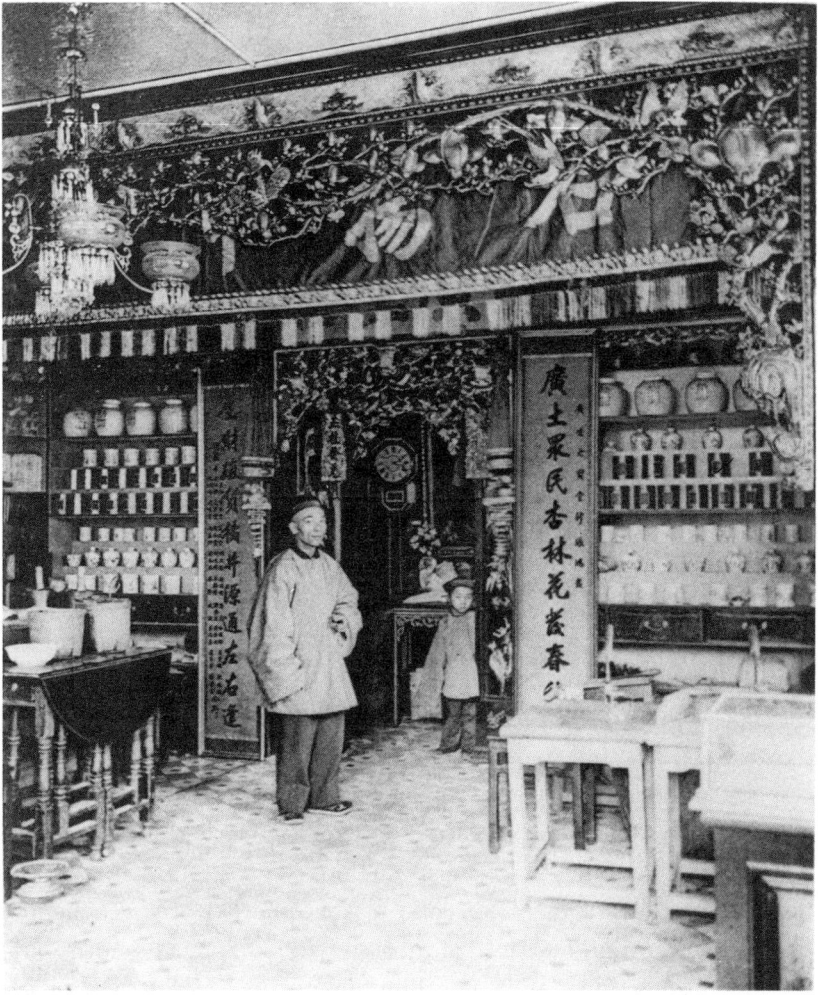

The interior of a San Francisco apothecary around the turn of the twentieth
century. Roy D. Graves Pictorial Collection, BANC PIC 1905.17500 v. 21:98—
ALB. Courtesy of the Bancroft Library, University of California, Berkeley.

was marked by an engraved, wooden sign bearing gold and vermillion
Chinese characters that spelled out the name of the resident physician,
Tung Fuk Tung. Simmons's account devoted much of its attention to
the contents of the pharmacy, "over 1,100 bundles, each marked with a
different character, and all brought from the Celestial Empire," and the

instruments used to process dried ingredients. He filtered his observations through a lens of Orientalism. His descriptions emphasized the stereotype of China as ancient and unchanging: "The scales show the great antiquity of the people. They still disdain to use other than those which have been in use for centuries. They have but a single plate and a long beam . . . similar to the old fashioned steelyard." Yet Simmons also noted, possibly with some surprise, the overlap between the Chinese and Western pharmacopoeia. He referenced common botanical and zoological medicines with similar applications and commented on their uses. As it turned out, his trip to the apothecary was but a small step into the unknown.[13]

By the 1870s, Li Po Tai's shop on Washington Square in San Francisco had become a regular stop on the travel writer's Chinatown excursion.[14] In 1875, *Lippincott's Magazine* published a "stroll" through Chinatown. Its author, J. W. Ames, professed no special knowledge of Chinese culture and engaged a police officer to escort him through the darker byways, into restaurants, opium dens, and the apothecary of the famed physician. Ames seemed at first taken aback by the banality of the shop's appearance. It looked to him like any other drugstore with its drawers and jars, but once the policeman opened a drawer for Ames's inspection, the difference was apparent: "[The drawer] is divided into four equal compartments, one containing partially charred bones of lions and tigers; another dried bugs . . . a third, some lentil-like seeds; and the fourth small fragments of bark."[15] The officer continued opening drawers while Ames marveled at their contents: rhinoceros-horn shavings, elephant's skin, "and the gallipots—quaint little earthen vessels with red labels in character—contain such sovereign remedies as alligator's gall, ass's glue, the flesh of dogs, and many other specifics that a scientific mind alone could appreciate." Later, gazing on medical charts of the human body with bemusement, Ames remarked on the visual depiction of the Chinese theory of channels: "Something not greatly unlike viscera were plentifully arranged in regular rows of parallels and generously piled up almost to the chin. For such an internal economy, no doubt the mixed tigers' bones and tumblebugs are tonic and effectual." He also noted the work of Li's apprentice, "naked to the waist . . . compounding some witch's brew." Ames reported that he left the shop, not with courteous thanks but with a cry of terror: "We closed the door with a bang and ran howling to the open air."[16]

As these early examples from Sacramento and San Francisco reflect, travelogues exhibited a morbid fascination with the Chinese pharmacopoeia. No tour of the apothecary was complete without comment on the most exotic and sensational ingredients. An 1893 article in the *Salt Lake Herald* prominently featured a large illustration captioned "Chinese Doctor Shaving Rhinoceros Horn for Medical Purposes," and called Chinese medicine "the strangest medical system in the world." Nearly a third of the article was devoted to listing the various insect and animal parts that made it into Chinese decoctions.[17] The *Los Angeles Times* too expressed a strange attraction to what it called "methods and remedies of remarkable repulsiveness." In a reprint of an article from a professional journal, the *Medical Record,* the newspaper shared with its readership a day in the life of a practitioner of Chinese medicine in China. The reporter portrayed him as "adorned with huge circular horn-rimmed spectacles and thin patriarchal chin whiskers, sitting behind his counter with his stock of remedies, which are necessary in practicing the healing art." The article went on to describe, in stomach-churning detail, how barbers-turned-surgeons and physicians cared for their patients:

> It is the custom for a Chinaman to visit his barber every week to have a general overhauling; first the head and face are shaved; second the ears are scraped and cleansed with a small brush made of duck's hair; third, the upper and lower eyelids are scraped with a dull-edged knife, all granulations being smoothed away, and then an application is made with a duck's hair brush of salt solution. This is the reason one will find so much blindness in China, as they take no antiseptic measures whatever; all instruments are held in the operator's mouth during the process of operation.

Concluding with the standard trope of the genre, the reporter listed the most shocking and bizarre Chinese remedies: spotted rhinoceros horn; tiger bones ground into wine and tiger eyeballs, livers, and blood; deer horns; gunpowder; and desiccated, pulverized cobra.[18]

An equally popular convention was to caricaturize the practitioner as an ancient, magical person. Accounts of Chinese medicine made
much of its origins in antiquity. Reporters often referred to the doctor as a disciple of "Aesculapius," the ancient Greek god of medicine
and healing.[19] When Lum Ling Wau opened shop in New York City,
the *New York Herald* announcement went a step further, calling him
both "Aesculapius" and a "Druid" in the same sentence.[20] *The World's*
biographical sketch of Choy Yeu Chong, a student of a "school of medicine that is 6,700 years old," included an eccentric history of Chinese
medicine with mention of the "Chinese Hippocrates," Shun Song, born
some 1,700 years prior and possessed of a fantastical physiology: "He
was transparent . . . He could watch his own heart pump blood through
his own arteries . . . Shun Song could take food and watch himself digest
it . . . With such a teacher, small wonder that Dr. Choy Yeu Chong de-
clares that American physicians know nothing."[21]

The Early Arrivals

Between the tiger eyeballs and Oriental wizardry, Chinatown travelogues altogether ignored the more prosaic but essential functions of the
apothecary as a business. The bespectacled, whiskered patriarchs described by tourists and reporters were merchants attending to the needs
of their immigrant communities. Due to the dangerous work that Chinese immigrants did in the United States and the discrimination they
faced, health-related services were in high demand. Reading Chinatown
travelogues and sensational journalism against other sources, including
personal and professional correspondence, advertising, material culture, and U.S. Census manuscripts, it is possible to construct a fuller
picture of the roles that Chinese medicine and its practitioners played in
late nineteenth- and early twentieth-century American Chinatowns.

By the time Indian laborers discovered gold in a millrace in northern California in 1848, well-traveled trade routes already connected the
port of San Francisco to the Pearl River Delta of Canton Province. After
many centuries of trade with Europe, Canton had a thriving market
economy and a population accustomed to traveling for work. News of
the California Gold Rush traveled quickly across the Pacific and hap-

pened to coincide with a particularly acute period of political and social upheaval in southern China. A series of natural disasters had exacerbated the region's chronic land shortages, which swelled the ranks of the landless and discontent.[22] Such conditions made a long oceanic voyage for slim prospects in a foreign land seem comparatively appealing.[23] Some twenty thousand Chinese prospectors arrived in the San Francisco Customs Shed in 1852 alone. The Cantonese provincial government further facilitated outmigration in 1859 by allowing foreign employers to recruit Chinese labor directly, and the imperial government made its approval official in the following year with the signing of the Treaty of Peking. Between 1870 and 1880, over 100,000 Chinese men and women immigrated to the United States.[24]

In these early decades, Chinese immigrants toiled in a variety of trades: domestic service, light manufacturing, construction, agriculture, and mining. The work was physical and dangerous. Railroad, construction, and mining companies hired Chinese laborers to do the least desirable and most treacherous jobs, often tunneling and blasting through granite mountainsides. Mineshafts caved in; ill-timed dynamiting claimed lives; and in the winter, frostbite took fingers and toes.[25] In remote worksites, Chinese laborers were at the mercy of their employers to provide basic necessities. In 1882, 10 percent of Chinese building the Canadian Pacific railroad died of scurvy.[26] Poverty and discrimination confined the Chinese to overcrowded and unsanitary living quarters, the perfect breeding ground for infectious diseases like influenza, cholera, typhoid fever, dysentery, and meningitis. Violence was pervasive. Within the community, rival Chinese gangs (or *tongs*) battled for supremacy.[27] Chinese people also became victims of interracial violence. Anti-coolie clubs mobbed and attacked Chinese workers. In Chinatowns, mining camps, coal pits, and railroad worksites across the United States, Chinese men were stoned, beaten, and burned.[28]

To prevent or recover from illness and injuries, the Chinese often self-diagnosed and self-dosed. They typically packed medicinal herbs and other traditional remedies in their luggage before their departure from home.[29] An 1882 article in the *San Francisco Chronicle* documented the arrival of a steamer at the Vallejo Street Wharf with hundreds of Chinese men, all "evidently believers in the Confucian art of healing,

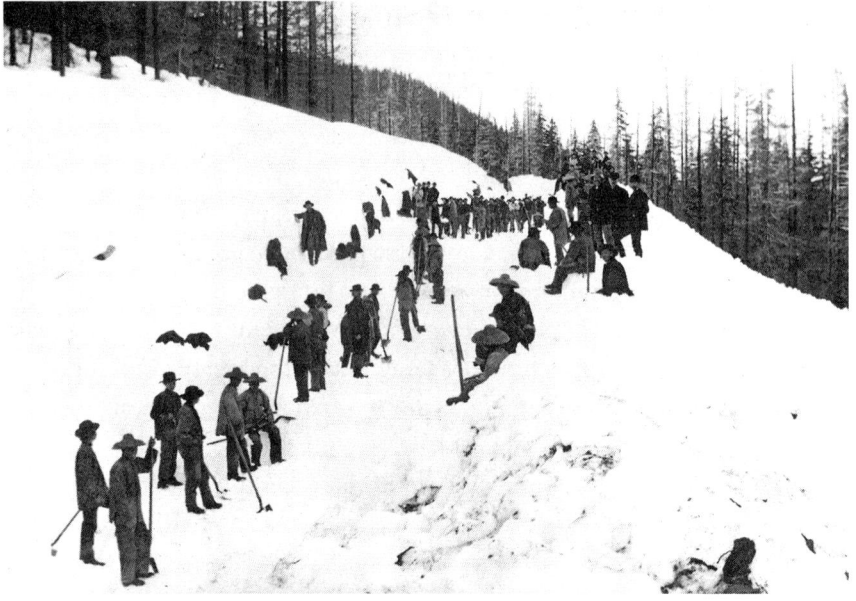

Chinese workers clearing snow from railroad tracks near the summit of the
Cascades, 1886. Courtesy of the University of Washington Libraries,
Special Collections, SOC0049.

for every trunk and bundle contained pills, herbs, and other indescrib-
able substances called medicine."[30] Moderately priced reference books,
printed in China, provided dosing guidelines for individuals without
formal training.[31] Chinese workers became adept at foraging around
their camps for familiar plants and animals with medicinal properties.
The finder kept his collection for personal use, sold it to local shops,
or shipped it home.[32] Chinese workers likely transplanted some species native to China such as *Hyoscyamus niger* (stinking nightshade),
a pain-reliever, and *Ailanthus atissima* ("Tree of Heaven"), a digestive.
Both were commonly grown in mining districts and could be used in
combination with other drugs to enhance their potency.[33] In Nevada's
Chinatowns and Chinese cemeteries, archaeologists have also recovered gingko nuts, a traditional preventative medicine.[34] Chinese men
and women might also seek out medical diagnoses and remedies at local temples. When consultation with Chinese and American doctors

failed to find a cure for Daisy Lee Chung Chow's chronic vomiting, her mother burned incense and prayed at a local shrine to a god of medicine in Kern County, California, in the 1920s. A Chinese fortune stick or oracle lot, selected at random, revealed a course of treatment for the young girl. Chow remembered that a friend of her mother's—perhaps a female herbalist—came to their home to prepare the remedy, which she credits for her recovery.[35]

Chinese workers may have had cultural preferences for their folk remedies, but they were also willing to experiment with medical practices they encountered in the United States. Glass vials recovered by archaeologists at Chinese workplaces and residences suggest trade with Native American herbalists and the consumption of American patent remedies, European American bitters, Vaseline, and aspirin.[36] Practicing Chinese physicians sometimes consulted with Western-style medical doctors for the most intractable cases. Louise Leung Larson recalled that her father, a Los Angeles doctor, Tom Leung, sought out care from an American doctor when his infant son, Taft, contracted a bad case of eczema. The family successfully treated the rash with the Cuticura brand of soap.[37] Some years later, when the elderly physician fell ill and failed to cure himself with herbs, he called in another American doctor who diagnosed him with kidney disease and prescribed a strict dietary regimen.[38]

It was not easy for Chinese patients to access treatment from American doctors.[39] European American doctors and clinics routinely denied care to Chinese immigrants or forcibly segregated them in special buildings designated for smallpox victims and lepers.[40] In San Francisco, the Chinese rarely received medical care in the city's two public hospitals. Historian Joan Trauner has analyzed hospital admissions data and noted that between 1870 and 1897, the Chinese accounted for between 5 and 11 percent of the total municipal population but only 0.1 percent of hospital inpatients at the City and County Hospital and the Almshouse. The city contemplated schemes to maintain the segregation of Chinese patients from the general population. In 1872, a state senator from San Francisco proposed a bill to tax the Chinese one dollar per capita to pay for a Chinese hospital, but ten years earlier, the courts had deemed such discriminatory legislation unconstitutional in *Lin Sing v. Washburn*, a case that rolled back a tax on the Chinese to pay for police services. The San Francisco Chinese Hospital bill did not pass.[41] In 1881, the San Francisco Board of Health resolved to bar the Chinese from admission to the City and County Hospital, located just a stone's throw from Chinatown on the corner of Francisco and Stockton Streets. Instead, they were sent to a separate clinic on the city's fringes at Twenty-Sixth and Army Streets, a site that also housed lepers.[42]

Medical discrimination against the Chinese was part of the expansion of public health bureaucracies in the late nineteenth century. From the 1870s to the 1940s, city health officers persistently slandered Chinatowns as sources of rampant infectious disease. Officials identified these areas' brothels and gambling houses, streets and sewers, people and rats as vectors for venereal disease, leprosy, smallpox, bubonic plague, and tuberculosis.[43] In San Francisco—California's largest city and the site of the largest Chinese immigrant population in the United States—regular physicians and their political allies experimented with medical investigation as a mode of social control. Beginning in 1854, state and local officials conducted investigations of Chinatown under the pretense of nuisance abatement. Their reports conflated the unavoidable environmental health hazards created by urban poverty with racial degeneration. Chinatown was dirty, overcrowded, and—consequently—susceptible to outbreaks of infectious disease, and public health officials portrayed these circumstances as tied inexorably to the alterity of the Chinese race and the dangers they posed to the city's European American majority. In reality, the Chinese had no higher rates of morbidity and mortality than other working-class San Franciscans, but as historian Nayan Shah has argued, "By 1880, the understanding of Chinatown as the site of filth, disease, and inhuman habitation had achieved a pervasiveness in public discourse as both scientific truth and common sense."[44] As smallpox swept through the city in 1869, 1876, and 1888, followed by fears of bubonic plague at the turn of the twentieth century, the Chinese became a ready target for the combined efforts of sanitarians and nativists. Western-style scientific medicine naturalized and justified public campaigns to dispossess and drive out the Chinese.[45]

In some places, the Chinese responded to medical discrimination by attempting to open and operate their own health care facilities. In

Chinatowns across the United States, *huigans* (organizations of immi-grants from the same provincial district in China) organized makeshift hospitals, with shelter and straw mats for their sick and elderly.[46] In 1873, when the county hospital in Elko, Nevada, refused to treat injured Chi-nese employees of the Central Pacific Railroad, they raised the funds to build a Chinese hospital and hired Ken Fung, a physician from Canton, to direct it.[47] For nearly twenty years, the Chinese Consolidated Benevo-lent Association of San Francisco (an umbrella association that united the city's Chinese Six Companies) and the Chinese consul-general dog-gedly petitioned the city to open a Chinese general hospital. They even went so far as to purchase land in the suburbs for the purpose, but the city denied their petition. During a smallpox epidemic in 1888, the San Francisco Supervisors' Committee on Health refused to authorize the construction of a Chinese hospital staffed solely by "Chinese doctors" because their "limited knowledge of medicines and surgery" made them incapable of "conducting a hospital without menacing the health of the neighborhood."[48]

Perhaps as a political expedient then, the first major Chinese hospi-tals in the United States incorporated Western-style therapies and hired Western-trained doctors. In 1899, the San Francisco Chinese leadership revised their request and proposed to rent a building within Chinatown for a hospital employing doctors with American or European diplomas. Ho Yow, the Chinese consul-general in San Francisco, praised the pro-posal for the city's Chinese hospital—named Tung Wah Dispensary af-ter a well-regarded hospital in Hong Kong—and insisted that the subor-dination of traditional practitioners to Western-style medical scientists reflected the preferences of the Chinese immigrant community. Ho told the *San Francisco Chronicle:* "The Chinese have seen here the benefits of western science and are glad of an opportunity to receive its benefits for themselves."[49] Ho's politics undoubtedly colored his statement to the press. Like his immediate superior, Minister Wu Tingfang in Washing-ton, D.C., Ho was a modernizer. Both Chinese diplomats had studied law at British universities before joining the Chinese diplomatic service. They had strong ties to prominent Protestant missionary societies and an intense desire to grow American investment in China. Westernizing Chinatown's medical culture was part of their multipronged effort to

enhance China's reputation among modern nations.[50] Meanwhile, in
New York, white missionaries and philanthropists formed a coalition
with Chinese merchants to raise money for a clinic in Brooklyn Heights.
Like its San Francisco counterpart, the Brooklyn hospital announced
its intention to combine "Chinese and Western methods" in treatment
and care.[51]

In 1900, these separate initiatives in San Francisco and Brooklyn
came to fruition. Their staff included traditional herbalists, but the direct managers were all Western-trained doctors, either Chinese natives
or former American medical missionaries to China.[52] A decade later,
when Chinese merchants in Portland, Oregon, raised money to open
a dedicated hospital for their immigrant community, they adopted the
same hybrid approach.[53] An organizational structure that ostensibly
placed scientific medical experts at the top combated the prejudices of
public health officials and non-Chinese neighbors, and Chinese patients
did use these hybrid institutions. The *San Francisco Chronicle* reported
that the San Francisco hospital treated over three thousand patients in
its first two years alone.[54]

The Chinese hospitals in San Francisco and Brooklyn struggled
nonetheless. When public health officials pinned the 1900 outbreak of
bubonic plague on Chinese laborers in San Francisco, the mayor's office
forced the clinic to become a lazaretto (a house to isolate victims of infectious diseases), staffed by Western-style medical scientists. Its image
never recovered.[55] Decades later, San Francisco's first Chinese hospital
was still remembered as little more than a "deathhouse" where patients
came only as a last resort. In 1906, the citywide fire that followed San
Francisco's historic earthquake destroyed the building, but Tung Wah
Dispensary rebuilt and eventually incorporated as the San Francisco
Chinese Hospital in 1925.[56] Across the country in New York, the Brooklyn hospital floundered, closing when it could not comply with New
York's medical licensing laws.[57] In the next decade, a Chinese hospital
in Manhattan, also funded by Chinatown merchants, failed for similar
reasons, and efforts to reopen the Brooklyn hospital were not renewed
until 1907.[58]

Beginning in the late nineteenth century, a select few Chinese
men and women studied scientific medicine at European or Ameri-

can medical colleges. American and British missionaries in China selected promising young Chinese men and some women for study
abroad with the hopes that they would return to their homeland to
proselytize equally for Christ and for scientific medicine. In 1847, Yung
Wing and Wong Shing were the first Chinese men known to matriculate
at an American medical college. Wong, unfortunately, fell ill and had to
return to China, but Yung completed his course of study and received
his diploma in medicine from Yale University in 1854.[59] In the 1880s
and 1890s, the first Chinese women graduated from American medical schools: Yamei Kin from the Women's Medical College of New York
in 1884, Mary Stone (Shi Meiyu; "Stone" was an English translation of
her family name) and Ida Kahn (Kang Cheng) from the University of
Michigan in 1892, and Hu King Eng from the Women's Medical College of Philadelphia at approximately the same time. All of them were
affiliated with missionary societies, and upon graduation each duti-
fully returned to China, where they assumed prominent positions at
Western-style hospitals.[60]

Some members of this pioneering generation of Chinese doctors remained in the United States after completing their studies, but
they did not strictly practice scientific medicine. Joseph C. Thoms, who
graduated from Long Island College Hospital in 1889, seems to have
been successful catering to the Chinese community of Brooklyn with
a mix of Western-style and traditional therapies.[61] Similarly, Wah Jean
Lamb, who went by the name "Dr. Lamb" among his European American patients, practiced Chinese herbalism after receiving an M.D. With
the assistance of missionaries in Canton, Lamb studied at the University of Southern California College of Medicine and graduated in 1896.[62]
Not long thereafter, he moved to Butte, Montana, where he hung out
his shingle as a traditional "Chinese herb physician." From at least 1905
to 1922, his advertisements in local newspapers included an easily recognizable illustration of a Chinese man wearing a Mandarin hat and
jacket. He promised to "cure all disease with his famous Chinese medicine, never before introduced into this country."[63] It is not clear whether
Lamb's American medical degree helped him when he applied for a license to practice medicine with Montana's Board of Medical Examiners
in 1901. The *Great Falls Tribune* noted that Lamb "was allowed to take

the examination" because he spoke "excellent English," but there is no record of his licensure until 1915.[64]

A rare exception, Jim (or Jin) Fuey Moy did practice Western-style scientific medicine among Chinese immigrants in the United States, but he does not seem to have been terribly successful at it. Moy paid his way through Jefferson Medical College in Philadelphia by working as a valet, clerk, and interpreter. In 1891, he returned to San Francisco, where he offered Western-style medical therapies to Chinese immigrants with a mixed reception. The *Philadelphia Record* noted that he "had a hard battle against their ignorance and superstition. When Chinamen are taken sick they have greater faith in the treatment of their native doctors or medicine men, and readily accept their wonderful decoctions of drugs and chemicals which are prescribed."[65] Although it is not possible to confirm or refute the assessment of the *Philadelphia Record,* we can say for certain that Jim did not stay in San Francisco for long. By 1893, he was back in New York, working with St. Bartholomew's Episcopal Church to combat anti-Chinese discrimination.[66] If Jim continued to practice medicine in New York or New Jersey, where he eventually relocated with his American wife and daughter, there is no record of it. Perhaps Jim found that racialized expectations of medical authority were too difficult to transcend. In California, Montana, and New York, it was easier for a Chinese man to present himself to the American medical marketplace as an herbalist. A Chinese M.D. would have struggled to secure the trust of patients conditioned to seek out Chinese people for Chinese medicine and European American people for Western-style scientific medicine.

For American-born Chinese M.D.s, nativity did not lower the barrier that race threw up. Born in San Francisco in 1882, the year of the passage of the first Chinese Exclusion Act, Shin Tive Pond Mooar Jee was likely the first American-born Chinese person to graduate from a major medical college when he received his diploma from the University of California, San Francisco, in 1908. He practiced medicine in the United States for fewer than four years before relocating permanently to Harbin, China, with his Chinese American wife, Mabel.[67] He left no record of why he moved to China, but it is not a stretch to think that he might have found Chinese hospitals and their patients more accepting of his authority as a medical scientist.

Setting Down Roots

In the absence of a trusted Chinese hospital or ready access to mainstream health services, Chinese herbalists provided essential services to their communities. As early as 1851, a Chinese herb shop operated out of a rammed-earth adobe building in Fiddletown, a mining community in Amador County, California. Chinese immigrant Fan-Chung Yee opened the Chew Kee Herb Shop to cater to Chinese miners working the Mother Lode. Even after Gold Rush euphoria waned, historians estimate that between five and ten thousand Chinese continued to reside in the vicinity of Fiddletown. Chinese miners became railroad workers, employed by the Central Pacific, and Yee's shop attended to their injuries and ailments.[68] In 1856, a San Francisco directory of Chinese businesses identified fifteen pharmacies and five doctors, and federal census manuscripts from 1860 counted over thirty Chinese druggists or physicians residing in the city.[69] In 1860, when the federal census counted 35,933 Chinese men and women living in the United States, census takers identified 189 as physicians, druggists, or doctors.[70] In aggregate federal census tables from 1870, 193 Chinese physicians were enumerated.[71] According to historian Liu Boji, every Chinese settlement in the United States had between one and four herbalists.[72]

It is difficult to estimate the total population of Chinese physicians in the late nineteenth-century United States with great precision. A decennial census only captures a moment in time. Given the mobility and high rate of return migration among Chinese immigrants, it is impossible to say how many doctors moved in, out, and around different states between census years. Moreover, as with all classifications of occupation, census enumerators identified individuals as doctors only if they "discharge[d] such duties to the exclusion of other gainful occupations or, at least, as their principal or sole professed means of support."[73] Thus, individuals who sold herbs and offered medical advice may or may not have been included in the count depending on how they self-identified and how the census canvasser perceived their princi-pal mode of employment.[74] While federal census takers probably failed to notice each individual practicing medicine, their count was probably not a gross underestimate. In 1870 and 1880, among the general popula-tion, the percentage of physicians and surgeons was 0.2 percent, com-pared to 0.3 percent among the Chinese. There is no reason to expect that the proportion of doctors in the Chinese immigrant community would be significantly higher than that of the general population.

Up until 1880, Chinese doctors were concentrated in California, where the population of Chinese immigrants and the need for their ser-vices were greatest. Census manuscripts from 1860 located only one Chi-nese doctor residing outside of California. Identified as a "Chinaman," he was a forty-five-year-old physician who lived in Jackson County, a gold-mining district in southern Oregon.[75] In 1870, the census recorded all but nineteen Chinese physicians and surgeons as residing in Cali-fornia. The scattered remainder were in Idaho, Montana, Nevada, and Oregon, not coincidentally the places that boasted the largest popula-tions of Chinese people after California (table 1). This pattern remained consistent in the 1880 census as Chinese populations fanned out to other states and territories (table 2).

Table 1: Chinese and Japanese doctors in the United States, 1870

State or territory	Number of Chinese and Japanese doctors	Total Chinese population
California	174	49,277
Oregon	8	3,330
Idaho Territory	6	4,274
Montana	3	1,949
Nevada	2	3,152

Source: U.S. Census, 1870 (Washington, D.C.: Government Printing Office, 1872), 1:719–765.
Note: These numbers include Japanese physicians since the census combined Chinese and Japanese native-born respondents in the same category. But given that the population of Japanese immigrants in the United States in 1870 totaled 55 people, it seems unlikely that they accounted for a significant number of the 193 physicians and surgeons enumerated in the census.

Table 2: Chinese doctors in the United States, 1880

State or territory	Number of Chinese doctors	Total Chinese population
California	196	73,548
Oregon	48	9,472
Nevada	25	5,402
Idaho Territory	8	3,366
New York	4	1,015
Wyoming Territory	3	913
Montana	2	1,756
Washington Territory	2	3,166
Arizona Territory	1	11,642
Colorado	1	601

Source: U.S. Census, 1880, Records of the Bureau of the Census, Record Group 29, National Archives, Washington, D.C., Ancestry.com; Department of the Interior, Census Office, *Compendium of the 10th Census,* part 1 (Washington, D.C.: Government Printing Office, 1882), 483. In her book *Dreaming of Gold, Dreaming of Home,* Madeline Yuan-yin Hsu identifies an entrepreneurial doctor from Taishan (Toishan) who opened an herb shop in Savannah, Georgia, in the 1870s, but he went unnoticed by the 1880 census. Madeline Yuan-yin Hsu, *Dreaming of Gold, Dreaming of Home* (Stanford, Calif.: Stanford University Press, 2000), 29.

Chinese doctors also clustered in Hawaii before it became a part of the United States. Chinese immigrants began arriving in the Kingdom of Hawaii in the 1850s, mainly as contract laborers on sugar plantations. The first Chinese doctor may have come to Hawaii as a medical officer for a British ship originating in Hong Kong in 1852.[76] He appeared in the public record when he applied for permission to care for Chinese patients in Honolulu. Purportedly educated in Macao, the doctor had developed a positive reputation among his countrymen, especially in the wake of a smallpox epidemic in 1853. In 1859, the medical board, a subsidiary of the Ministry of the Interior, refused to issue him a license, which sparked outrage among Honolulu's Chinese merchant class.[77] Eventually, the medical board reversed itself.[78] By 1860, the medical board had licensed three Chinese physicians.[79] Such decisions

proceeded on an ad-hoc basis until 1880, when the king and the Legislative Assembly officially licensed "any native of China" with good
standing and authority to practice medicine in the Hawaiian kingdom.[80]
By 1887, the *Hawaiian Gazette* reported that the new law had licensed
twenty-eight physicians in total.[81]

Chinese doctors also immigrated to Mexico and Canada. Indeed,
New Spain had likely been their first place of arrival in the Americas. In
colonial Mexico, Chinese healers found employment as *barberos* ("barbers"), a quasi-medical profession. In 1635, Spanish barbers filed a petition with Mexico City's council objecting to unfair competition with
"*chino* slaves." The colonial government responded by restricting Chinese barbers in several ways. No longer could they practice in the cen-
trally located Plaza Mayor nor could Spanish barbers take them on as
apprentices. They were also subject to special, limited licensing. Nonetheless, Chinese barbers continued to practice in Mexico City, with or
without a license, up until the nineteenth century, and their reputation
as blood-letters—one of the barber's essential services—created a permanent niche for them in the Mexican medical profession as phleboto-
mists.[82] Outside of Mexico and what would become the United States,
British Columbia was a major destination for Chinese immigrating to
North America. By 1880, the Canadian census identified 6 Chinese physicians serving a community of over 4,300 Chinese men and women.[83]

In the most remote corners of the United States, Chinese doctors
catered to the needs of Chinese miners, timber workers, and ranch and
farmhands. In California, only 73 of 196 Chinese doctors counted in the
1880 census lived and worked in San Francisco. The remaining 123 lived
in various mining towns and trading outposts across the state (table 3).

Rural parts of Nevada, Oregon, and Idaho similarly boasted significant numbers of Chinese physicians in the late nineteenth century.
The 1880 federal census identified twenty-five Chinese doctors living in
Nevada, and historian Sue Fawn Chung estimates that some fifty-seven
worked in the territory between 1860 and 1890.[84] Beginning in the 1850s,
major mineral discoveries on the Carson River drew Chinese immigrants from California to what was then Utah Territory. They primarily found work in the mining and timber industries. Mormons hired
Chinese laborers to dig irrigation ditches in the Carson Valley and then

Table 3: Chinese doctors in California by county, 1880

County	Number of Chinese doctors
San Francisco	73
Sacramento	17
Butte	16
Placer	12
Tehama	7
Alameda	6
Los Angeles	6
Amador	5
Siskiyou	5
Tuolumne	5
Santa Clara	4
Nevada	3
San Joaquin	3
Inyo	2
Trinity	2
Yuba	2
Merced	2
Mono	2
Calaveras	2
San Diego	2
El Dorado	1
Fresno	1
Kern	1
Madera	1
Mendocino	1
Monterey	1
Napa	1
Plumas	1
San Bernardino	1
Santa Barbara	1
Sierra	1
Solano	1
Stanislaus	1
Ventura	1
Yolo	1

Source: U.S. Census, 1880, Records of the Bureau of the Census, Record Group 29, National Archives, Washington, D.C., Ancestry.com.

permitted them to stay under the assumption that they would leave when surface-level (or placer) deposits dried up. Defying expectations, the Chinese continued to work their claims for several decades.[85] In the 1860s and 1870s, the Chinese of Nevada migrated north and east, following the Central Pacific Railroad and the major gold discoveries in Elko County. Not surprisingly, the distribution of Chinese doctors in Nevada reflected the distribution of the Chinese population. Nevada's capital, Carson City, which was the major commercial center and transportation crossroads of the territory and then state, boasted six Chinese doctors in the 1880 federal census. Virginia City, the closest urban center to the Comstock Lode, and a nearby town of Gold Hill were home to five more Chinese doctors according to the 1880 census. Another cluster of five lived near the silver- and lead-rich hills near Eureka, and a few were scattered across mining boomtowns like Tuscarora and Treasure Hill.[86]

Chinese miners made their way to Oregon as early as 1851, when gold was first discovered in the Rogue River Valley, and their numbers increased with the series of discoveries around the Blue Mountains and Snake River in the 1860s and 1870s. In 1862, eastern Oregon experienced its own gold rush when miners on their way to the Florence mines in Idaho stumbled on placer deposits in Canyon Creek. Within a month, hundreds of other prospectors descended on the area. A year later, Canyon City was established with 1,500 residents and soon achieved a reputation as a thriving waystation for gold miners traveling throughout eastern Oregon and Idaho. As was the case in California, panning for gold quickly gave way to more capital-intensive forms of mining, and soon labor gangs were working in deep-vein mines, blasting the sides of mountains with water and dredging riverbed gravel as waged employees of ever-larger mining companies. By the 1870s, the Chinese were among them, with perhaps as many as a thousand of them making their homes in an encampment adjacent to Canyon City. They took jobs with mining companies or lit out on their own, to pick through the gravel left behind by hydraulic and dredge operations or to work the meager remnants of the placer deposits.[87]

Eastern Oregon Chinese miners were subject to the same kinds of racialized violence and acts of terrorism that their compatriots faced elsewhere in the United States, and after a fire devastated Canyon City's

Chinatown in 1885, city officials seized on the opportunity to cast out the community. Some seeking safety in numbers moved away to mining towns in Washington and Idaho with larger Chinese populations, but about five hundred or so decamped farther down the creek in "Lower Town," later renamed John Day for the river nearby.[88] In 1870, the Chinese population of Grant County—where Canyon City and John Day are located—numbered 946, the highest it would ever be. Three doctors were among them. Ten years later, the population had declined slightly to 905 but added another physician.[89] In 1880, the census identified two local physicians, Chi Wah and Ah Look.[90] Nearby counties like Baker and Union also boasted a handful of Chinese physicians, likely employed by mining companies to attend to the needs of Chinese laborers under contract with them.[91]

On John Day River, in mining and timber country, Ing Hay set up shop in the 1880s. "Doc Hay," as he was known to his English-speaking patients, became the best remembered of the United States' Chinese herbalists. Between 1888 and 1948, Ing operated an apothecary in a building formerly occupied by a trading post and fort on the Dalles Military Road, connecting the Columbia River to the interior of eastern Oregon and Idaho. Because the building bears a resemblance to southern Chinese farmhouses, some speculate that it was constructed by Chinese immigrants who worked on the road in the 1860s. By 1871, Chinese miners were using the building as a general store called Kam Wah Chung and Company. In 1888, Ing and two other Chinese immigrants—Lung On and Ye Nem—pooled their resources to take over the business from another Chinese immigrant, Shee Pon.[92] Among the three partners who assumed control of Kam Wah Chung in 1888, very little is known about Ye, who quickly sold his share to the other two and vanished from the written record. Lung, fluent in both Chinese and English, left a fuller accounting of his life and that of his partner, Ing, through his correspondence with other Chinese merchants and non-Chinese acquaintances as well as through business documents.

In many ways, Ing was a typical Chinese immigrant. He had immigrated to the United States in 1883 with his father and made his way to John Day as a gold prospector, arriving in 1887. With the ink barely dry on the 1882 Chinese Exclusion Act and little certainty of how its

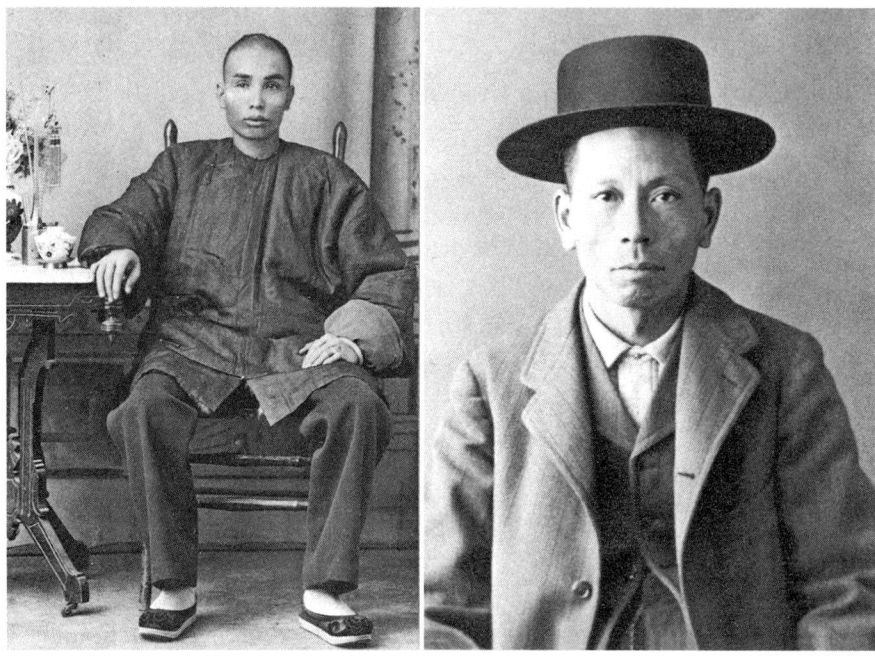

Herbalist Ing Hay (left) and his business partner Lung On. Courtesy of
Kam Wah Chung State Heritage Site Archival Collection, Oregon Parks
and Recreation Department.

terms would be applied, twenty-one-year-old Ing left his wife and two
children in Taishan, in southern China. He and his father followed five
of Ing's uncles, who had settled and flourished in Walla Walla, Washington, in the 1860s and 1870s. Ing and his father entered the United States
via Port Townsend, where Chinese arrivals were subject to relatively less
scrutiny by American officials. Although he had a few years of training
in Chinese medicine (probably as an apprentice in a Chinese drugstore),
Ing did not initially apply his experience in the United States. In the few
years he stayed in Walla Walla, he worked as a miner and laborer, not as
a doctor. When his father opted to return to China in 1887, Ing pressed
on, moving from Walla Walla to John Day.[93] Ing Hay had good reason
to go to John Day. Most of the miners who clustered in there were also
from Taishan, spoke the same dialect, and shared the surname, "Ing."
They considered themselves part of one extended family.[94] Local lore re-

calls that Ing Hay learned pulsology and herbal medicine from an older Chinese resident of John Day, "Doc Lee," whose presence was not noted in the 1880 census. The story goes that Doc Lee, recognizing Ing's innate sensitivity and aptitude for diagnosis by pulse, took him on as an apprentice and bequeathed to him a book of medicinal herbs and prescriptions now on display at the restored Kam Wah Chung building.[95]

Like Ing Hay, Lung On also left behind a family in China to immigrate to the United States. He arrived in San Francisco in 1882 and was evidently fluent in English by 1887. He was charismatic and educated, able to read and write in classical Chinese. By all accounts, Lung and Ing had a tense but productive partnership. Lung was a gambler whose proclivities threatened to undermine the business, but his bilingualism made him invaluable.[96] While Ing tended to patients, Lung interfaced with English-speaking business owners and officials, assisted Ing in the pharmacy, and drove him to house calls in a horse-drawn buggy.[97]

Idaho, like Oregon and Nevada, drew a significant population of Chinese laborers to work in mining and railroad construction, and by the late nineteenth century, southwestern Idaho was home to the second-largest population of Chinese immigrants in the United States, following San Francisco. The territorial capital, Boise, located at the crossroads of the Oregon Trail and major routes into the mineral-rich Boise Basin and Owyhee mines, boasted a large and bustling Chinatown on Idaho Street between Seventh and Eighth Streets. Although the 1880 federal census enumerated eight Chinese physicians residing in mining camps near Boise, it did not identify any living in the city itself.[98] The two most famous Chinese physicians in Boise, Chin Man Sui and C. K. Ah Fong, did not migrate to the city until the 1890s, but both achieved such local success and notoriety as to become the subject of short biographies and, in the case of Ah Fong, the inspiration for an exhibit at the Idaho State Historical Society.

Census manuscripts note that Chin immigrated to the United States from China in 1872, at the age of twenty-two and just three years after his marriage.[99] Crossing over the Oregon-Idaho border, he built a medical practice in what would become White Bird, the site of the first battle in the Nez Perce War of 1877. Conflict with Indians disrupted Chin's business and eventually drove him from White Bird to Boise, where he established another clinic in its Chinatown. There he served Chinese and non-Chinese patients until his death in 1916.[100]

Chin's notoriety was eclipsed by that of Ah Fong, who sold herbs and offered medical advice from 1892 to 1927 out of a pair of apothecaries in the heart of Boise's Chinatown. As "Ah Fong Chuck," he immigrated to the United States in 1867 at the age of twenty-two, purportedly with some education in medicine. He came with his father, Whey Fong, who was also a doctor. U.S. Customs officials made an error while processing his immigration documents, and Ah Fong Chuck became C. K. Ah Fong. Ah Fong and his father's motivation for emigrating may have been political. They came from a merchant family at odds with the Manchu leadership in Canton and were somehow involved with anti-Manchu protests that unleashed the Taiping Rebellion and Hakka-Punti Wars in the 1850s and 1860s. The father and son initially set up shop in San Francisco, but perhaps finding competition among Chinese physicians too fierce, in 1875 Ah Fong made his way to Idaho, where he offered his services to the Chinese miners in the boomtowns of Rocky Bar and Atlanta.[101] He stayed there until 1892, when a hotel fire spread and destroyed much of Rocky Bar.[102]

Ah Fong restarted his business in Boise's Chinatown. He opened up an apothecary at 824 Idaho Street, occupying the ground floor of a building owned by a local Chinese *tong*. Because of his family connections to the medical trade in China, Ah Fong was able to develop a thriving wholesale business. He imported traditional medicines from Canton, Siup-ki, and Shanghai, and distributed them to Pacific Northwest Chinese apothecaries as well as to individual mail-order customers residing across the greater Rocky Mountain West and south to Mexico.[103] To expand his retail operations, he opened a second branch of his store on Seventh Street. Ah Fong remained in Boise for the rest of his life. He was married and widowed three times over and raised two biological children and two more adopted ones. Upon his death at the age of eighty-two in 1927, he left his eldest son, Herbert, and grandson Gerald to carry on the family business.[104]

The 1880 census takers did not always recognize Chinese physicians in their population counts. Although it is difficult to document such omissions, one can assume that every sizeable Chinese population

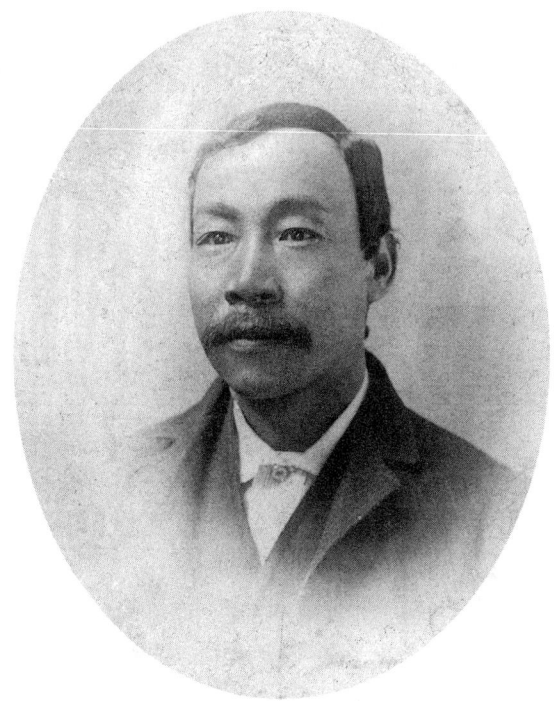

C. K. Ah Fong, 1893. Image no. 70-178-1.
Courtesy of Idaho State Archives.

had a purveyor of traditional medicines. For example, in Utah Territory, where the 1880 federal census counted 502 Chinese people, someone must have assumed responsibility for importing and distributing Chinese medicines even if the census taker failed to identify him. Census manuscripts from 1880 identified the vast majority of Utah Chinese as laborers or launderers, but four were categorized as shopkeepers and another seven as merchants. Perhaps Hong Lee, identified by the census taker as "keep[ing] store" in the town of Terrace in Box Elder County, Utah, stocked Chinese herbs. Forty-seven years old in 1880, Hong lived in a community of 165 Chinese men and 13 Chinese women not far from Promontory Point, where the "golden spike" united the Union Pacific and Central Pacific Railroads in 1869. Many of the Box Elder County Chinese had come to Utah with the transcontinental railroads and stayed on after their completion to work in maintenance. Census manuscripts list Hong as living alongside a tailor, Wong Tschong, and a cook, Ching Winn. Nearby was a launderer, Yong Pou, and a grocer, Ching Moon. Did these four men provide the basic provisions for the community of laborers: food, clothing, and medicine? Or possibly the duty fell to Gun Wau or Kin Long, men who owned "Chinese Stores" in nearby Ogden, a major railroad hub and point of disembarkation for freight and travelers coming from San Francisco.[105] They would have been well positioned to receive shipments from San Francisco herb wholesalers. Gun Wau is perhaps the more likely candidate of the two Ogden merchants; his name was similar to that of another Chinese physician who practiced in Pittsburgh in 1889 as well as to a name given to a chain of Chinese-style drugstores that spread across the Midwest in the 1890s.[106] By 1885, the Salt Lake City newspaper the *Daily Tribune* recorded the presence of Mun Yook, who "hung out his shingle on Fifth Street" in Ogden and promised to cure "outside" sickness, meaning anything that could be visually observed such as broken bones and skin disorders.[107] Other doctors appeared in the public record in the 1890s, primarily in Utah's major population centers like Salt Lake City, Ogden, and Brigham City.[108]

Community Care

Despite the sensationalism of San Francisco Chinatown travelogues, Li Po Tai's business took place in a rather mundane setting. His Washington Square shop occupied a brick building, converted from a resort and restaurant into an office and clinic. In the old restaurant kitchen, Li's assistants prepared his prescriptions while the dining hall served as a combination reception area and exam room for male patients. Women were escorted into a small adjoining chamber for private consultations.[109] Li ran the most famous and successful apothecary in nineteenth-century San Francisco's Chinatown, and his establishment was befittingly substantial. His contemporaries often worked out of smaller spaces: in rented rooms above storefronts or in their family's parlors (usually while a wife or assistant compounded drugs in the kitchen). Some Chinese doctors made house calls like their American competitors.

For their patients, the main difference between a visit to a Chinese herbalist and one to an American physician was not the office environment but the presence or absence of a pharmacy. American pharmacists and physicians defined themselves as separate professions, decoupling the compounding and sale of drugs from clinical evaluation and diagnosis.[110] For practitioners of Chinese medicine, these functions remained lodged under one roof, often under the supervision of a single person.

In the late nineteenth century, Chinese physicians like Li primarily practiced pulsology and herbalism. This therapeutic emphasis reflected the demographics of Chinese immigration. In China, there were multiple strata of health care providers: At the top were the formally educated doctors, who trained under the auspices of the Imperial Medical Academy in Peking (Beijing) and were guaranteed employment caring for the emperor and his extended family. Such individuals had little reason to immigrate overseas. At the bottom were informally trained or self-taught male and female healers, itinerant drug peddlers, and midwifes. They were likely among the laboring classes that immigrated to the United States, but they may have largely conducted their medical work out of the public eye, in ways not easily captured by the historical record. An occasional mention of a Chinese midwife or a shamanic healing might appear in local lore or legal records, but without the financial means to rent an office or run an advertisement, these healers left behind only traces of their existence. Among overseas Chinese medical practitioners, the most visible were the middling class of merchant-physician. Many of them had apprenticed at a Chinese drugstore, where they usually learned to make a single, proprietary remedy and to diagnose patients by taking their pulse.[111]

In our own time, acupuncture is the modality most commonly associated with traditional Chinese medicine in the United States, but it was a negligible part of the nineteenth-century doctor's repertoire. Acupuncture and its frequently paired therapy moxibustion (or moxacautery) were ancient treatments that had fallen out of fashion in nineteenth-century China. In 1822, the emperor forbade the Imperial Medical Academy from teaching acupuncture, fearing that the needles—which in the nineteenth century bore some resemblance to scalpels—might be used in an assassination attempt against him or his family.[112] By the early twentieth century, acupuncture persisted only among lower-class street surgeons.[113] Consequently, very few Chinese merchant-doctors had any significant contact with, let alone training in, acupuncture.[114] Nonetheless, some Chinese doctors in the United States did perform acupuncture and moxibustion as a secondary business. Boise doctor Ah Fong, for example, was renowned for his expertise in diagnosis by pulse and herbal remedies, but artifacts and medical texts recovered from his estate suggest that his services may have included acupuncture and moxibustion as well.[115] Thomas W. Wing recalled that his father, Sue Narm Shun (who went by the name N. S. Sue among his English-speaking patients), was primarily an herbalist but occasionally offered acupuncture (with needles) or acupressure (with touch, heat, or magnets) as well as cupping to his patients in Modesto, California, in the 1920s.[116]

In traditional Chinese apothecaries, a doctor examined and diagnosed but did not compound remedies. Historian Paul D. Buell has noted that this custom remained prevalent among Chinese doctors in British Columbia.[117] At some of the larger American apothecaries, such an arrangement may have been possible. For example, in San Francisco, Li Po Tai hired a fleet of druggists to handle the preparation of medicine, whereas in John Day, Oregon, Ing Hay seems to have done that work with the assistance of his business partner Lung On.[118] Druggists and their assistants ground dried substances with a mortar and pestle, weighed them carefully, and combined and packaged them.[119] Like American pharmacists, some Chinese herbalists offered mail-order services for patients unable to meet face to face. Patients wrote letters describing their ailments or filled out preprinted "symptom sheets," and the doctor sent back packages of medicine along with detailed instruction sheets. Sometimes mail-order prescriptions would include an unusually long list of ingredients to address ambiguous descriptions of symptoms.[120]

The overseas Chinese formulary would have likely been composed mostly of medicinal herbs and vegetables with rarer, more expensive animal products like deer antler and tiger's bone used only sparingly.[121] An inventory of medicinal ingredients recovered at Kam Wah Chung was 91 percent botanical, 6 percent zoological, and 3 percent mineral.[122] For the most part, Chinese medicines were sourced in China because of the specificity with which each ingredient had to be cultivated and processed, and Chinese doctors imported medicines from Hong Kong or Canton through the port of San Francisco. By 1878, there were eighteen wholesale herb companies in San Francisco.[123] Chinese doctors who knew one another might trade or purchase small quantities when needed, and there are some indications of exchange between Chinese doctors and non-Chinese merchants for items such as opium.[124] There is ample evidence—both anecdotal and archaeological—that the Chinese in America grew and foraged for local sources of medicinal ingredients. In 1898, a newspaper in Washington, D.C., reported that Lee Poit, recently transplanted from California, had given up trying to compete in the crowded field of laundry and retail and was instead growing "many queer vegetables and herbs" on four acres of land that he rented near Terra Cotta Station, on the Baltimore and Ohio Railroad. He sold his produce to the Chinese businesses in the district.[125] After Appalachian and Midwestern sources of wild ginseng had been depleted, Chinese doctors in the United States seem to have turned to cultivated varietals of the medicinal root.[126] J. B. McCloskey, an American farmer who studied commercial ginseng production in Korea, opened his own farm on two acres in Oxnard in 1904 and became the major supplier for Los Angeles–area Chinese physicians.[127]

Zoological-based medicines seem to have been sourced nearby as well. An 1880 advertisement for Sacramento druggist and apothecary Loy Fook Wan read, "Wanted—Bear Galls," and in 1900 the *Los Angeles Times* noted a lively business in "bear feet speculation" among members of the Chinese community.[128] In 1902, one of Ing Hay's white customers in eastern Oregon attempted to repay his debts by offering up a gland (probably a gall bladder) from a bear he caught.[129] The Chinese also collected all manner of reptiles and amphibians—snakes, lizards, frogs, and toads—to supplement dried, imported varieties.[130] A San Francisco newspaper noted that Los Angeles herbalist Hop Lee hunted horned toads in the Sierra Madre foothills for his Chinatown pharmacy.[131] Sometimes doctors substituted local species that seemed similar to what would have been available in China. In Boise, Idaho, C. K. Ah Fong famously used rattlesnake (a North American reptile) in traditional Chinese tinctures to treat arthritis, and amid other Chinese health-related artifacts from Lovelock, Nevada, archaeologist Sarah Heffner has found bobcat bones that may have been used in place of expensive, imported tiger bones.[132] As Li Wing Fawn explained to the *Los Angeles Times* in 1896, "We shall not confine ourselves exclusively to the importations from the Orient, but shall seek out also the very many valuable medicinal herbs growing in our own country [the United States]."[133] Chinese doctors were not so bound by tradition that they failed to adapt their formularies to their new environment.

Where self-care failed, ailing immigrants first looked to their local herbalists for relief. Chinese physicians were often the first line of defense against outbreaks of epidemic disease. In 1869, an editorial in the *Daily Alta California* noted that the smallpox epidemic sweeping through San Francisco caused no fatalities in Chinatown due to the ministrations of a Chinese physician and asked:

> Is it not worthwhile to examine into the matter and see if we cannot gain some hints from the Chinese which would be valuable as a means of saving the lives of our own people? . . . It is easy enough to sneer at a man and call him a barbarian, quack, or humbug; but in a time like this we cannot afford to do so, if there is any chance of his being able to teach us what we desire to learn. Civilization has been indebted to China for many of the greatest arts and inventions and may it not be worthwhile to ascertain whether we cannot yet learn something of inestimable value from her people?[134]

Chinese doctors offered care not only for their own community but also for the general population. In the winter of 1891 and 1892, an outbreak of influenza struck gold prospectors in Rocky Bar, Idaho. A county newspaper reported that Ah Fong's patients experienced an unusually high recovery rate. He quickly gained a local reputation as a gifted healer among Chinese and non-Chinese patients alike.[135]

Public records—written by regular physicians and their political allies—typically obscured or denigrated Chinese medicine. Reading against the grain of these politically motivated texts, however, it becomes clear that public health officials were aware of the work that Chinese doctors did for their communities and did not exclude them out of hand. In 1878, an outbreak of leprosy in a San Francisco jail occasioned the meeting of a county physician and a Chinese doctor named Loo Chan Foey. The county physician, a Dr. Blach, read a paper before the local medical society meeting in which he described the "native treatment" furnished by Loo.[136] In Chicago, officials were divided over the utility of traditional Chinese medicine in matters of public health. The city's health commissioner told a local newspaper that "their drugs are efficacious . . . there is virtue in their pharmacopoeia," while a colleague in the same department retorted, "Don't make any difference. [A Chinese doctor] can't practice medicine in Illinois unless he passes an examination and gets a license."[137] Collaboration with practitioners of traditional medicine made sense for public health officials seeking to contain epidemic disease with minimum disruption to their broader constituency. In February 1900, Wong Chut King, a lumberyard worker in San Francisco, suffered fever, aches, painful discharge, and eventually a lump in his groin area, so he consulted two Chinatown herbalists. Unfortunately, neither doctor recognized the early signs of bubonic plague, and Wong became patient zero in the 1900 epidemic that struck San Francisco.[138] By working with practitioners of Chinese medicine, public health officials could potentially minimize the effects of malpractice.

Many Chinese apothecaries offered far more than drugs. Preservationists who made an inventory of the Chew Kee Herb Shop in Fiddletown, California, revealed the diverse uses to which it was once put by the local Chinese community.[139] As one would expect, there were medical textbooks, including works on medicinal remedies and physiognomy, as well as a mortar, scale, vials, and bottles used to prepare, measure, and package prescriptions for sale. The inventory also clearly indicated that the shop was a home; items recovered included all manner of kitchenware and some dried food, a toothbrush, toys, makeup, and jewelry. Hunting and fishing licenses, sewing equipment, and some basic carpentry tools suggested a self-sufficient household. Other items showed that the shop was a site for recreation: dominoes, dice, tan chips, chess pieces, and playing cards were recovered along with tobacco, tobacco papers, and a rice wine still.[140] Along Dry Creek in the foothills of the Sierras, Chew Kee was apothecary, home, and community center all at once.

Kam Wah Chung in John Day, Oregon, was likewise a center for community life, religion, and recreation. All across eastern Oregon, Kam Wah Chung was known to the Chinese as a place to worship at a Buddhist shrine, to drink tea, to gamble, and to smoke opium.[141] Under Ing Hay and Lung On's management, Kam Wah Chung's shelves were stocked with goods imported from Canton and Hong Kong as well as from wholesalers in Portland, Seattle, St. Louis, and Chicago.[142] Lung brokered labor contracts between Chinese craftsmen, cooks, and other workers and English-speaking employers.[143] Admired for his penmanship, he wrote letters and prepared other documents, then arranged to have them sent home to China. The local post office used Kam Wah Chung as a site for storing undeliverable letters from China, making the store a kind of quasi-post office.[144] During the era of exclusion, both legal and extralegal immigration services were available at Kam Wah Chung. The company vouched for "merchants" exempt from the law's prohibitions and coached new arrivals on how to navigate the elaborate series of exams and interrogations required of Chinese immigrants.[145] Lung, who cultivated a close relationship with a U.S. Customs officer in Portland, Oregon, also seems to have prepared false documents and identification papers for Chinese immigrants seeking to circumvent exclusion.[146] The company supported Chinese immigrants financially by investing in their gold mines, and on occasion made personal loans. For example, Ing Hay paid for his nephew Ing Tow to learn English in Walla Walla, Washington.[147]

Los Angeles herbalist Tom Leung offered similar forms of community assistance in the early decades of the twentieth century. His daughter Louise remembered stirring in the night to the sounds of hurried whispers and the clandestine arrival of "dirty and disheveled" Chinese men, who would be sheltered as a relative or student in the family herb business. "Much later," she writes, "we learned that these men had been smuggled into the country; they could not enter legally because of the immigration laws."[148] Leung facilitated the illegal entry of not only blood relatives but also political dissidents. In China, he was part of the opposition to the nationalist revolution and backed a constitutional monarchy with the Qing emperor at its helm. After his immigration to the United States, he continued to support that group by offering money, room, and board to young members so that they might study at Pomona College and the University of Southern California.[149] Leung also—unwisely—invested in some friends' business, sinking $15,000 into a fishery that eventually failed. When he could not recover the loan, Leung appealed to the Bing Kong *tong*, but the Chinese gangsters were no more successful than he.[150]

Chinese herbalists positioned themselves to act as go-betweens in the trans-Pacific labor market. As merchants, they had the professional contacts, the social standing, and the English-language skills necessary to transact business with American customs officials and non-Chinese-owned companies. As community doctors, they had the personal connections and, perhaps, trust of their countrymen. In the 1860s, Wo Sing cared for a Nevada community of Chinese miners and served simultaneously as their labor broker for the North Bloomfield Mining Company.[151] An Oregon doctor, Wing Lee (also known as Zang Liang Rong Li), simultaneously ran a Portland drugstore and a semi-successful mining operation in southern Oregon in the 1880s. To work the mines, he arranged for the immigration of twenty-six Chinese men.[152] In that same decade, a public scandal involving a San Diego doctor who also went by the name Wo Sing (likely an alias for a man really named Lu Chung and Tom Li Chung) provides further evidence of the multiple roles that Chinese herbalists played within their communities. In the wake of Chinese exclusion, the San Diego Wo became a human trafficker, smuggling Chinese miners from Ensenada, Mexico, across the border via boat to San Diego. Immigration officials intercepted the sloop in the bay. Its Portuguese captain identified Wo as the ringleader of the "Chinese underground railroad," and authorities arrested him in Los Angeles in April 1890.[153] In the end, the courts could not prove his intent to aid and abet the illegal landing of Chinese workers and acquitted him.[154]

In New York City, Jim Fuey Moy used his English fluency to spread awareness of anti-Chinese discrimination and racial violence. Between 1893 and 1900, Jim was the superintendent of the Chinese

Guild at St. Bartholomew's Episcopal Church on the Lower East Side of Manhattan. The Chinese Guild offered basic services to immigrants, arranged for legal representation, and—like Chew Kee and Kam Wah Chung—provided a center for intellectual and social life.[155] Jim spoke out against the renewal of the Chinese Exclusion Act in 1893 and called for justice after the savage beating of a Chinese launderer in 1895.[156] When a Chinese worker called Long Tong was identified as a leper and confined to North Brother Island in 1896, Jim went before the New York Board of Health to protest that Long was misdiagnosed and suffered from some other, noncontagious disease.[157] Like San Diego's Wo Sing, Jim also had his brush with the law when a federal grand jury indicted him in 1911 for smuggling Chinese workers from Mexico and Jamaica into Massachusetts.[158] To his countrymen in the United States, the Chinese doctor wore many hats: healer, defender, and trafficker.

Sharing Knowledge

In San Francisco, Li Po Tai's shop was a medical school for two generations of Chinese physicians. The 1870 federal census found Li living above his business, with more than a dozen male and female assistants, ranging in age from ten to fifty. The census taker identified nine of them as "druggists."[159] Many of Li's assistants went on to open their own shops in other cities around the San Francisco Bay or farther afield. Tom Foo Yuen (or "Foo" as he was called), Li's nephew by marriage, and Li's son Li Wing (who went by "Wing") successfully expanded the family business to southern California, setting up a shop first in Redlands and then in Los Angeles in the 1890s. In Los Angeles, they named their business the Foo and Wing Herb Company and made it a chain with offices in Oakland and Boston, where Foo trained and employed his four sons.[160]

In 1899, Foo invited another cousin, Tom Leung, to work in his Los Angeles shop as an assistant. Promotional materials for their partnership claimed that Leung descended from a "race of physicians" dating back six generations in his family, and that he held a diploma from the Imperial Medical Academy of Peking, but his wife, Bing Woo, later contradicted that account. She recalled that the family had been involved with local Chinese government and trade.[161] Foo and Leung dissolved

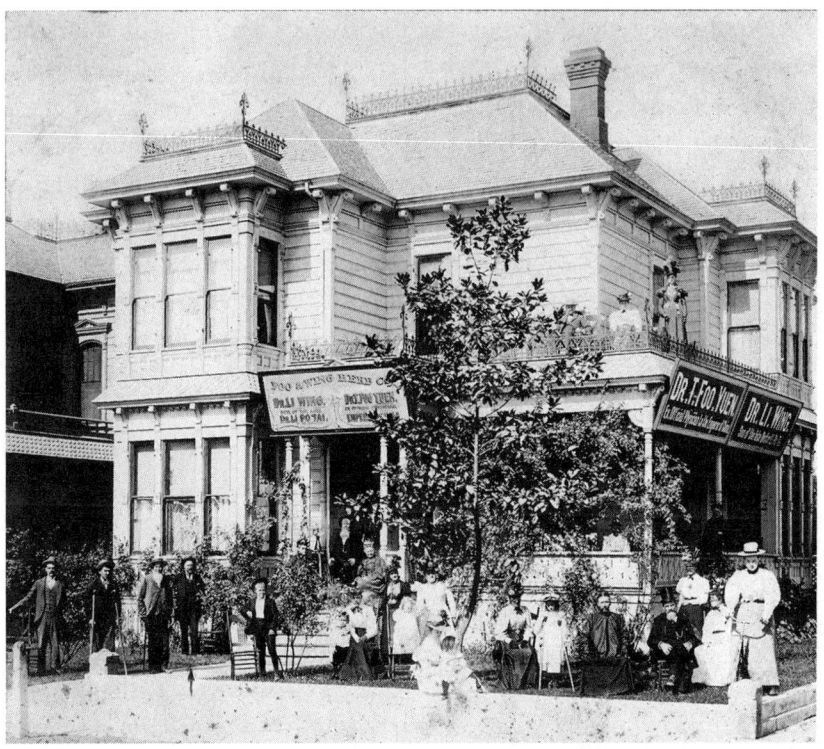

Herbalists, assistants, and family members in front of the Foo and Wing Herb Company store, 903 South Olive Street, Los Angeles, around the turn of the twentieth century. Courtesy of the Huntington Library, San Marino, California, Hazard-Dyson Collection.

their partnership on less than amicable terms when the younger man opened his own herb shop a few miles from the original Foo and Wing location and failed to cut his cousin a favorable share.[162] At the new location, Leung put his wife and children to work: his eldest daughter, Lillie, wrote English business letters; his eldest son, Taft, met with patients; and his wife filled prescriptions. Leung also dispatched a cousin, Chuck Ga Sook, to San Diego to open a branch of the family business.[163]

Meanwhile, Foo began to teach herbalism to Chinese Christian preachers in Los Angeles, and in 1925, when he was around seventy-five years old, he persuaded one of them, Je Yuen, to move with him to Spokane, Washington, and open the Foo Yuen Herb Company there. Je temporarily abandoned his pregnant wife, Yee Ching, in San Francisco, but soon after she delivered their fourth child in 1926, she joined them, and the elderly Tom Foo Yuen trained both Je and Yee as herbalists. Eventually, their children learned to work alongside them, and the Foo Yuen Herb Company became a fixture of the Chinese community of Spokane until the couple's retirement in 1957.[164] In both China and the United States, the herb business was a family business.

While some Chinese physicians learned herbalism only after their arrival in the United States, others had at least some training in the medical arts before they left China.[165] According to family lore, N. S. Sue was considered the most intelligent among his five brothers, and so they elected to pay for his studies in medicine. After hearing that a Chinese physician could earn a good living in California, the brothers scraped together enough money to purchase a stake in a Chinese restaurant in Stockton, California, so that Sue could immigrate as a merchant—and circumvent the Exclusion Act—in the 1890s. Sue eventually went on to open his own medical practice in nearby Modesto in the first decade of the twentieth century.[166] Los Angeles herbalist Yitang Chang (Yick Hong Chung) initially learned herbalism at home in Canton Province and honed the craft as an apprentice in his father-in-law's Hong Kong apothecary. He eventually returned to Canton to start a successful business, hiring his nephews as assistants.[167] Chang's status as a merchant allowed him to immigrate to the United States in 1900. He disembarked in San Diego, where his wife had a family member, but quickly made his way to Los Angeles, where he became a partner in the Dun Sow Hong Company, an herb shop. According to his biographer, Haiming Liu, Chang's investment in Dun Sow Hong not only enabled him to continue his medical practice but protected his exemption from the Exclusion Act and made it safe for him to bring his eleven-year-old son, Elbert, over from China.[168]

Letters written to Ing Hay from other herbalists in Oregon and California suggest that the connections among herbalists were necessary not only for education but for the exchange of goods and advice. An "herbist" in Portland wrote to Ing in 1905: "I have heard for a long time all the miracles you have done . . . I am ashamed to say, although I am also a person of the same profession, I am nothing compared to you."

The Portland-based doctor, Lao Chi-Kwang, went on to describe how one of his patients recommended Ing's treatment for a "foot disease," which included lancing and bleeding the affected site. Lao invited Ing to Portland, all expenses paid, to teach him "the method of using the needle, where and how to pierce, along with the prescription."[169] Ing also solicited advice from fellow practitioners on complicated cases of throat disease or hemorrhoids.[170]

In cities with more than one Chinese doctor, apothecaries tended to group on particular streets or intersections. The concentration of Chinese herbalists was both an artifact of Chinese immigrants' residential segregation as well as a demonstration of the importance of industrial clustering, where companies locate themselves within walking distance of one another. Proximity allowed the small businesses to share supplies or expertise, and it likely facilitated their recruitment of customers, both Chinese and non-Chinese. In San Francisco, anyone looking for Chinese medicine would have known to go to Washington Square. In Los Angeles, Chinese herb shops lined Marchessault and Main Streets off the central plaza. Chinese doctors often occupied the same office space, either simultaneously or sequentially. In 1892, when a Dr. Woh was compelled to return to China, he announced that he would turn over his shop on South Main Street to a Dr. Bow. Between 1891 and 1893, that same address—227 South Main Street—was occupied by doctors S. N. Kwong and Wong Fay.[171] City directories and classified advertisements reveal that successive herbalists maintained certain addresses, much like a restaurant space might change ownership but not function over time. In Los Angeles, 208 Marchessault Street was rented by a series of Chinese herb dealers between 1904 and 1934: S. N. Kwong, Rukiss Fong, Dy Chun Tong Company, and finally Chew Fun and Company.[172]

Competition and opportunity drove Chinese physicians to move frequently, sometimes at great distances. They followed gold and mineral strikes or ventured into unserved communities. Wing Lee immigrated to San Francisco in the early 1860s, and over the next two decades set up a series of practices first in California, then Idaho, then Washington, then back to Idaho, and finally to Oregon, where he opened shops in Dayton, Portland, and Salem in the early 1880s.[173] Another Oregon doctor, Chang Gee Wo, first disembarked in New Orleans in 1885, and according to his advertisements, "after spending several years in different cities to decide what he preferred, he finally located in Denver, Colorado." Four years later, he moved his practice to Omaha, Nebraska, where he married an American-born woman of English descent, Sarah Celestine Starbuck, called Sadie. Their two children, Celestine and Hendricks, were born in Omaha.[174] He also operated offices under his name in Chicago, Milwaukee, Billings, and Walla Walla, but it is not clear if he ever resided in any of those cities.[175] Chang achieved some notoriety in 1893 when he helped sponsor the construction of a Chinese theater, "joss house" (Chinese temple), and bazaar on the Midway at the Chicago World's Fair.[176] In 1900, Chang moved to Portland, Oregon, where he had close connections with a Chinese drug wholesaler. In 1920, the census indicated that he lived in a predominantly European American neighborhood on San Rafael Street in Portland with his interracial, mutigenerational family: his wife and children; his daughter's young son, Kenneth; two of Sadie's elderly relatives (her father and aunt); and Chang's brother Chungeho, who worked as a druggist in his shop.[177]

Chan Doo Sung was even more peripatetic. As an eighteen-year-old in 1916, he emigrated from Canton to the United States on a student visa and apprenticed with his uncle in an herb shop on Clay Street in Oakland. Originally founded in the late 1890s by Chan's grandfather, Chan and Wing (also called Chan and Kong) was a successful franchise of Chinese herb shops, with each branch owned by a different member of the extended family.[178] In Oakland, Chan Doo Sung met Aster Lee, a Chinese American born in San Francisco in 1899.[179] Chan and Lee married in 1921 or 1922 and began their lives as itinerant doctor and pharmacist. Chan did the diagnosis, and Lee prepared and packaged the prescriptions. Their first three children, Edward, Florence, and Lyman, were all born in San Francisco. After Florence's birth, Chan opened his first shop in Sacramento in 1928, only to leave a year later for Fresno and then Bakersfield. A year after that, the family decamped to Redding, then Anaheim. Another four moves in 1931, first to Medford, Oregon, and then to Yakima, Washington, brought another child—Anna—before short stints in Aberdeen, Washington, and Dunsmuir, California. The family of six then moved to Pueblo, Colorado, in 1932 before swinging back to California to set up shop in San Rafael, Petaluma, Napa,

Sonora, and Vallejo, all within the next two years. Another son, Keylor, was born in 1935 in Walla Walla, Washington, before the family moved to Salt Lake City in 1936. The following year took the family to Idaho, first Idaho Falls and then Twin Falls, where the youngest child, Paul, was born. Another move took them back to California, but after less than a year in Santa Cruz, the family made its twenty-first and final move to Tucson, Arizona, in 1940. Why did Chan and Lee move so frequently? Chan claimed that it was customer demand. In a 1938 interview for the *Idaho Evening Times* announcing the opening of a new office, Chan explained that "he was prompted to open offices in Twin Falls because

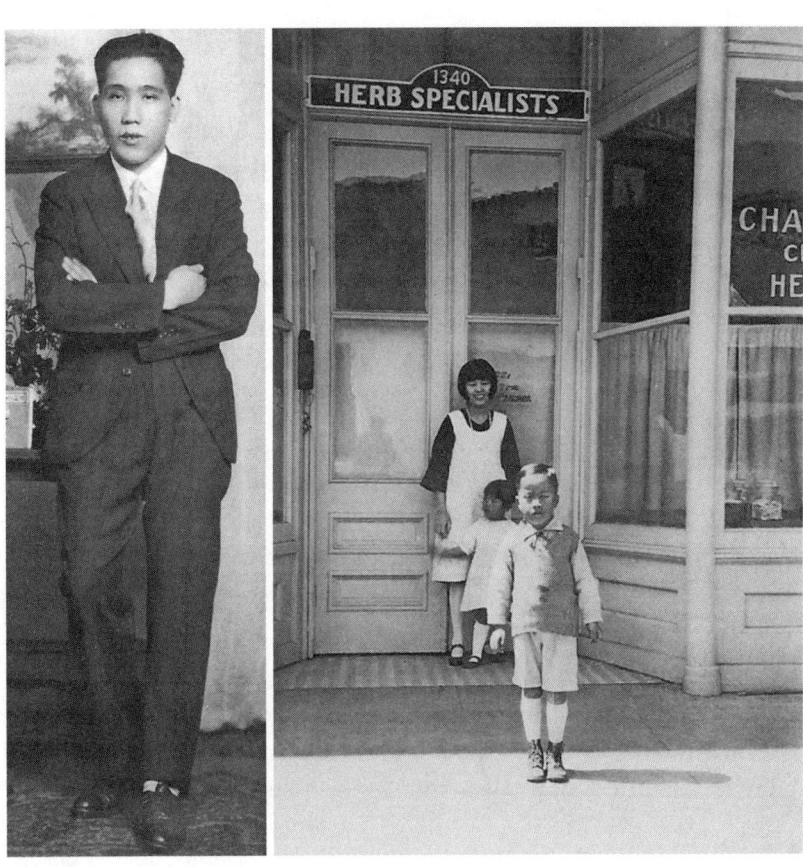

Chan Doo Sung in 1928 and Aster Lee with two of her children, Florence and Lyman, outside the family herb shop in 1930. Courtesy of Anna Don.

of the numerous patients from this district coming to Idaho Falls or going to Salt Lake for treatment."[180] His daughter Anna attributed their frequent moves to the opposite: competition with other herbalists and a lack of patients. "With so many mouths to feed, I'm sure he felt desperate to be able to provide for his family, and he probably felt the only way out was to move," she said.[181] Whatever the reason, Anna recalled that each time they moved, her father's first stop in their new hometown would be the local newspaper, where he ran an advertisement, stamped from a metal plate. The address changed but the rest remained the same: an image of a prototypical Chinese scholar-official wearing a Ming Era costume and holding a sign that read, in all capital letters, "HERBS."[182]

Conclusion

In twenty-one cities across the American West between 1927 and 1940, Chan Doo Sung continued a tradition that had begun in the 1850s. Chinese doctors like Chan, linked by real and fictive kinship networks, sustained their community in sickness and in health. The Chinese immigrant community depended on Chinese doctors, their knowledge and connections, both within the United States and overseas in China. At the same time, however, Chan's near constant relocation represented an important change that had taken place in the American practice of Chinese medicine. When he moved his family to a new place, Chan deliberately set up shop outside the local Chinese enclave to have better access to non-Chinese patients.[183] His choice reflected the fact that Chinese medicine was not just for Chinese people. The widespread consumption of Chinese medicine by European American patients was also evident at Li Po Tai's funeral procession, with its racially diverse mourners. In the late nineteenth and early twentieth centuries, practitioners of Chinese medicine continued to play a vital role in their immigrant communities, but, as the next chapter describes, with increasing frequency they catered to the needs of English- and Spanish-speaking patients as well.

Translated

Fong Poy wanted to be a dentist. Growing up in Canton Province in the 1880s and 1890s, Fong helped his father make bamboo shell lanterns, which had been the family business for nearly one hundred years. Lantern-making kept the family fed and clothed, but Fong's father had higher ambitions for his children, and he sent Fong (and later a younger son) to learn English in the United States in 1900. The teenager first went to live with his cousin Walter Fong, the pride of the family. A Stanford graduate, lawyer, clergyman, and instructor of Chinese language, Walter lived in Berkeley with his wife, Emma Ellen Howse, a woman of English descent, and their two infant sons.[1] When Walter and Emma traveled abroad, Fong went to live with his mother's brother Wan See Mon, who served the Chinese diplomatic corps in San Francisco as an herbalist, but Fong demonstrated no affinity for medicine.[2] Much later, Fong recalled that he would tease his uncle and the other herbalists and pull on their long queues.[3] With Walter and Emma's encouragement, Fong Poy enrolled in the Berkeley public schools and set his sights on attending dental college in San Francisco after graduation. Then, in 1910, the summer before his senior year at Berkeley High School, a bicycle accident permanently derailed Fong's academic progress. With a cracked jaw and a row of broken teeth,

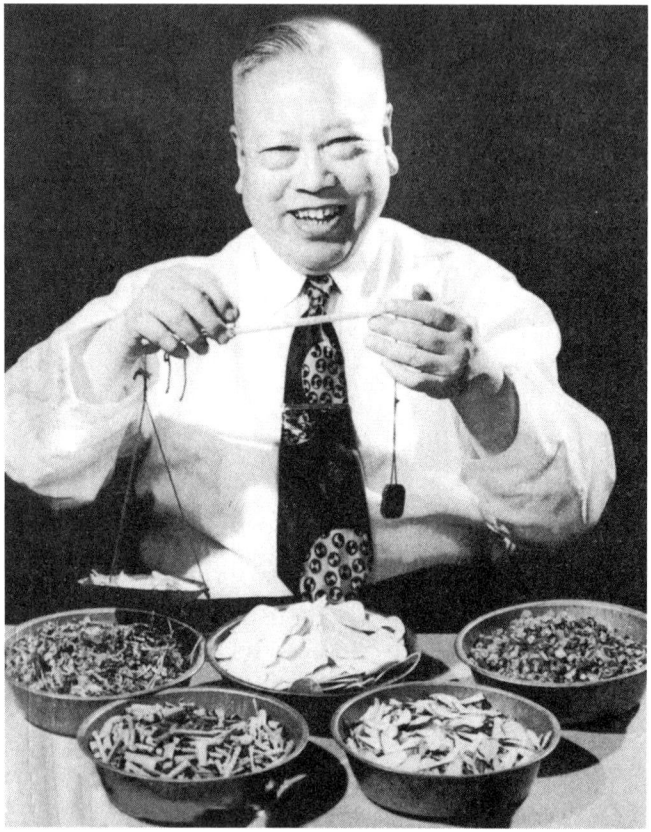

Fong Wan as shown on the cover of his advertising booklet,
Herb Lore, 1950. Courtesy of Calvin Fong.

he could barely speak for six months. By that point, Walter had passed away. Emma, widowed with two children, quickly remarried one of her husband's colleagues, Yoshi S. Kuno, a professor of Asian languages at the University of California, Berkeley. Although Emma continued to sign Fong's report cards and to identify herself as his guardian after Walter's death, it was perhaps too much of a burden to have the young man convalesce in her home. Fong returned to San Francisco to live with his uncle, the herbalist, and he never went to dental school. Instead, he was drawn into the world of traditional Chinese medicine.[4] He changed his name from Fong Poy to Fong Wan, in honor of his uncle and mother, and up until his death in 1968, he ran a thriving herb business with part-nerships in Santa Rosa and Oakland.

Throughout his career, Fong Wan served a principally non-Chinese clientele, patients he called "Occidentals." He was fluent in English, having nearly graduated from Berkeley High School with more than passing grades in all subjects, so communication was not an issue. Fong located his apothecaries on the outer edges of Chinese neighbor-hoods and took out advertisements in English-language newspapers: the *Santa Rosa Republican* and *Press Democrat,* the *Oakland Tribune,* the *Berkeley Daily Gazette,* the *San Francisco Chronicle,* and others around the bay. They featured glowing testimonials from patients with Western names and, occasionally, a photograph of their distinctly Western faces. At a location two blocks outside of Santa Rosa's small Chinatown, Fong offered free consultations to non-Chinese patients.[5] In 1916, Fong rented a stately Victorian mansion on Eighth Street in Oakland and began to build up his practice in the city. Eight years later, he purchased a home on Tenth Street, where he transformed the first floor into an opulent apothecary and clinic, and he put his family to work. His sons—Rich-ard and Edward—joined his nephews, chopping and wrapping herbs for sale in the shop or by mail order while his former guardian, Emma, and her son Chester wrote advertising copy. Fong Wan—always dap-per in a three-piece, Western-style suit and hat—handled all consulta-tions, diagnoses, and prescriptions with his "Occidental" patients.[6] By the 1930s, Fong Wan had made himself into a twentieth-century version of Li Po Tai. He was a local celebrity in the Chinese and non-Chinese communities of the greater San Francisco Bay area.

By marketing his services to "Occidental" patients, Fong Wan followed in the footsteps of at least two generations of Chinese immi-grant doctors before him. In the late nineteenth century, Chinese doc-tors freely entered the American medical marketplace. With few and poorly enforced medical licensing laws, American patient-consumers could choose among an eclectic assortment of health practitioners and practices. As early as the 1850s, but increasingly in the last decades of the nineteenth century, Chinese doctors sold their services to non-Chinese patients. For some, like Fong Wan, European American men and women came to comprise the overwhelming majority of their practice.

Through different business strategies, Chinese doctors bridged the linguistic and cultural divide with non-Chinese patients and combated the negative stereotypes that circulated in public health reports and the popular press. They naturally promised to deliver superior therapeutic efficacy but did not stop there. Their outreach to European American patients also emphasized cultural congruencies between Chinese and Western medical knowledge systems. Although a synthetic drug industry had started to develop in earnest in the late nineteenth century, the ailing still primarily consumed plant-based, raw or minimally processed remedies. The prevalence of similarly procured and produced herbal medicines in the Chinese pharmacopoeia would have seemed comfortingly familiar. Chinese herbalists also promised noninvasive procedures. Modern surgery had experienced significant technical and sanitary improvements in the nineteenth century, but it was still a risky proposition for most patients.

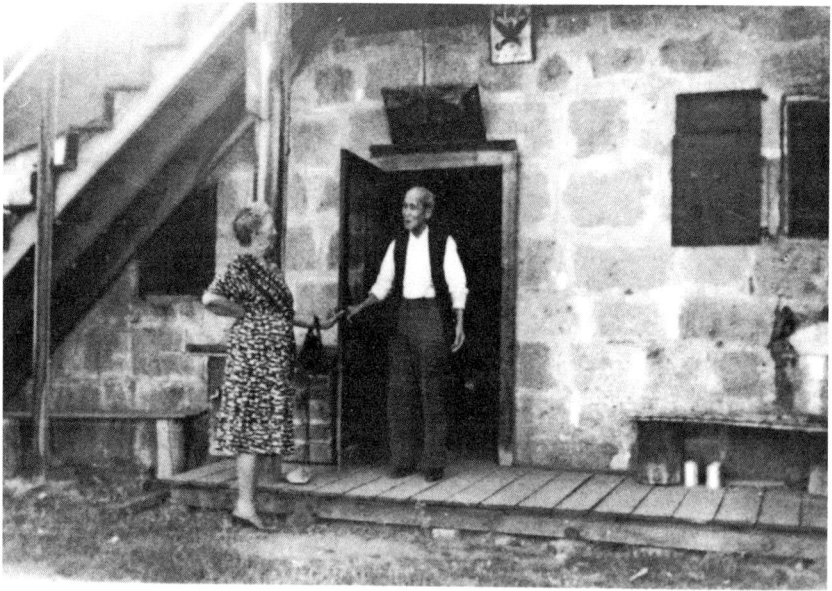

Ing Hay outside Kam Wah Chung with one of his patients, Maude Truesdell, around the turn of the twentieth century. Courtesy of Kam Wah Chung State Heritage Site Archival Collection, Oregon Parks and Recreation Department.

Finally, Chinese herbalists offered services that fit into the economic niches already occupied by Chinese immigrants in the United States. In places where Chinese immigrants concentrated, nineteenth-century Americans became accustomed to entrusting their physical wellbeing to Chinese people. Many elite and even some ordinary Americans hired Chinese men and women to launder their clothing and maintain the cleanliness and order of their households. Chinese fishers and farmers peddled goods that Chinese cooks prepared for meals served at non-Chinese tables. The physical labor associated with preparing food and preparing herbs was alike: measuring, grinding, boiling, and steeping. Domestic service and health care often brought Chinese men and women into intimate contact with non-Chinese customers.

"The Doctor Speaks Good English"

Chinese doctors adopted various tactics to recruit non-Chinese patients. They began with simple English-language signs, displayed outside of Chinese drugstores as early as the late 1850s. In 1857, a newspaper called *Wide West* reprinted an article from the *Sacramento Bee* with a description of Sutterville, California's "Doctor Lola," a "China Doctor" promoting his services with an English-language sign. Unable to afford the rents in Sacramento, Lola had set up shop in nearby Sutterville. Equipped with an English-to-Chinese dictionary, Chinese medical books, and a stock of botanical and zoological medicines, he had established a good reputation among non-Chinese patients. The reporter for the *Sacramento Bee* noted, "While we were in Lola's offices, several white persons, residing in the neighborhood, came in, and we learned from them that . . . [he] had very good success indeed in curing diseases."[7] According to historian Haiming Liu, by 1858, "an herbalist named Hu Junxiao (Tsun Yuen Wo) in San Francisco Chinatown used English language signs on his shop to attract Caucasian patients."[8]

The first English-language newspaper advertisements for Chinese doctors appeared not long after that. In 1860, the *Sacramento Daily Union* began to run classified ads for "Gom Wa, Chinese Doctor," located at I Street between Front and Second, and for "Dr. Offo, Chinese Physician," who saw patients in an office on Front Street between I and

J Streets.[9] In 1860, a Marysville, California, newspaper reported that an "almond-eyed Galen" administered the "juices of three large lizards" to cure a rheumatic miner.[10] By 1865, that newspaper was printing advertisements for several Chinese physicians practicing in Marysville.[11]

Chinese doctors, like other health care providers in the American medical marketplace, exercised a great deal of freedom in their advertising claims and messages. When Chinese doctors reached out to non-Chinese patients in the late nineteenth and early twentieth centuries, medical advertising was almost entirely unregulated.[12] Chinese doctors advertising in English-language media adopted techniques developed and perfected by makers of proprietary (also known as patent) medicines. Peddlers of nostrums and drug sellers claiming a patent on a unique compound had been part of the American medical marketplace since its colonial era, but in the decades after the Civil War, industrialization expanded the market for proprietary medicine. Mechanized agriculture increased the production of domestic and imported medicinal plants. A national network of railroads carried them great distances to a growing number of drug manufacturers.[13] Medical advertising took a giant leap forward in this era as well. Public interest in the Civil War had expanded the readership for newspapers and magazines, and proprietary medicine manufacturers capitalized on the medium to promote their products in an increasingly crowded market.[14] While makers of proprietary medicine had been cultivating what historian T. J. Jackson Lears has called "a carnivalesque commercial vernacular" since the eighteenth century, the late nineteenth century witnessed a boom in the aesthetic quality, sophistication, and sheer quantity of medical advertising as technical advances in printing made it possible to run eye-catching, illustrated advertisements.[15] Patent medicine advertisements might feature patient testimonials or offer a free trial or money-back guarantee through various forms of printed ephemera, such as handbills, booklets, trade cards, almanacs, and calendars.[16] In pictures and texts, patent medicines celebrated the exotic and the ancient, invoked the laws of nature, and highlighted the metaphysical links between body and soul.[17] Chinese doctors made use of all of these techniques. Those who were literate in English could have easily seen them in any local newspaper, and perhaps they did.[18]

As with makers of proprietary medicines, Chinese doctors often described their remedies as "miracle" cures. "Wonderful, marvelous, miraculous!" claimed an 1890 advertisement for Chang Gee Wo's Omaha, Nebraska, practice.[19] At his Los Angeles office and sanitarium, a Dr. Wong promised that his "marvelous" herbal remedies would fight diseases that "have resisted all other efforts of modern medical science for months, or even years." According to an 1899 advertisement, "Dr. Wong can tell a patient more by his pulse diagnosis than any reputable American physician after an examination."[20] Of another Los Angeles doctor, Wong Him, a 1905 advertisement declared in boldfaced letters, "His deeds border on the miraculous."[21] In an Arizona paper in 1914, Chin Mai Fong told tales of patients who had "recovered as if by magic."[22] These elements worked together to distinguish the value proposition of Chinese medicine from that of regular medicine, but they did not distinguish Chinese medicine from proprietary medicine.

What set advertisements for Chinese medicine apart from manufacturers of proprietary remedies was not the overall marketing approach but the specific ways in which Chinese doctors consciously employed Orientalist stereotypes. As early as the 1880s, print advertisements for Chinese physicians and herb companies began to include images, most commonly a representation of the practitioner wearing an easily identifiable Oriental costume. One of the earliest examples is an 1882 advertisement for Los Angeles doctor Hoy Kung, which included a simple line drawing of a man in a traditional Chinese jacket and trousers holding a flower.[23] In an economy of images, the illustration conveyed the racial identity of the doctor and his expertise in botanical medicines. Chinese physicians did not portray themselves in Western dress until 1903, and images of the stereotypical Mandarin scholar continued to appear regularly in advertisements throughout the 1930s.[24] In so doing, Chinese doctors made themselves the embodiment of an Oriental aesthetic that was popular among the American middle and upper classes.

When illustrated advertisements became more common in the 1890s, Chinese herbalists often displayed their tools: a mortar and pestle, a reference book, a box of herbs. Occasionally, advertisements included extra Oriental flourishes such as Chinese calligraphy, dragons, or pagodas. In 1896, Los Angeles partners Doctors Wong and Yim began to advertise their sanitarium for "nervous and chronic diseases." The Chinese sanitarium offered not only diagnosis and herbal remedies but also lodging. The advertisement featured a stately looking Victorian building with a carriage and elegantly dressed patients ascending the front stairs.[25] Located at 713 South Main Street, it was a few blocks southeast of Chinatown, probably to attract a non-Chinese clientele. By 1907, Tom She Bin (or Ben) had taken over the business from Wong and Yim, using the same illustration but adding some Chinese elements: a dragon flag and a Mandarin scholar floating above the roofline.[26] The pairing of those images—Victorian manor and Orientalia—conveyed simultaneously the luxury of a health resort with the otherworldliness of the Oriental.

Up until the 1870s, San Francisco Chinese doctors were the most likely to promote themselves in English-language newspapers, perhaps because there were more of them, and stiffer competition drove them to recruit patients outside their co-ethnic clientele. By the last decades of the nineteenth century, doctors in Sacramento and the Sierras, Los Angeles, New York, and Portland and Astoria, Oregon, were also experimenting with advertising in English.[27] In cities with large Latino populations, Chinese doctors sometimes appealed to potential customers in Spanish as well. In Los Angeles, the Chinese quarter was adjacent to the central Mexican plaza, so it is not surprising that herbalists reached out to Spanish-speaking patients. An 1881 three-line advertisement for Dr. Chin Quong Zie in Los Angeles included a single Spanish phrase, promising that "*todos los infirmidas se curado aqui.*"[28] In the following decade, a local competitor, Tom She Bin, began printing trade cards and running newspaper ads with Spanish and English versions side by side.[29] Among Los Angeles herbalists, the practice persisted well into the twentieth century. Historians George J. Sánchez and Juily Iyn Vo Phun have documented Chinese physicians' efforts to attract Mexican workers in Los Angeles in the 1920s and 1930s by promising low-cost herbal remedies.[30] In 1948, Los Angeles herbalist Garding Lui wrote a tourist guide to his city's Chinatown in which he noted his colleagues' preference for hiring a "Mexican girl" as a nurse: "Where there is a large patronage of Spanish or Mexican people, a Mexican girl is needed who can write and interpret Spanish."[31]

Early English- and Spanish-language advertisements commonly addressed the Chinese doctor's ability to communicate. In 1865, San Francisco doctor Fung Sheuk ran an ad in the *San Francisco Chronicle* asserting, "The Doctor speaks good English."[32] In the same year, "Dr. Jim," also of San Francisco similarly advertised, "Dr. Jim speaks English."[33] By 1865, Li Po Tai was advertising in the *Daily Alta California*. Although Li purportedly spoke English, his early advertisements highlighted that his office "engaged the daily services of Charles T. Carvalho, the Chinese interpreter for the Courts."[34] An article for the same newspaper described Carvalho as "the only man in California capable of speaking both English and Chinese 'like a native.'" The occasion was noteworthy enough to receive front-page attention.[35] An advertisement for Los Angeles doctor Hoy Kung related his credentials differently: "Late from Canton, China," it read, "where he was employed as a physician for the leading white families," the implication being that Hoy had been able to converse freely with them.[36] In 1887, Dr. Him Wo Hong, also of Los Angeles, made a simple promise: "English and Spanish spoken."[37] Such claims reassured potential patients that the exotic foreign doctor would understand their complaints.

Around the time of the passage of the first Chinese Exclusion Act in 1882, English-language advertising for Chinese doctors increased in frequency and expanded in geography. Advertisements proliferated in Los Angeles newspapers and, by the end of the 1890, they had fanned out to places like Helena, Montana; Omaha, Nebraska; Milwaukee, Wisconsin; and other parts of the Mountain West and Midwest. At the same time, some Chinese doctors began to move their offices and drugstores out of their traditional ethnic enclaves to other corners of the city, possibly targeting areas with less dense competition. Los Angeles physician Tom She Bin opened a San Francisco branch in 1894 on Market Street, not far from City Hall.[38] In the same city, between 1910 and 1912, a cluster of Chinese doctors set up shop in a neighborhood west of Chinatown around the intersection of Fillmore and Geary.[39] Wong Wing ventured farther afield into a predominantly Latino part of town when he established a business on Valencia Street, just a few blocks from the Mission Dolores.[40] In Los Angeles, Chinese doctors followed a similar pattern of geographic dispersion after 1882, gradually spreading south and west from the historic Chinese neighborhood near the plaza around the turn of the twentieth century and then expanding more adventurously in the 1920s and 1930s into Hollywood, Long Beach, and Santa Monica.[41] In 1948, Garding Lui noted that Los Angeles herbalists often avoided setting up shop in the city's Chinatown: "The herbalists like to get in a prosperous residence district . . . near a settlement composed chiefly of Germans, Italians, Mexicans, Scandinavians, Irish, English, and Scotch descendants."[42] Moving out of Chinatown and advertising in English-language newspapers fulfilled the same goals: increasing the visibility of Chinese medicine in non-Chinese communities. It may have also physically distanced Chinese doctors from Chinatown's association with infectious disease. Although it is difficult to link the timing of specific epidemics to business relocations, it is reasonable to think that for some doctors, practicing outside of Chinatown assuaged their patients' potential concerns about contagion.

Why did Chinese doctors recruit non-Chinese patients so aggressively beginning in the late nineteenth century? Perhaps they anticipated a decline in their co-ethnic customer base due to Chinese exclusion, or perhaps quite simply enough time had passed for Chinese doctors to acquire the language skills and cultural literacy necessary to market their services to non-Chinese patients. By the 1880s, many doctors—like Li Po Tai—had lived the majority of their adult lives in the United States and, as travel accounts and newspaper articles suggest, were at least proficient in English. Los Angeles doctor Tom Leung, who had immigrated to the United States in 1899, hired his neighbor, a horticulturalist named Paul Howard, to tutor him in English. According to Leung's daughter and biographer, he never became fluent but he spoke well enough to converse with his English-speaking patients.[43] In 1903, Leung's cousin Tom Foo Yuen and his business partner Li Wing promised readers of the *Los Angeles Times* that their employees were both "familiar with the needs as regards the health, the language, the ways, and habits of Americans."[44]

Chinese doctors surmounted linguistic and cultural barriers by seeking out business partnerships with native English and Spanish speakers. These partners assumed responsibility for interfacing with American patients, in the reception areas or exam rooms, or through

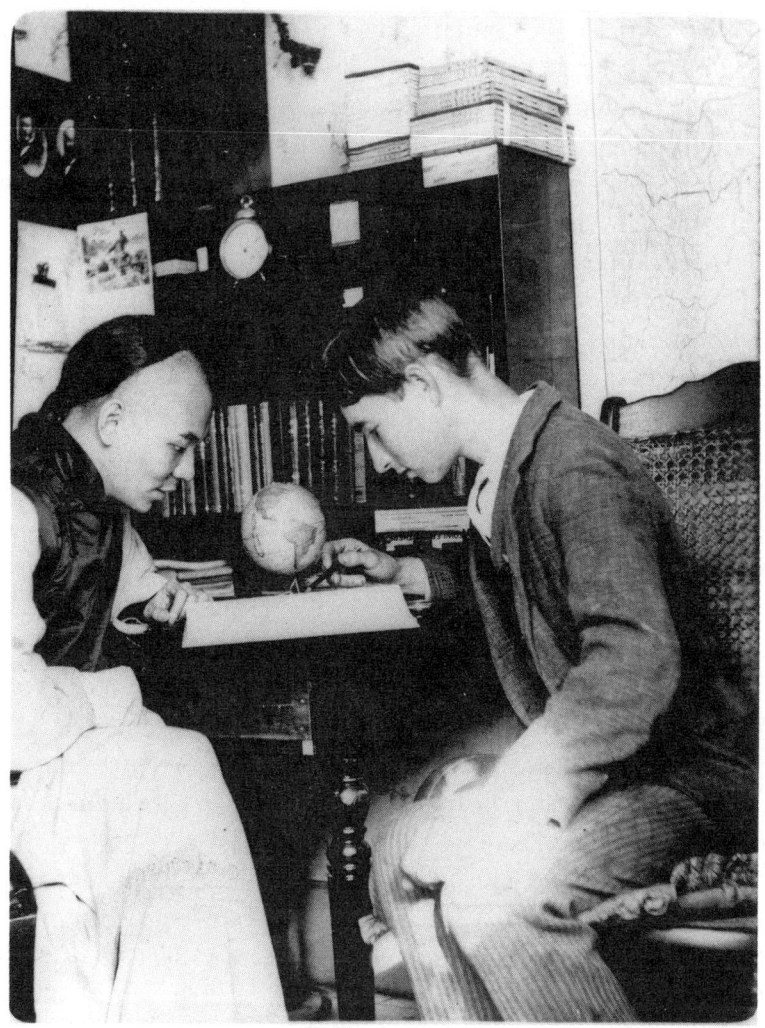

Tom Leung with his neighbor and English tutor John Howard.
Courtesy of Jane Leung Larson.

other forms of public outreach such as writing advertising copy, newspaper editorials, and recruiting patients directly.[45] In other cases, business associates seem to have offered assistance to Chinese doctors navigating American immigration laws and other discriminatory policies. In
Los Angeles, Yitang Chang formed a partnership with a chiropractor,

A. Z. Holmes. Holmes purportedly spoke some Cantonese, at least enough to greet patients on arrival, and he served as a translator at Chang's herb shop downtown.[46] Holmes and other white business associates of Chang also occasionally testified for the Chang family at immigration hearings.[47] Years later, Chang's son Arthur recalled that the family was only able to rent their home at 917 Hill Street, a primarily white neighborhood, by putting Holmes's name on the lease.[48]

Arrest records sometimes revealed partnerships that otherwise would have gone unnoticed. When police arrested Jim Lee for practicing without a license in 1890, they also took in two American men employed by him: C. A. Jansen worked as the office manager and B. A. Wilt as the advertising manager and interpreter. Investigators discovered that Lee's business was in fact one branch of a chain of herb stores operating under the name of "Gun Wa," all directed out of a Denver headquarters by "a man named Smith," who posted bail for the trio.[49] A federal inquiry into the firm's mail-order business implicated a Chicago advertising agent named G. M. Paine and another non-Chinese proprietor, Detroit-based W. H. Hale, both of whom were later arrested for mail fraud.[50] Oddly, another doctor going by the name "Gun Wa" had been arrested the year before with his European American manager C. A. Bernard in Pittsburgh, but they do not seem to have been affiliated with the Midwestern chain.[51]

European American partners enhanced the credibility of Chinese medicine and assuaged the concerns of non-Chinese patients. An 1890 advertisement for the Gun Wa chain encouraged patients to have their ailments diagnosed and prescriptions filled by mail, showing an illustration of the "correspondence office" in which five European American men and one European American woman, all clothed in Western dress, huddled over desks and ledgers beneath a sign bearing Chinese characters. Not a single Chinese face appeared in the advertisement.[52] In a 1907 advertisement, "Oriental Doctors" including Wong-San, urged the residents of Bakersfield to learn of "Oriental Medical Secrets that have been hidden from the eyes of the white man for untold centuries," but assuaged potential cultural concerns with the promise that they would be "assisted by the German-American Doctors."[53] When Dr. Chin Man Sui advertised in English-language newspapers in Boise, Idaho, in 1911, he included a photo of himself, dressed in traditional Chinese clothing, seated beside his European American secretary, N. Von Santen, dressed in a Western suit and tie.[54] Perhaps such images were meant to comfort prospective non-Chinese patients that a familiar face and culture would greet them when they paid a visit to the "exotic" doctor.

Over the course of his career, Tom Foo Yuen contracted with several American business managers, who worked primarily as advertising agents for his herb companies. Foo's managers initially knew him as their doctor. The first was Levi Carter of Ceres, California, of whom little is known. In a testimonial printed in an 1896 advertisement, Carter identified himself as a one-time patient of Foo's.[55] Burton C. Platt became Foo's next business manager. Platt got his start in the dairy business and somehow branched out from there to representing Chinese physicians. Prior to contracting with Foo, Platt had worked as an agent for a "Dr. Wong," one of the longest-practicing physicians in Los Angeles.[56] Like Carter, Platt claimed to have met Foo first as a patient:

> I resolved to find, if possible, a thoroughly educated Chinese physician in this country. If I could not find one here I would go to China. At this time I was in a very weak condition, scarcely able to walk three blocks. In company with my brother I went to San Francisco. This was the 15th of November, 1892. I consulted Li Po Tai and remained under his care until his death in the following March. In the meanwhile I had become acquainted with T. Foo Yuen who was then assisting in his uncle's practice. After Li Po Tai's death I persuaded Dr. Foo to come to Southern California, my prime motive being to place myself under his care, as I was satisfied, from what I had seen of his skill in San Francisco, that he was an even greater physician than his distinguished uncle.[57]

Through the Redlands dairy industry, Platt had developed business connections in southern California and encouraged Foo to open an herb shop there in 1893. First in Redlands and then in Los Angeles, Foo worked closely with Platt, who seems to have been primarily responsible for advertising and other forms of public outreach with the

English-speaking community. Platt deflected attacks on Foo and Chinese medicine in the English-language press. In 1895, at the regular session of the Southern California Medical Society, its president, P. G. Redmondino, read a satirical paper entitled "Why American Doctors Should Employ Chinese Practices." Redmondino described the "barbarous and benighted" theories that underpinned Chinese medicine and characterized the formulary as an absurd and disgusting assemblage of insects and reptiles as well as human and other animal excrement. With tongue firmly planted in cheek, he declared, "The more recherché in its nastiness and mysticism, the greater the virtue the drug is believed to possess. Fluid as well as solid excrements of all sorts enter largely into their most expensive compounds, and these the Chinese practitioners industriously and conscientiously cram down the throats of either Chinese or American patients."[58] On Foo's behalf, Platt launched a media campaign to defend Chinese medicine, publishing several articles in the *Los Angeles Times* that included glowing testimonials from European American patients.[59]

Foo's legal woes offer further insight into the nature of his business relationship with Platt and a subsequent agent. The death of a patient, Curtis Barney, revealed that Platt also did patient recruitment: "Platt, acting as an agent for a Chinese doctor . . . called upon him and said that for a certain sum, the doctor would have him up and around in nineteen days."[60] As an agent, Platt collected payment for Foo and Wing's prescriptions, a fact that became apparent when Foo sued Platt for embezzlement in 1896.[61] When Foo and Platt parted ways that year, Platt remained in the business of "Oriental Medicine." Twenty years later, he resurfaced in court records when he was arrested for practicing medicine without a license. From the report of his arrest, it is clear that Platt modeled his therapeutic practices on Chinese practices of pulsology. An advertising pamphlet submitted as evidence identified him as the "vice-president and general manager" of the "American Institute of Oriental Medicine," subordinate to T. G. Hing, a Chinese herbalist based in San Jose.[62] Meanwhile, Dr. Foo fared no better with his next business manager, William Maybury (or Mayberry). Their relationship ended in a lawsuit as well with Maybury suing Foo for breach of contract. In April 1896, Foo had agreed to pay Maybury a salary of one hundred

dollars per month to handle advertising for Foo and Wing and promised to make him the "sole [west] coast agent" for the business, imply-
ing Foo employed other managers in a similar capacity. Three months
later, Maybury found himself summarily replaced by another agent and
evicted from a property he rented with Foo and Wing.[63] Foo seemed to
have more success with Maybury's successor, a man named W. A. Hallowell, who remained with the company for at least a decade, running
errands and somehow serving as an interpreter despite his apparent inability to speak Chinese.[64]

Although there is no reason to believe there was a shortage of capital within the Chinese community, herb companies occasionally took
on white investors. Dr. Wong, the once-employer of Burton C. Platt,
drafted articles of incorporation in 1901 under five trustees: three Chinese and two non-Chinese. Identified as "S. White" and "John T. Jones"
both of Los Angeles, the latter were minor investors, contributing $100
each, compared to Wong You Ting at $6,800 and Wong Ting Cheung
and Dong Soon, both at $1,000.[65] When the Chinese American Herb
Company of Los Angeles incorporated in 1904, the *Los Angeles Times*
named its five directors, A. Z. Holmes (the one-time partner of Yitang
Chang), Julia Holmes, J. B. Earley, J. R. Weller, and J. E. White, not a
single one Chinese. Two years later, the *Los Angeles Herald* covered the
incorporation of the Toy Kee Herb Company under the direction of Toy
Kee, William Waller, Phoebe Lankersley, O. M. Walter, and F. F. Pratt.[66]
The articles did not explain why.[67] Perhaps European American business
partners offered some combination of connections, capital, and credibility to Chinese physicians competing in the American marketplace.

When the assistance of European American interpreters and
business managers was not sufficient, Chinese doctors relied on one
another. Doctors who worked closely with one another or who were
members of one extended family used the same advertising copy and
images. By these means, Chinese doctors were able to leverage a little
cultural knowledge across their professional community. Los Angeles
doctors Woh and Kwong worked out of the same offices, next door to
the *Times* building on First Avenue, and their 1890 print advertisements
were identical (again, with the exception of the name), right down to
the sketch of a Chinese scholar in Mandarin dress.[68] Foo and Wing Herb

Company commissioned an engraving of a photograph in which Foo demonstrated pulsology on his business partner, Hallowell, and printed versions of it in their display advertising. Not long thereafter, they seem to have loaned out the engraving's central figure—Foo himself—for use in the advertisements of another Los Angeles herbalist, Tom She Bin, who may have been a member of the extended family.[69] Chan and Kong, an herb franchise founded in Oakland in the early twentieth century, shared the same basic template for its advertisements.[70] Advertising copy was not always shared with consent. In 1865, "Dr. Jim" of San Francisco ran an advertisement in the *Daily Dramatic Chronicle* that copied language verbatim from an advertisement for Dr. Fung Sheuk. Fung's original advertisement read, "The public are hereby notified that several other Chinese Physicians, with little reputation or skill, have located themselves in the vicinity of DR. FUNG SHEUK, with a view of diverting his practice to their emolument." Dr. Jim was likely the target of the insult. The offices of Fung and Jim were in close proximity to one another, Fung on the northwest corner of Washington Square and Jim catty-corner to him. Jim took his revenge by swapping his name for his rival's in his plagiarized version of the advertisement.[71]

"Exotic Cures"

In 1870, San Francisco doctor Li Po Tai appeared in the pages of the *Wellsville Free Press,* a newspaper circulating in a small town near New York's border with Pennsylvania. With astonishment and consternation, a correspondent for the newspaper reported that Chinese medicine had become quite popular on the West Coast among "white patients," who assumed the Chinese formulary "contain[ed] some remedies unknown to western physicians." The correspondent described his visit to Li's offices at the end of a "long dirty passage," with a "lady who believed herself to be in an incipient consumption." Readers of the *Wellsville Free Press* learned of the mysterious process by which patients were admitted and medicines administered, and of the many iron pots that lined the walls, each containing some unknown elixir. Li conducted a short interview with his patient, prescribed a course of treatment, and advised abstinence from dancing and other exertions. Throughout the report, the correspondent remained skeptical. Of his "lady friend," the correspondent wrote, "Whether it was the medicine or the advice (I strongly suspect the latter, for it was strictly followed), my lady friend soon recovered her health, and is, of course a firm believer in the medical abilities of the Chinese."[72] The implication was clear: the popularity of Chinese medicine among European American patients defied logical explanation.

Accounts like the one in the *Wellsville Free Press* became increasingly common as practitioners of Chinese medicine expanded their presence in the American marketplace in the late nineteenth century. The readers of this newspaper and other English-language dailies may have been surprised by the popularity of Chinese medicine because they were most likely to encounter tales of the immigrant doctors as victims or perpetrators of crimes. Newspapers lavished attention on herbalists when they crossed paths with opium addicts and jealous mistresses, high binders and shadowy organizations, the more sordid and salacious, the better.[73] Real and imagined connections between Chinese herbs and death by poisoning made for exciting newspaper copy and confirmed stereotypes that associated the Chinese with barbarity. In 1883, the *New York Times* published an article on a "Coroners' Manual" outlining Chinese methods of murder and suicide by poison: "The commonest poisons are said to be opium, arsenic, and certain noxious essences derived from herbs. But besides these other things are taken by suicides and given by murderers to cause death." The article went on to describe a special "Golden Silkworm . . . reared by miscreants" in the southern provinces and the preferred method of suicide among wealthy Chinese men: swallowing gold or silver to effect suffocation or internal bleeding.[74] San Francisco's *Daily Call* attributed the murder of Chinatown doctor Ng See Poy to so-called Chinese high binders, a secret society of Chinese American assassins, blackmailers, and assorted criminals.[75] "Highbinders at War" read the headline after the 1893 murder of Ah Yok, a Fresno-based doctor.[76] In 1898, when Los Angeles doctor Bow Son was discovered shot in the stomach on Marchessault Street, the *Los Angeles Herald* covered the case in gruesome detail and linked his eventual demise to the activities of a "notorious San Francisco gambler and procurer" hell-bent on avenging Bow's "alleged theft of a Chinese female."[77]

A few years later, Oregon doctor Lee Sing Nom received another flurry of attention when he was assassinated at the corner of Fourth and Pine in Portland's Chinatown. Chinese witnesses to the attack claimed that it was a white assailant who killed Lee, but white firefighters from a station two blocks away conjectured that the assassination stemmed from a rivalry among the "Chinese companies," neighborhood organizations that controlled Chinatown affairs. The firefighters' testimony trumped that of the Chinese until a white witness, Gus Whalley, came forward to explain that two drunk white men had followed, harassed, and eventually assaulted Lee in the streets. Lee "came to his death, not from the blow struck by his assailant, but by striking his head against a sharply-pointed rock in the street when he was felled to the ground." The county coroner corroborated that testimony, and the assailants were charged with manslaughter, not murder.[78]

Chinese doctors were perhaps especially targeted for robbery because of their relative wealth and standing within the immigrant community.[79] In 1901, when Sacramento doctor Lue Que Hing (Suey Quong) was shot and killed in the Chinese quarter, the detectives claimed that the murder had "grown out of highbinder disputes in San Francisco over gambling privileges."[80] The 1905 murder of Lin Moon Chuck, scion of a wealthy Oakland family, seemed to combine all tropes of the genre of the murdered Chinese doctor. The *Oakland Tribune* claimed, "the murdered man was fond of numbers of women" and aroused the jealousies of his countrymen, who attacked him on Washington Street and strangled him with his own queue. The article went on to describe Lin as a "lady killer," driven from his practice in Portland "on account of his fondness for other men's wives," and it predicted that "the murder of Lin Moon Chuck will lead to a highbinder war of great proportions."[81]

Muckrakers were convinced that Chinese physicians were nothing more than dope dealers in disguise.[82] Chinese doctors openly imported, prescribed, and sold medicinal-grade opium, which was less potent and addictive than narcotic-grade opium.[83] Some Chinese doctors may have trafficked in the narcotic, but it is difficult to say how many with any certainty. What is clear, however, is that campaigns against Chinese immigration and campaigns against opiate addiction were complementary and deployed in service of one other. The therapeutic use of opium dated back to antiquity, but the perils of addiction only became a public concern in the late nineteenth century when rates of addiction seemed to spike.[84] Reformers blamed the growing numbers of Chinese immigrants to the United States for the uptick in American addicts. In the last decades of the nineteenth century, anti-opiate reformers called for not only restrictions on opium imports but also the exclusion of the Chinese men and women they closely associated with the drug.[85]

Given their proximity to legally imported opium, it is not surprising that Chinese doctors drew the unwanted attention of reformers. In Butte, Montana, the *Anaconda Standard* reported that "although the number of 'old and established' Chinese doctors who have been in the city for several years is already large, new ones are constantly coming in, and . . . a goodly share of their income is derived from the sale of opium and other opiates to depraved whites, of both sexes."[86] A critical account of Boston's Chinatown noted that "the air in the dark dismal stairways leading to the doctor's apartments was laden with the fumes of opium, and to an ordinary person it was almost suffocating."[87] In the kingdom of Hawaii, the *Hawaiian Gazette* interpreted the assembly's decision to license Chinese physicians as an underhanded scheme to promote and monopolize the flow of opium into the islands:

> It is wonderful how quickly the Government has changed its mind with regard to Chinese doctors. A short time ago it was quite difficult for a Chinese doctor to obtain a license to practice now there is no difficulty whatever about the matter. We understand that there are no less than twenty eight licensed Chinese physicians. Why this change in the spirit of the dream? It is not far to seek. Chinese physicians are available for prescribing opium for any diseases of their countrymen and this helps forward the sale of the drug in which the Government is interested. Anything to boom up the sale of opium by the licensed monopolists.[88]

In 1887, new legislation expressly prohibited Chinese physicians from prescribing opium in Hawaii.[89] Up and down the Pacific Coast and across the Midwest, Chinese apothecaries and doctor's offices were subject to police raids on suspicion of being secret opium dens.[90] Li Po Tai was among the many arrested and fined for "keeping a Chinese opium resort."[91] Salt Lake City police officers arrested See Lum Kee in 1885 for selling opium out of his shop on Commercial Street but could only prove that he shared a smoke with a young witness named John Spencer.[92]

Despite all reports of a repulsive formulary and the dubious morality of its practitioners, Chinese medicine continued to attract white patients, which some observers attributed to a virtual epidemic in foolishness and gullibility. When Ling Law opened shop on Union Square in San Francisco in 1870, the *San Francisco Chronicle* covered the occasion as evidence of the success of the "Chinese Quack" in their city: "There are plenty of victims for the Chinese Quack, with his wonderful medicines, which will do everything but cure fools of their folly."[93] San Francisco's *Daily Alta California,* describing Li Po Tai's formulary, disparaged both the doctor and his patients, "for whose medical prescriptions in the shape of dried toads, medicated snails, and bottled slugs, many white gudgeons have displayed great voracity."[94]

In 1880, the *Chronicle* considered Chinese doctors more generally as it endeavored to understand the appeal of their services in an article entitled "Celestial Quacks: The Implicit Confidence Placed in Them by Many." In a crude kind of undercover reporting, the reporter feigned sickness to expose the exorbitant fees exacted for baseless diagnoses and imaginary cures. The reporter riffed on common stereotypes of the Chinese in his portrayal of the unnamed doctor. Like "Ah Sin" in Bret Harte's "Heathen Chinee," a much misinterpreted and popular satire of anti-Chinese racism published in 1870, the unnamed "Celestial Quack" was equal parts conniving and ridiculous. He was also, after "much profitable intercourse with credulous and ignorant white people," possessed of "contempt for our race, which he took little trouble to conceal." The *Chronicle* reporter quoted the doctor speaking in Pidgin English, clumsy and all too transparent in his schemes to exact ten dollars per week to cure pretend ailments. Although the writer luxuriated in descriptions of the exotic Chinese formulary, his primary question was why white patients paid for the services of the "Asiatic impostors?" The article first conjectured that Chinese medicine held particular appeal for the terminally ill: "In health the average citizen sneers at the methods of the Chinese empiric: but tortured by incurable disease he flees to the Mongolian quack for the comfort denied by competent white practitioners. The Mongolian quack humors him to his full bent with promises of restored health, and the poor victim cheerfully bestows his last dollar on the impostor."[95]

But desperation alone could not account for the popularity of Chinese medicine among a class of people presumed to know better. It was well known at the time that business tycoons like Leland Stanford and Mark Hopkins frequented Chinese doctors, and the reporter for the *Chronicle* noted the presence of "leading citizens" awaiting appointments with the Chinese doctor.[96] So, he called on another stereotype: a common association between decadence and "the Oriental." In this sense, the *Chronicle* article became both an attack on Chinese medicine as well as a critique of Gilded Age San Francisco society. The reporter quoted a "well-known American physician" as saying, "You would be surprised . . . were I to tell you the names of the people who patronize these Chinese quacks. It is no uncommon thing to see handsome carriages drive up to their doors." The pills prescribed by these doctors were, purportedly, "coated in gold leaf" for the "aristocracy of Jackson Street."[97] These were gilded pills for the Gilded Age.

In the 1880s and 1890s, most explanations for the popularity of Chinese medicine among non-Chinese patients continued to focus on those same factors as the 1880 *Chronicle* exposé: the patients' gullibility or desperation and Chinese medicine's fashionableness. In 1890, Butte, Montana's newspaper, the *Anaconda Standard,* marveled that there were some forty Chinese physicians in residence with a majority of revenues from white patients: "As in every American city, there is a very large percentage of people that liked to be duped."[98] When the newspaper sent a reporter to observe the preparation of a Chinese prescription firsthand, he wrote, "The weird witches of Macbeth never brewed a more strange decoction than did 'Dr.' Charley for this ailing celestial," and the writer attributed Charley's success to the naiveté of his white patients:

These Chinese doctors, who simulate a knowledge of the human system and its needs in case of debility, are doubt-less patronized by many white people who imagine them in

possession of some secret remedies of which regular physicians are ignorant. But such a belief is only founded upon the
most asinine stupidity. The alleged Chinese healers surround
their methods and business with a sort of oriental mystery and
secrecy, which leads many to think them able to diagnose and
cure diseases in a more skillful manner than white doctors.[99]

Nearly twenty years later, the success of Chinese medicine continued
to perplex the *Anaconda Standard,* which ran an article concluding that
"exotic cures are more appealing than familiar ones, and the desperate
more likely to ignore cultural barriers."[100] Remarking on a "local boom
in Chinese doctors," the *Los Angeles Times* surmised in 1890, "There is a
fashion in medicine, as well as in bonnets, and fashions, as we all know
are sometimes very peculiar."[101]

Some critics explained the popularity of Chinese medicine with
American Orientalist stereotypes: if Chinese doctors were innately devi-
ant and feminine, so must be their patients. Following a wave of arrests
of Chinese doctors practicing medicine without a license in Los Angeles
County, coverage of the trials became opportunities for newspapers to
underscore the exoticism and gendered deviance of these "irregular"
physicians. The *Los Angeles Times* reported the arrest and arraignment
of Tom Leung. The article lingered over the details of Leung's appearance ("faultlessly dressed, wearing a frock coat and silk hat") and soberly
noted, "Women have been used to get evidence."[102] When Leung was
arrested yet again a few years later, the same newspaper lavished attention on the "fancy costumes" worn by Leung and his fellow physicians:
"The Chinese were arrayed in robes of wonderful richness, and the appointments of the rooms carried the impression of Oriental mystery."[103]
In a 1907 sting operation conducted by the Los Angeles Police Department, a "woman detective" went undercover to get evidence that G. S.
Chan was prescribing medicine without a license. The detective became
more of a curiosity for the newspaper than the Chinese herbalist, who
turned out to be far less exotic than the spectators attending the trial
hoped he would be. Chan arrived in court "attired in garments of the
latest [Western] fashion. . . . The spectators looked for the long, plaited
hair and swishy clothes and were . . . disappointed." Bessie K. Hall, the

undercover detective, on the other hand, happily provided lurid details for the newspaper, which reported that she "was married in Bakersfield but has not been living with her husband for some years past."[104]

Female patronage of Chinese doctors seemed to confirm their potential for duplicity and debauchery. In 1907, the *Los Angeles Times* reported contemptuously on women's affinity for Chinese doctors:

> The oriental "healer" business has increased wonderfully in Los Angeles in the last three years. Chinese "physicians" who formerly were barely able to make a living came here and waxed fat and rich. The places conducted by some of these smooth-tongued Celestials have been patronized largely by women. They scent to find something "romantic" in visiting the yellow quacks and having a "doctor" with long finger nails, a little round, black cap, with a red topknot, and loose, flowing robes, "prescribe" for their ills.[105]

The *Los Angeles Times'* depiction of the apothecary managed to mock both Chinese physicians and their white, female patients. Chinese doctors were foppish and effeminate, and their patients were fools. Decadence and luxury hinted at something nefarious: "Most of these places are beautifully furnished with oriental draperies, teak-wood furniture, Chinese porcelains, and other fittings calculated to create an impression of culture and wealth."[106] Female patients were, in effect, entranced by Chinese doctors. The *Los Angeles Herald* concurred: "It seems the seductive influence of the sweet smelling drugs which the long nailed celestials prepare is not to be resisted by the fair sex."[107] This susceptibility linked an innate feminine weakness and irrationality to women's inability to make sound decisions for their own health care.

Male patients were not exempt from accusations of deviancy. When Louis Potter, a prominent New York sculptor, died in Seattle in 1912, the coroner identified the cause of death as poison in the form of peach-tree extract prescribed by a Chinese doctor. Articles about the sculptor's death lingered over the "mystical" details of Chinese medicine. "Potter," the reporter lamented, "apparently had great faith in his oriental physician." The article went on to describe the state of the body: "Dr. Snyder [the coroner] said that in addition to the abrasions of the skin into which the oriental herbs were rubbed and a strong plaster applied, Potter apparently had been taking a strong medicine . . . Six large bottles of the black fluid had been consumed in eight days. The Coroner has not determined the nature of the concoction."[108] The intrigue was only compounded by the presence of a "mysterious companion," a woman who would not divulge her identity but who admitted that she was not the sculptor's wife: "The Coroner described the woman as 'apparently highly intellectual.'"[109] Newspapers covering the Potter death subtly intimated a connection between dangerous Chinese medicine and the dissolute lifestyle of artists and "intellectuals."

In Defense of Chinese Medicine

Defenders of Chinese medicine countered such demeaning depictions and encouraged regular physicians to consider Chinese medicine as an opportunity to expand the knowledge base of medical science. In an 1887 paper published by the *American Journal of Pharmacy,* ethnographer Stewart Culin explained that the "accounts of travelers" had depicted the Chinese formulary as "grotesque and childish," but in fact, scientific studies had shown that "many of their drugs are not without great value, [that] a large number of them, in fact, [are] nearly identical with those of our own pharmacopoeia, and that many important discoveries have resulted from the centuries of experiment upon which their practice of medicine is founded." Culin urged his audience of pharmacists to visit Chinese apothecaries in American cities and to study their *materia medica* as he had done in his hometown of Philadelphia.[110] Patient testimonials and anecdotal evidence also pointed toward the fact that Chinese medicine worked, at least some of the time. In 1916, the *Los Angeles Times* reprinted an article in the *Boston Transcript* covering judicial proceedings against a Chinese herbalist practicing without a license. The trial revealed that the herbalist had successfully treated a number of "influential and socially distinguished" patients, who testified on his behalf. "In the present state of uncertainty about medicines," the reporter wondered, "what is really the matter with herbs?" He also described "the extreme skill of the Chinese physicians" in diagnosis by pulse and encouraged the readers of the *Boston Transcript* to trust in Chinese medicine.[111]

Yet even advocates of Chinese medicine struggled to explain its worth without relying on the framework and vocabulary established by its detractors. Thus, the defense of Chinese medicine in the English-language press tended to rely on the same well-rehearsed tropes of American Orientalist discourse. Cured of malaria by Chinese medicine in 1886, a reporter for the *New York Sun* recounted his meeting with Ying Tsi Hing in purple prose:

> I slowly climbed a high old-fashioned winding staircase the other day in a queer old-fashioned house in Clinton place, and rapped once on the open door at the top of the landing. The door opened in upon a gaudily papered room, the atmosphere of which was heavy with the odor of burning opium. A curtain of red Chinese silk was stretched on a wire across the middle of the room dividing it into two compartments. The upper half of the open door was of glass. A red oil curtain was drawn across the panes on the inside. Upon the glass ware some Chinese characters in blood-red paint and under them this inscription in English in more red paint: Dr. Ying Tsi Hing, resident Chinese physician, from 10 A.M. to 4 P.M.

The patient had exhausted all other remedies, and, under the advice of a friend, went to consult the "Chinee doctor," certain that he "couldn't compound anything worse than the stuff I had been taking." The *Sun* reporter described Ying as "decidedly picturesque" and dressed in a costume "like the magician's garb in juvenile fairy tales."[112] With the assistance of a Chinese translator, the reporter made his condition understood and was eventually cured by Ying's decoction, but the testimonial was presented almost as an afterthought, decidedly secondary in importance to the presentation of Orientalist fantasies.

In an 1899 article for *Lippincott's Magazine,* William Tisdale decried travel writers who described Chinese physicians in terms more befitting a haunted house than a place of business: "Newspaper writers in

search of a sensation . . . thread narrow alleys and climb dark stairways
to find him in his secluded den, and relate thrilling stories of wrinkled
mummies who felt their quickly-beating pulses and wrote prescriptions
for sharks' fins, or spiders' eggs, or dried toads and lizards. These fairy
tales go the rounds and are read by thousands who shudder at their
imaginary horrors."[113] Tisdale was careful to distinguish trained Chinese physicians from pretenders, and he spoke highly of diagnosis by
pulse: "Whether it is based on some form of chicanery or upon science,
it is certainly successful."[114] Yet even as Tisdale commended Chinese
medicine for its efficacy, he could not resist embellishing his praise with
references to the mystical and supernatural. The ability to diagnose by
pulse, he claimed, was "analogous to the sixth sense which the blind
sometimes possess."[115] Tisdale's article alternated between describing
the apothecary as an ordinary American doctor's office and lingering
on the most exotic details of the doctor's costume and herbal formulary. The equivocation reflected a fundamental uncertainty about how
to extol the virtues of Chinese medicine. Did it work because it was like
American medicine or because it was not? Tisdale's ambivalence was
reflected in how he excerpted his interviews with white patients. He included the full gamut of responses, from those who "freely assert that
the Chinese system of medicine is more rational" than regular medicine
to those who marveled at what "these degraded heathen can do with
their herbs, which our own doctors with all their skill and knowledge
cannot."[116] Tisdale found ways to promote Chinese medicine by both
denying and affirming its racial otherness.

"Dread of the Knife"

For non-Chinese patients, Chinese medicine was neither a ruse nor a
fad, nor was it necessarily an outlet to express their own deviancy. While
travel accounts and sensational journalism may have portrayed Chinese
medicine as foreign and mysterious, its surface-level correspondences
with European American herbalism may have made it seem familiar to
non-Chinese patients. When seeking help for her daughter's infected
finger from Ing Hay, Mrs. Fred Deardorff wrote, "I have been using
flax seed poultis [*sic*] and white of egg but without much results."[117]

Historians and biographers have also noted that Chinese medicine's noninvasive approach to diagnosis and treatment likely appealed to patients fearful of surgery.[118] Another of Doc Hay's patients, Mrs. M. J. Baker, expressed just that sentiment. She suffered from a tumor on the left side of her neck and wrote beseeching him to treat it with herbs: "I would be so glad if you could reduce that as the [doctors] are wanting to cut it out and I have such a dread of the knife."[119] In Butte, Montana, a white female patient voiced her support for Chinese physician Ah Kong by calling all white doctors "butchers" in a public testimony.[120] Chinese doctors were well aware of their patients' phobias, and English-language advertisements frequently featured the noninvasive nature of diagnosis and treatment: "No knife! No pain!" Quan Tong declared. "Without operations or knife," Loo Chun promised. "Why operate?" Tom Leung asked.[121]

Capitalizing on their reputation for gentle herbal remedies and noninvasive procedures, Chinese doctors marketed their services to patients afflicted with venereal disease. Advertisements claiming "private diseases" as a specialty began to appear in English-language newspapers in the 1890s.[122] Such a specialty made good business sense. Given the prevalence of vice in frontier towns, Chinese doctors probably encountered more cases of sexually transmitted diseases than typical. Historian Paul D. Buell has studied handwritten "recipe" books from Seattle herbalists and argues that the numbers of prescriptions for gonorrhea and other sexually transmitted diseases were significantly higher than the numbers found in traditional Chinese herbals.[123]

Even in the late nineteenth century, the etiology of venereal diseases was still poorly understood. Some doctors believed gonorrhea was endemic in women and diagnosed all vaginal discharge as gonorrheal. Physicians sometimes counseled the afflicted that abstaining from sexual contact during treatment was sufficient, not realizing that the disappearance of symptoms did not mean the elimination of the disease.[124] Western pharmacy's early mass-produced antimicrobial Salvarsan was not widely available until the 1920s, and sulfa drugs were not developed until the 1930s. Thus, in the nineteenth and early twentieth centuries, a patient with a venereal disease might be treated with mercury, arsenic, or bismuth, either through topical application, inhaled vapors, or intravenous or intramuscular injection. Other treatments included the injection of near-boiling water or the bludgeoning of the genitalia. In the early twentieth century, the German chemical prophylaxis Viro became more common in the United States, but it required men to insert a tube of silver protein salt into the urethra after intercourse and apply a topical formaldehyde-based cream on the outside of the penis before and after intercourse.[125] It is no stretch to think that American men and women may have preferred to buy a packet of herbs to treat their "private diseases."[126]

"The Diseases of Women"

Before they claimed expertise in private diseases, Chinese doctors touted their ability to restore women's fertility and other "natural" functions.[127] Middle-class white women were particularly important targets for such advertising, not only because their affluence made it possible to purchase herbal remedies but also, as historians Sarah Stage and Linda Gordon have argued, because their culture dictated that women's bodies were most acutely in need of medical intervention.[128] Stage has described how "female invalidism" became an aesthetic ideal in the Victorian era. The performance of illness—whether consuming vinegar and arsenic to appear afflicted with tuberculosis or feigning nervousness and fainting spells to seem emotionally fragile—became a popular mode of expressing middle- and upper-class femininity.[129]

By 1880, Chinese doctors were regularly advertising treatments for gynecological disorders in their print advertising.[130] In 1897, Foo and Wing published a 238-page advertising book (later revised and expanded to 326 pages) entitled *The Science of Oriental Medicine*, which emphasized herbs' capacity to defend natural womanhood against "modern ways of life." The book attributed women's ailments—from irregular periods to cancers—to excessive food, alcohol, and parties; "overwork and anxiety"; and the use of contraceptives, which *The Science of Oriental Medicine* called "various perversions of marriage." Chinese herbs, Foo and Wing claimed, were "particularly adapted" to counter the poisonous effects of modern living and modern medicine.[131] In his advertising booklet entitled *Things Chinese*, Chang Gee Wo similarly spoke out against modern birth control and other interventionist medicine for their detrimental effects on women's health: "Why is it that the women of the twentieth century are not strong, healthy, and robust as the women of the first part of the nineteenth century? And why not mothers of a large family of strong, rosy-cheeked, and healthy children as their mothers and grandmothers had been before them?"[132] The answer, according to Chang, was modern medicine's tendency to "unsex" women by encouraging them to interrupt menses, seek abortions, or otherwise alter their reproductive systems.

Chinese doctors promoted philosophical and cultural aspects of their practice in ways that simultaneously appealed to women's traditional and modern identities. When Chang Gee Wo spoke directly to female patients through promotional books, his depiction of femininity cleaved closely to the Victorian ideal of "true womanhood," which identified domesticity (along with piety, purity, and submissiveness) as the source of women's social power and moral authority. While a woman might express her domesticity as a wife, daughter, or sister, the mother was the ultimate manifestation of Victorian femininity.[133] At the same time, however, Chang portrayed Chinese women, and by extension Chinese culture, as more modern than their American counterparts in some ways. He claimed that "the women in China do not lace or wear corsets as many of those further advanced in civilization do." For some American women, the implication that Chinese medical knowledge liberated the female body from confining, Victorian fashion might have been appealing. Business cards from the 1910s advertising Kam Wah Chung likewise aimed to sell not only "medical herbs, groceries, Chinese goods and general merchandise," but also a vision of modern femininity.[134] Each card portrays a white woman: "Dorothy" gaily ice skating, "Jestine" posing in a fur-trimmed coat, "Mildred" playfully tipping a hat, and "Clara" looking regal in finely draped robes and upswept hair. These were not images of the eastern Oregon ranching and farm wives who patronized Kam Wah Chung but perhaps representations of what they aspired to be.[135]

When the popular press portrayed women as overly susceptible to "Oriental quackery," it failed to recognize the ways in which Western-style medical science failed to meet the needs of female patients.

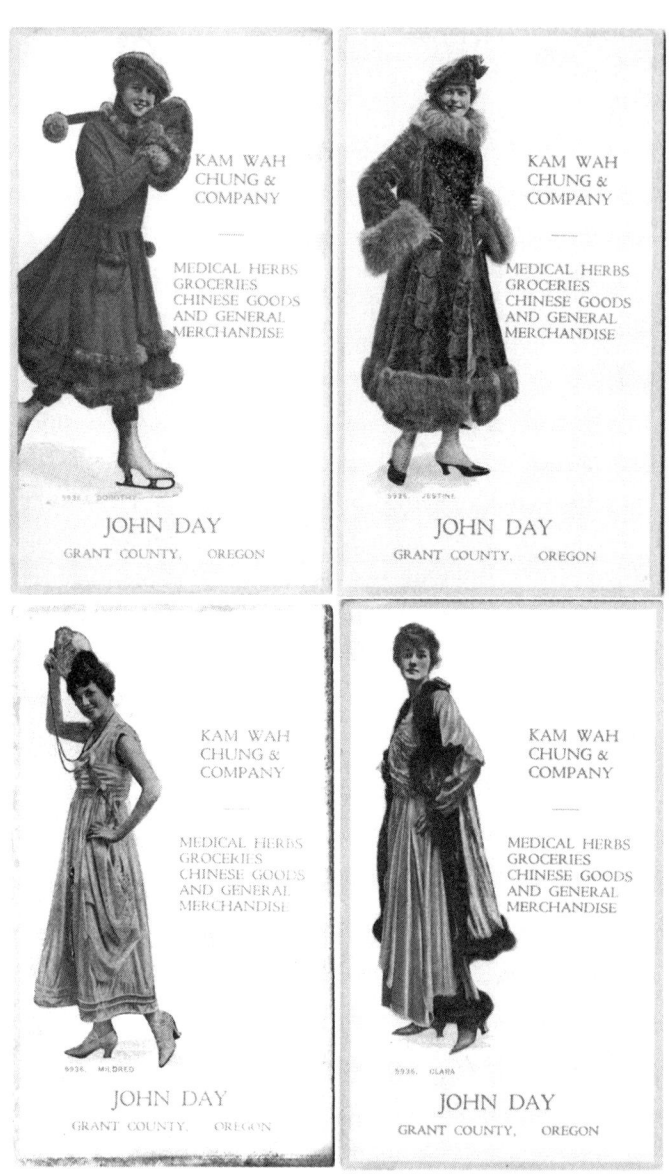

Trade cards from Kam Wah Chung, 1910. Courtesy of
Kam Wah Chung State Heritage Site Archival Collection,
Oregon Parks and Recreation Department.

Chinese medicine likely appealed to women on many levels. The distance and discretion offered by Chinatown offices may have been important for some, but the many women who signed letters of support or testified on behalf of Chinese doctors in court certainly did not have anonymity at the top of their minds. Testimonials attributed to female patients appeared in English-language advertisements as early as 1869.[136] A 1909 advertisement for the Hop Wing Chinese Herb and Tea Company of Los Angeles included not only a portrait and testimony but also the home address of a female patient named Lottie Baskerville, who claimed to have been cured of stomach and liver trouble by Dr. Hung Chun Hong.[137]

The prevalence of herbal remedies and noninvasive procedures in Chinese medicine may have been attractive to women because they had good reason to distrust regular medicine. Throughout the nineteenth century, American women were both major consumers and practitioners of irregular medicine. Irregular doctors often defended women from physically and psychologically damaging procedures championed by their regular rivals.[138] In 1869, the *Pacific Medical and Surgical Journal* reported that Li Po Tai recommended that a woman shave her head and "blister it" (perhaps a reference to the practice of moxibustion) to remedy a prolapsed uterus.[139] While that recommendation may not have seemed particularly pleasant, it was probably preferable to a hysterectomy or colpocleisis (the surgical closure of the vagina) that regular surgeons typically prescribed.[140]

In Western-style scientific medicine, gynecology was a surgical specialty. Interest in women's sexual function flourished during the Victorian era, but gynecologists struggled for legitimacy in the medical profession. Cultural prohibitions on immodest touching between men and women limited doctors' ability to assess and diagnose. The modern vaginal speculum was developed in the 1840s but not widely used for fears that it would arouse the patient.[141] Surgical interventions may have seemed like a way to elevate the urgency and thus the status of gynecological science. In the late nineteenth century, unnecessary removals of the uterus and ovaries were often prescribed, despite high mortality rates.[142]

Chinese doctors explicitly denounced gynecological surgeries in their advertising. The 1902 edition of *The Science of Oriental Medicine* included a chapter specifically addressing "The Diseases of Women" in which Foo and Wing decried gynecological surgeries as a "fad pure and simple."[143] In *Things Chinese,* Chang Gee Wo wrote, "In the majority of cases, when a woman succeeds in mustering up sufficient courage to submit to a local examination, she is informed that an operation is necessary, and if she consents to undergo the fearful suffering that must always attend anything of that kind, she arises to find, only too frequently, that she has but added to her misery." Chang declared that his herbal remedies would eliminate menstrual pains, making operations unnecessary.[144]

For European American women apprehensive about the prospect of physical intimacy with a male Chinese physician, some advertisements promised the presence of white female assistants and receptionists. Boston-based doctor Pang Suey employed two white women, May Matherson and Emma F. Goodwin, in his office. They seem to have assumed responsibility for communicating with white patients, who comprised an estimated 90 percent of Pang's business. When he died in 1917, his apprentice Gouy Shang (Shong) took over his practice, and Matherson and Goodwin remained on his staff.[145] In Los Angeles, Tom Leung hired a series of English-speaking secretaries—mostly women—and he credited one of them, Willa Brooker, with attracting new clientele to his office at 719 South Main Street. Brooker was the daughter of a woman employed as a nanny to Leung's eight children.[146] In Portland, Oregon, the Chinese Medicine Company went a step further and offered the services of Mrs. S. K. Chan, an herbalist who promised to handle all examinations of female patients. Chan enjoyed an elite status among Portland's Chinese community. She was married to the Reverend Chan Sing Kai, a Methodist who led services in Chinese and English at the corner of Second and Alder Streets, and one of their daughters, Mary, had married Seid Gain, remembered as the "leader of the native-born Chinese" in Portland and son of prominent local businessman Seid Back.[147] Early advertisements for the company portrayed a bespectacled Mrs. Chan on equal footing with her business partner and fellow doctor C. P. Huie.[148] By 1907, Chan had struck out on her own and was advertising her services to women out of her home on Clay and Third, several blocks south of Chinatown.[149]

Diagnosis by pulse may have attracted a female clientele as it promised a minimum of physical contact between doctor and patient. In China, male physicians might examine women through a veil, sometimes going so far as to tie a string around the patient's wrist so that the vibrations of the pulse could be observed without any touching at all. This tradition was intended to preserve the virtue of the woman, and it was translated for Victorian Americans who were similarly sensitive to improper contact, especially between white women and nonwhite men. Women who sought care from male Chinese physicians could be assured of limited physical contact during their exam. Modesto doctor N. S. Sue kept an ivory carving of a woman's body on the desk in his office so that his female patients might point to the site of their affliction.[150] An 1894 advertisement for Chang Gee Wo's Chicago office promised to cure "all diseases of women without examinations or instruments."[151]

In English-language advertisements for Chinese doctors, images showing the practitioner conducting diagnosis by pulse on a non-Chinese patient became popular around the turn of the twentieth century.[152] Such images instructed the patient on what to expect when they submitted to an examination by a Chinese physician.[153] Advertising in the Los Angeles Times in the first decades of the twentieth century, Tom Foo Yuen and Tom Leung showed a doctor in traditional Chinese garb, seated and practicing diagnosis by pulse on a white male patient. The drawing reproduced a photograph that appeared in a 1902 edition of their advertising booklet, The Science of Oriental Medicine, and it inspired a nearly identical advertisement featuring a drawing of a white woman.[154] The patient is clothed and coiffed in a way that bespeaks of Victorian affluence and respectability. There is no hint of impropriety in the relationship between the male Chinese doctor and female white patient. Whereas in the original ad, the male patient's and doctor's faces were slightly turned in, suggesting the possibility of making eye contact, the female patient and her doctor connect only at the wrist. The woman's face is tilted toward her doctor, but the doctor looks out toward the viewer and unquestionably does not meet her gaze. Diagnosis by pulse required no disrobing, no intimate touching, and—as this particular ad

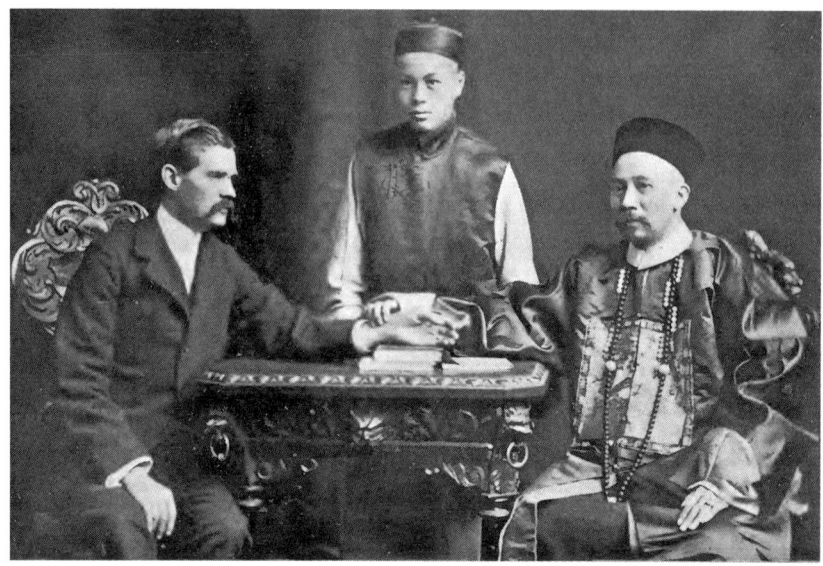

"The above cut represents a pulse diagnosis. The figure at the right is T. Foo Yuen, President of the FOO & WING HERB COMPANY, that in the center is his son, Tom How Wing, the figure at the left is W. A. Hallowell, Jr., one of the friends of this corporation." Frontispiece of *The Science of Oriental Medicine*, 1902. Hathi Trust Digital Library.

suggested—not even locking eyes. Chinese doctors held out the promise of obstetrical examinations and treatments that freed women from fear of pain and humiliation.

The promise of noninvasive procedures may have encouraged white women to seek out Chinese doctors for assistance with childbirth. Professional obstetricians—usually formally educated or apprenticed-trained white males—had come to rely heavily on interventions beginning in the late eighteenth century. Obstetrics introduced forceps to facilitate the passage of the baby through the pelvis and pain-relieving medication, such as opium, chloroform, or ether.[155] Some women welcomed the services of the "male physician-*accoucheur*" over a midwife who might encourage labor to take its course. Others, however, justifiably feared the interventions of the overeager physician, whose use of forceps might result in lacerations or infection.[156]

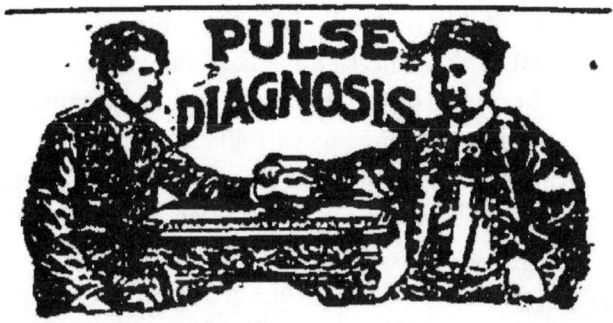

GIFT—BOOK—A Guide to Health and How to
Keep Well, by Dr. T. Foo Yuen and his
brother, Dr. T. Leung. Give a diagnosis without asking a question. Costs nothing.
THE FOO & WING HERB CO.,
903 S. Olive st.   Los Angeles, Cal.

For Centuries
Chinese Herbs
HAVE RELIEVED AND CURED
All Kinds of Diseases

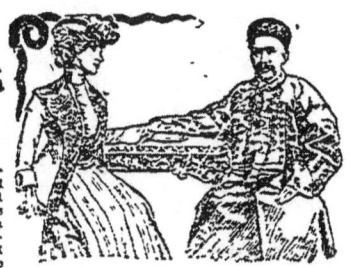

The distinguished men at the head of the
Foo & Wing Herb Company have had
many years' experience in the Orient and
in this country. Hundreds of Americans
testify to the return of splendid health
after taking the herbs especially imported by this company. Testimonials tell
of marvelous cures. Read for instance
the following:

Pasadena, Cal., Aug. 22, 1912.

T. Leung, Gen. Man., The Foo & Wing Herb Co.,

903 S. Olive St., Los Angeles, Cal.

Dear Sir: I wish to express to you the great benefit that I received from your Herb Remedies. After six years of Treatment with
the "Old Schools of Medicines," and when all hope of recovery was
gone, I put aside my prejudices and began taking your Herb Remedies, and they have saved my life. I wish to recommend your treatment to all who are ill. You may use my name for reference if you
so desire.   Yours cheerily,

(Signed) C. M. MELICK, Pasadena, Cal.

R. F. D. No. 1.

SEND FOR THEIR FREE BOOK

THE FOO & WING HERB CO., Inc. 1897
T. Foo Yuen, Pres.   T. Leung, Gen. Mgr.
903 South Olive St., Los Angeles,
Chinese Herbs, Rice and Tea for Sale.

Foo and Leung advertisements, *Los Angeles Times,* 1904 and 1912.

At the turn of the twentieth century, then, midwifery remained a thriving segment of the American medical marketplace. By the 1920s, midwifes had begun to organize schools and professionalize, but up until that point, they were informally trained by other midwifes, principally women, and often people of color.[157] Chinese women and some men joined their ranks. A Chinese woman known as Mrs. Chow Sing Huey served as a midwife for European American, Paiute, and Chinese mothers in Carson City, Nevada.[158] In Kern County, California, the local midwife, Mrs. Jung Sing, was fondly remembered as "the wise old lady of Chinatown."[159] Chinese doctors' involvement in pregnancy and childbirth often only came to light when tragedy struck. In 1899, Lin Tong of Albany, Oregon, was arrested for practicing without a license when he misused forceps to deliver the infant of a longtime patient. The child survived but suffered serious lacerations to its scalp and required stitches. Lin was later exonerated when it could not be proven that he had handled the instrument.[160]

With regard to pregnancy, Chinese doctors were philosophically pragmatic. The study of women's diseases and recommendations for childbirth had been part of the mainstream Chinese medical canon and training in the imperial palace since the Song Dynasty (960–1279). Imperial scholars, steeped in Confucian philosophy, considered the health of wives and mothers as crucial to the health of the empire, which was founded on a familial model.[161] In the late Qing period, printing houses across China distributed affordable and simplified medical texts, which would have been available to Chinese doctors immigrating abroad.[162] Popular publications included manuals on women's health, most famously the writings of the Bamboo Grove monks, members of a monastery in Xiaoshan, Zhejiang Province, who famously specialized in *fuke* (women's health), and the *Treatise on Easy Childbirth*, both of which advocated noninterventionist approaches such as herbal remedies and prayer to cope with infertility, childbirth, and the termination of pregnancies that risked the health of the mother.[163]

Chinese medicine's approach to pregnancy distinguished it from American medical science, which seemed designed to discourage women from making choices about their reproductive life. In the realm of birth control, regular physicians were not always reliable sources of information or service. According to historian Linda Gordon, "Most of the moderates as well as the extremists [among American doctors] emphasized the debilitating effects of sexual indulgence, defined normal sexual intercourse as that leading most directly to male orgasm, and opposed contraception."[164] Certainly, there were individuals who privately performed abortions or offered advice on avoiding pregnancy, but in public statements, regular doctors tended to link birth control with female promiscuity. As early as the 1850s, the American Medical Association joined a movement to suppress women's access to birth control and abortions as part of a larger "social purity" campaign that elevated regular physicians' status as the arbiters of not only human health but also morality. Up until the 1860s, abortion before fetal movement ("quickening") had been mostly unregulated, and abortions after fetal movement considered high misdemeanors in cases of maternal death. Between the 1860s and 1880s, regular physicians supported new state laws that criminalized abortion and made it illegal to circulate information about birth control across state lines.[165] Progressive Era birth-control activists like Margaret Sanger largely operated without the approval of mainstream medical authorities. It was not until the era of the Great Depression that regular physicians publicly supported efforts to educate women on family planning and agreed to provide contraception at specially designated clinics.[166]

At a time when abortion was illegal and the AMA officially opposed its practice, Chinese doctors terminated unwanted pregnancies for their patients. Locals in eastern Oregon recalled that Chinese doctor Ing Hay provided abortions by rubbing sandpaper, a coin, and an onion over the patient's navel in his office and then prescribing an herbal tea to be consumed at home.[167] Salt Lake City doctor Yee Foo Lun was arrested for practicing without a license after performing "a criminal operation on a young woman"—euphemistic language for an abortion—at a local hotel in 1913.[168]

The most famous case of a Chinese abortionist was T. Wah Hing (Yee Lok Sam) of Sacramento. By some accounts, the original family name was Yee, which was poorly transliterated as "T." The Sacramento family was possibly related to Fan-Chung Yee, the proprietor of Fiddletown's Chew Kee Store.[169] T. Wah Hing's family history—like many

Chinese immigrant families of his generation—is difficult to trace. The man he claimed to be his father was also a doctor called T. Wah Hing, who according to the Bureau of the Census was born in China in 1848 and immigrated to the United States in 1870. That timing is difficult to square with the family's assertion that the son, also identified as Wah Hing by census takers, had been born in California in 1869.[170] It may have been a simple error, or it may have been evidence of an illegal entry into the United States that made the younger Wah Hing the "paper son" of the elder. Between 1886 and 1891, the elder T. Wah Hing practiced medicine in Nevada, first in Virginia City, where he was arrested for being an unlicensed doctor, and then in Reno.[171] By December 1891, he was back in California and advertising his services in Sacramento.[172] In 1897, his son Yee Lok Sam took over the family business and adopted his father's name. When the census taker recorded his household in 1900, both of the Hing's (as they were known), the younger's wife, and that couple's two children were all living together in their home and office on J Street, between Seventh and Eighth Streets.[173] Over time, the younger Hing developed a reputation as a savvy businessman, a property holder, and a member of the Chamber of Commerce. Local lore claimed that he had successfully saved the wife of a California governor when she suffered complications after childbirth (although that accolade was sometimes attributed to his father or to their relative Fan-Chung Yee).[174]

In 1909, Hing the younger was roughly forty years old and charged with feticide. The indictment claimed that Hing had used a "long tongue-shaped instrument made of a hard and nonflexible substance ... about fifteen inches in length and shaped like a common round lead pencil" (possibly a curette or uterine sound) to induce a miscarriage in Lottie Phillips. Phillips was reportedly about three months pregnant but had only been married a month to a local clerk, William Phillips, who may or may not have fathered the fetus. On June 25, 1908, she and her mother, a Mrs. Toomey, visited Hing at his home and office on J Street. Toomey stayed in the reception area while Phillips received a private consultation in an adjoining room. Phillips later testified that Hing asked her why she wanted to terminate her pregnancy, and she replied that her torso had been badly burned in an accident; as a result, she did not think she could breastfeed the child. Hing asked for a payment of twenty-five dollars, then directed the patient and her mother to another building on nearby L and Sixth Streets, where they were greeted by an unidentified woman. Twenty minutes later, Hing joined them, took Phillips upstairs, presumably where he performed the abortion, and then sent her home to recuperate. Later that evening, Lottie's husband, William, went to Hing's office on J Street to purchase some pills at his wife's request. He testified that he gave the doctor all the money he had with him: five dollars—far less than Hing had requested.[175] Phillips then returned to his wife, who seemed to pass a large amount of tissue that may have been the fetus around one or two o'clock in the morning.[176] The following day, Lottie Phillips's condition worsened. It is not clear from newspaper coverage or the court transcript if she suffered from excessive bleeding or some other complications, but she was admitted to the county hospital and eventually recovered. Her doctors there encouraged her to file a complaint against Hing.[177]

Hing's case went to trial in November 1909. His defense insisted that no one but Lottie Phillips had seen Hing use the instrument to perform the abortion, and that her testimony was in fact an effort to blackmail the physician. Moreover, the attorneys argued that Hing was not even in Sacramento on the day in question, and they produced eyewitnesses and a ledger with his signature from a hotel in Marysville, over forty miles away.[178] The prosecution countered with evidence from a Sacramento post office showing that Hing had signed for a letter on the same day and could not have been in Marysville.[179] The original proceedings against Hing ended with a hung jury, but a second trial was quickly convened. The *Los Angeles Times* described the retrial as a "carnival of perjury."[180] The Phillipses' upstairs neighbor Gertrude Hill testified for the defense that Lottie's miscarriage had been self-induced. Another woman, identified in newspaper coverage as Mrs. George Gillespie, was discovered to have asked Hing to pay her $250 in exchange for persuading the Phillipses to abandon the case against him. After she failed to do so, she promised to produce a letter that she had transcribed from a dictation by the illiterate William Phillips, a letter that she claimed would exonerate Hing of all wrongdoing. Unfortunately, the letter went missing.[181] Hing tried to pin the crime on other unnamed doctors and a female nurse referred to as Miss McCarger, who may have performed abortions on C Street, but when the defense witness called to testify to that fact took the stand, he failed to corroborate the story and accused Hing's attorneys of attempting to bribe him.[182] On December 15, 1909, Hing was convicted and subsequently served three years in prison at Folsom. Upon his release, he returned to Sacramento and continued to practice medicine for more than twenty-five years.[183] In that time, he was arrested repeatedly for practicing medicine without a license, for drug fraud, for land fraud, and again for feticide. A 1917 indictment for feticide was set aside, and after another in 1922, he was exonerated.[184] Prosecution did not dissuade him from terminating pregnancies for women in need. It is impossible to say how many Chinese physicians included abortions in their roster of services, but the example of Hing demonstrates how for patients without recourse to mainstream medical care, Chinese physicians provided life-changing and life-saving treatment and procedures. Those services, along with the perception of therapeutic efficacy, familiarity of herbalism, and widespread aversion to surgery, made Chinese medicine appealing to non-Chinese patients.

The Intimate Economy

In Hornitos, a rural town in Mariposa County, California, the 1860 U.S. Census identified a Chinese woman named Mary Keng (also known by her married name, Mary Westfall) as a "doctor," but other records identified her as a cook. She was probably both.[185] For non-Chinese consumers of Chinese services, accepting domestic service and food preparation was a short step from seeking health advice. In California, Chinese labor had been prevalent in the service economy since the Gold Rush era, when Chinese men in sex-imbalanced mining districts assumed responsibility for work typically associated with women such as laundering and cooking.[186] As Chinese populations spread out across the American West in subsequent decades, affluent Californians and other westerners continued to employ Chinese cooks, servants, and gardeners despite reports that linked infectious diseases to the Chinese. In 1876, the same year that health officials identified Chinatown as the source of a smallpox epidemic in San Francisco, a special congressional committee investigating Chinese immigration estimated that approximately

7 percent of Chinese people living in the United States cooked, cleaned, and otherwise cared for the homes and bodies of non-Chinese people. In San Francisco, the site of the most vigorous public health campaigns against the Chinese, about 14 percent of Chinese workers were engaged as domestic servants in European American homes.[187] Across the American West, Chinese farmers provided food for non-Chinese tables. By 1879, in Portland, Oregon, Chinese vegetable peddlers had become a fixture in the urban landscape. They cultivated small plots in Tanner Creek Gulch in the southwest quadrant of the city and sold their produce door to door.[188]

It may seem contradictory that in the same period that regular physicians and public health officials began to identify Chinese enclaves as sites of infectious disease, middle-class and affluent Americans opened their homes and submitted their bodies to the care of Chinese men and women. White Americans may have weighed concerns about contagion against the chronic shortage of labor that characterized western economies in the late nineteenth century. They may have distrusted the still-developing science of public health. In 1876, when San Francisco health officials blamed a smallpox epidemic on the inhabitants of Chinatown, public opinion remained divided. The *Sacramento Daily Union* defended the Chinese, noting that throughout the crisis, their neighborhood remained disease-free: "It is rather doubtful whether justice has been done to the Chinese in ascribing [smallpox's] introduction to them."[189] While the reasons remain opaque, it is clear that by the end of the nineteenth century, Chinese hands regularly produced and handled food products consumed by American bodies.

American patients were accustomed to thinking about food as medicine. Hippocrates, the ancient founder of Western medical traditions, had done some nutritional theorizing that still resonated two millennia later; he was believed to have said, "Let thy food be thy medicine and thy medicine be thy food."[190] Affluent and ordinary Americans shared a common faith in the health-giving power of food. Domestic medicine guides comingled instructions for compounding herbal medicine with regular foodstuffs, and American cookbooks featured recipes for foods guaranteed to restore the sick to health.[191] Food fads seemed to proliferate in the late nineteenth century as self-proclaimed dietary experts and their acolytes promoted extreme regimens based on vegetarianism, high-fiber cereals, severe caloric restriction, and other imaginative combinations of foods. Industrializing economies raced to supply consumers dedicated to achieving health through diet.[192]

Thus, the old Chinese adage "food is medicine" translated easily into American health customs. By the early twentieth century, it was common for long-form advertisements for Chinese medicine to include lengthy discussions of diet and cooking. *The Science of Oriental Medicine* devoted fifty-two of its nearly three hundred pages to questions of diet and listed wholesome, disease-preventing foods and recipes.[193] *The Science of Oriental Medicine* explained that Chinese medicinal herbs were essentially common vegetables. Consuming them was as natural as eating regular food.[194] An advertisement for Portland herbalists Yee and York that circulated in nearby Walla Walla, Washington, promoted medicine with "the elements of natural food" to assuage the fears of potential patients: "You need not be afraid to take our medicine as it is compounded from roots, bark, flowers, and berries."[195] On the one hand, selling Chinese medicine as food could also work to dispel preconceived notions of exotic or stomach-churning ingredients in the Chinese formulary. Yet, it also reflected a core principle of traditional Chinese medicine extending back to the Bronze Age. Ancient medical texts prescribed specific diets to nourish *qi* (氣), an individual's life force.[196]

In the 1930s, Oakland doctor Fong Wan included a chapter entitled "The Herbalist and His Suggestions Regarding Drinking and Eating" in the advertising book that he sent to mail-order customers. He counseled his patients to consume "nourishing soups" as well as bamboo leaves, bean sprouts, and other vegetables. He also offered instruction in cooking various Chinese and Chinese American dishes, from a simple preparation of rice to *chop suey,* bean curd cakes, and noodles.[197] The section on diet included a recipe for shrimp omelet, which may have been a clever attempt at crossover marketing; Fong Wan and his Chinese partners had a side business selling shrimp in nearby Richmond, California. In this way, Fong Wan went beyond Foo and Wing. He used his herb business to launch a broader enterprise in Chinese comestibles, first as the proprietor of the Fong Wan Shrimp Company. Its advertisements used the language of human health to sell crustaceans:

"During the cold season, we should eat shrimps as seafood to build up the vitality of the body and to enable it to resist colds and prevent them from settling down on the bronchial tubes and lungs. Those persons who have secured shrimps from FONG WAN, renowned herbalist, have reported that shrimps as food, have relieved them of coughs, congestion, and have discharged phlegm out of their bronchial tubes."[198] Fong was a proud investor in a pair of Oakland restaurants, the Nanking Café and the New Shanghai Café, which boasted a "beautiful circular bar, large dance floor . . . and plenty of space for you to enjoy yourself and walk around."[199] Fong encouraged his patients to eat out at his restaurants, promising "the wholesome and delicious Chinese Herb dishes are unequaled in body-building value by any other foods."[200] Fong's success was evidence that American consumers agreed.

Conclusion

Through various means, Chinese immigrant doctors successfully expanded their practices beyond Chinatown's borders in the late nineteenth and early twentieth centuries. They borrowed advertising tactics from makers of proprietary medicines, found ways to overcome linguistic barriers, and offered support to one another. Herbalists became an extension of a larger service economy where Chinese men and women provided intimate, bodily care to non-Chinese consumers. By the end of the nineteenth century, Chinese medicine was firmly ensconced in the American medical marketplace, occupying a space similar to that of unorthodox medical therapies for its patients. Because of that association, Chinese doctors became subject to the same kind of scrutiny and discrimination that other irregular doctors faced when Western-style medical scientists expanded their control of the American medical profession in the late nineteenth and early twentieth centuries, a period historians often call "the long Progressive Era." The prosecution and defense of Chinese medicine in Progressive Era America is the subject of the next two chapters.

F · O · U · R

Chinese Quacks

I n the fall of 1878, California healers engaged in a legal experiment. Two years earlier, California had passed its first "Act to Regulate the Practice of Medicine in California," known more colloquially as the "Anti-Quackery Act." It stipulated that anyone practicing medicine in the state had to present a diploma from a "legally chartered medical school in good standing" for authentication by the Board of Examiners. To test the law's constitutionality, E. J. Fraser, the president of the Homeopathic Medical Society, offered himself up for arrest. He was followed swiftly by a trio of irregular practitioners, including Samuel H. Hall.[1] As Hall stood for trial at San Francisco's Criminal Court, he fingered another local physician practicing without a license: the celebrity Chinese herbalist Li Po Tai.[2] Li was the first of many Chinese doctors arrested under the Anti-Quackery Act. In the next year, six other Chinese physicians practicing in San Francisco were charged under the same law. All were convicted, paid their fines, and went back to work as if nothing had happened.[3]

California's 1876 Anti-Quackery Act was at the forefront of a nationwide movement to regulate medical practitioners through public licensure. Beginning in the late nineteenth century, states organized one or more medical boards. They took responsibility for interviewing applicants, receiving fees, and issuing certificates to practice medicine and surgery in the state. Elite, formally trained physicians, with the support of national professional organizations like the American Medical Association (AMA), used their dominance on state boards to make their medical education the standard for licensing. Beginning in the 1890s, state boards administered mandatory licensing exams that focused on recent medical science and pharmacology.[4] Those exams contributed to the gradually consolidating meanings of medical science and helped distinguish regular from irregular medicine.[5] Doctors practicing without a license faced the threat of fines and short prison sentences.[6]

Regular physicians assisted law enforcement with the arrest and conviction of unlicensed doctors by studying, surveilling, and entrapping "quack" doctors in their midst. Chinese physicians were doubly vulnerable to such campaigns. Unlicensed and socially marginalized by nativist groups, they became prime targets, particularly in California and the West, where they were a more visible segment of the medical market. Although many Chinese physicians claimed to have degrees from Chinese medical colleges, their qualifications carried little weight among American professional societies. Arrests for practicing without a license became an expected part of doing business. With very few exceptions, Chinese herbalists did not acquire medical licenses nor did state boards create alternative examinations for Chinese doctors as they did for homeopaths, chiropractors, and osteopaths. Through the legal persecution of Chinese doctors, practitioners of scientific medicine asserted their power over the politics of public health and the American medical marketplace. At the same time, however, new licensing statutes compelled Chinese doctors to develop fluency not only in American medical cultures but also in its laws. Their acts of resistance, compliance, and circumvention revealed the limits of regular medicine's power in the Progressive Era.

Making Regular Medicine

The Progressive Era movement for medical licensing was in fact a renewal of efforts that had stalled a half-century earlier. University-educated American physicians, often trained at European medical colleges, had long aspired to achieve the degree of exclusivity, authority, and market dominance that their European counterparts enjoyed.[7] Beginning in the mid-eighteenth century, elite physicians promoted the organization of public licensure. In 1760, New York City became the first American municipality to establish public examinations and licensing for physicians, with fines for those who practiced without the approval of the city. Other jurisdictions soon replicated New York's institutions. Licensing was good for both the state and the licensee; licensing fees generated revenues for public coffers, and doctors could use the official credentialing to attract patients. However, competing incentives compromised early efforts at regulation. On the one hand, stricter licensing standards concentrated market control; on the other, flexibility permitted more practitioners to claim professional status and pay membership dues, tuition, and licensing fees, all of which enlarged the capacity and visibility of regulatory bodies. For much of the nineteenth century, medical societies, faculty, and public officials chose to maximize revenues and accept the costs of relatively unconstrained competition.[8]

Yet even the feeblest attempts at regulation ran up against resistance. Inspired by the anti-elitism and anti-monopolism of the Jacksonian era, the herbalist Samuel Thomson and his followers successfully led repeals of public licensure laws in the 1830s and 1840s. For irregular practitioners like the Thomsonians, there was more at stake than mere licensing fees. Regular and irregular physicians were well aware that economic (and political) power flowed from public acceptance of their professional sovereignty. Licensing lent institutional legitimacy to the physician's claim to authority. Thomsonians worried that such public regulation or the lack thereof might erode the authority they held with patients.[9]

By rallying against regulation, Thomsonians refused to accept the antidemocratic and exclusionary definition of "scientific medicine" that early licensing laws implied. While Thomson and his followers privileged personal experience and lay authority over professional expertise, they nonetheless located the basis of their expertise in rational observation and experimentation. Thomsonians carefully differentiated themselves from supernatural healers. They made no pretense of channeling magical, spiritual, or religious powers. In the preface to Thomson's 1831 book *New Guide to Health,* "a friend" described the development of his therapeutic system:

> Dr. Thomson began his practice as it were from accident, with no other view than an honest endeavor to be useful to his fellow creatures; and had nothing to guide him but his own experience . . . His whole studies have been in the great book of nature . . . His first enquiry was to know of what all animal bodies were formed, and then to ascertain what caused disease; after being satisfied on this head, the next was to find what medicine was the best calculated to remove disease and restore health. For this he looked into the vegetable kingdom, where he found a large field for contemplation and for the exercise of his enquiring mind. Here by an invention of his own, that of ascertaining the qualities and power of vegetables by their taste, he was enabled at all times to find something to answer the desired purpose; his apothecary's shop was the woods and the fields. In his practice it has always been his first object to learn the course pointed out by nature, and has followed by administering those things best calculated to aid her in restoring health.[10]

As a therapeutic system, Thomsonianism embraced the same kind of systematic study of nature and pathology that characterized Western-style scientific medicine at that time. Nearly two-thirds of the 337 pages of the *New Guide* detailed how Thomson arrived at his understanding of the human body through experimentation and how he applied that understanding to cure disease. In an extended autobiographical section, Thomson explained his rigorous plan of research and practice: "I took nature for my guide, and experience as my instructor: and after seriously considering every part of the subject, I came to certain conclusions concerning disease and the whole animal economy, which thirty years' experience has perfectly satisfied me is the only correct theory."[11] Thomson not only painted himself as the archetypal American individual and autodidact, venerated in the culture of the Jacksonian era, but also as a true scientist in the tradition of the Enlightenment.

Indeed, much of what went by the name of "science" in the late eighteenth and nineteenth centuries would not seem terribly scientific to us now. When Benjamin Rush treated victims of yellow fever by bloodletting in 1793, he believed his treatment had a scientific basis. He had observed the positive effects of bleeding his patients and linked those observations to a theory of human health. In the early nineteenth century, when Samuel Thomson prescribed purgatives and hot baths to restore heat to the body, he claimed that empirical research had led him to conclude that cold caused disease. Similarly, in the mid-nineteenth century, when French chemist Louis Pasteur and German physician Robert Koch studied microorganisms in laboratories and postulated that "germs" were the cause of disease in animals and humans, they too spoke with the authority of science. As John Harley Warner argues in *The Therapeutic Perspective*, "Medicine did not simply become more scientific during the nineteenth century; what was considered science, and what was not, changed."[12] Eventually, the meanings of science in the medical marketplace narrowed, and the social and cultural authority it conveyed concentrated more squarely on elite, formally trained regular practitioners, but at the end of the nineteenth century, scientific medicine was still struggling to win its battle for supreme authority.

In the meanwhile, American political culture was becoming more accepting of regulation and bureaucracy. That regulatory impulse emerged from concerns about monopoly. Regulation promised to reign in the tendency of large-scale, industrial monopolies to restrict freedom of competition. Early state and then federal experiments regulating railroads quickly spread to other industries by the second half of the nineteenth century. The expansion of the regulatory powers of the state in the Progressive Era reflected the growing appreciation for government action as an effective countervailing force to monopoly.[13] Ironically, then, by seeking increased regulation of the medical profession, regular physicians used an anti-monopolist apparatus to extend their monopoly of the medical marketplace.

Spearheading the battle to regulate the medical marketplace was the AMA. Although the association did not truly flourish until the late nineteenth and early twentieth centuries, it had been in existence since the 1840s. In 1846, in response to the repeal of licensing statutes, New York physicians organized a national convention to coordinate regular physicians across jurisdictions. They aimed to restrict the medical marketplace to regular physicians by discrediting what they deemed "unscientific" medical practices and by promoting scientific standards for medical education and licensing. The AMA had limited success in its first fifty years: it managed to place a few of its members in key government and military positions, it appealed to schools to raise their degree requirements, and it temporarily enforced a code of ethics that barred its members from collaborating with irregular physicians.[14] Yet, as a private and voluntary association, the AMA had limited coercive power. Eventually, the AMA accepted some cooperation with eclectics and homeopaths, two medical sects that had similarly organized professional societies and schools. While these three groups held very different conceptions of the science of human health, they had common concerns about competition with self-taught medical practitioners. All three sects wanted to drive students to their colleges and professionals to their organizations, and in the 1870s and 1880s, they worked together to lobby for occupational licensing statutes making a medical diploma a prerequisite for practicing medicine. Early licensing did not differentiate among medical diplomas, rendering regular, eclectic, and homeopathic educations largely equivalent.[15]

This period of sectarian harmony did not last long. In the nineteenth century, new discoveries and technologies revolutionized what practitioners of scientific medicine could perceive and understand about the nature of human health. Early instruments had limited observation beyond the human senses, but over the course of the nineteenth century, new technologies would enable a select few students of human health to gather better evidence and narrow the meanings of scientific medicine.[16] In 1816, René Laennac made use of the first stethoscope, which enabled physicians to diagnose various cardiac and respiratory conditions.[17] Between 1800 and 1850, French physicians and surgeons working together were able to connect symptoms presented in clinic with the conditions of the body revealed at autopsy. This partnership laid the groundwork for modern clinical methods and statistical observation. By the second half of the nineteenth century, German universities had revolutionized laboratory science, funding and promoting a new generation of specialists in physiology, embryology and cytology, nutrition, and pharmacology.[18]

As the field of scientific medicine became more technical and technologically driven, it began to take on disciplinary characteristics still prevalent today. The ability to make better measurements led to the adoption of objectivity and universalism as central tenets. The sphygmomanometer, a device used to measure blood pressure, is one example of such a shift. In traditional Chinese medicine, pulsology depended on the physician's subjective experience of the pulse. The sphygmomanometer, first developed in 1896 by Scipione Riva-Rocci, removed the physician's subjectivity and permitted scientists to obtain objective measurements of blood pressure in clinical studies, to define a normal range, and to link diseases to abnormal readings of the pulse.[19] The expertise and skill necessary to operate new instruments and interpret data also meant that professional medicine became increasingly specialized. Different research centers and hospital departments proliferated, staffed by scientists trained to study and treat specific systems within the body.[20] By 1900, objectivity, universalism, and specialization increasingly defined regular medicine.

Microscopy led to what is arguably the most important conceptual revolution in regular medicine: the germ theory of disease. In the 1820s, English wine merchant Joseph Jackson Lister invented a new microscope that allowed scientists to observe the structure of tissues, the interior of cells, and other microbiological elements at a higher resolution. Over the next seventy years, scientists continued to improve the technology of microscopy and the associated methods of fixing and staining specimens for observation. Pasteur and Koch used these techniques to observe the growth of bacterial colonies and postulate that microorganisms called "germs" were the source of disease.[21] Beginning in the 1870s, the successful containment of infection and infectious diseases through sanitation and hygiene, and in 1909 the discovery of Salvarsan, an antimicrobial, gradually made the germ theory of disease a unifying principle for scientific medicine.[22]

Regular physicians, with their formal, often university education, already constituted an elite group, but by the end of the nineteenth century, new technologies and the knowledge they produced further widened the gulf between scientific medicine and its rivals. The science of human health could not be democratic in an era when observation and experimentation depended on access to expensive instruments and the training to interpret the data they captured. The evidence that microorganisms caused disease came from laboratories where trained professionals observed bacteria through microscopes, made cultures, and experimented on animals.[23] Surgeons and physicians experimenting with antiseptic sprays to reduce postoperative infections corroborated their findings.[24] Stethoscopes and eventually sphygmomanometers allowed trained physicians to make objective measures of the pulse and blood pressure, and to link those measurements to health outcomes.[25]

The emergent intellectual consensus among medical scientists became a platform from which to launch a larger reform in medical colleges. In the wake of the Civil War, American higher education generally underwent a process of greater professionalization and increased its enrollments. With a larger pool of qualified applicants, medical colleges could raise degree requirements, recruit accomplished researchers to teach basic science and clinical specialties, and screen potential students for their scientific aptitude. Changes in the American political economy further encouraged the standardization of scientific medicine based on the use of new technologies. Around the turn of the twentieth century, life insurance companies employed and trained thousands of physicians to perform exams using stethoscopes, x-rays, and other devices; the companies then used the data in actuarial calculations. Railroads and other corporations, the military, and government agencies employed physicians and equipped them with new diagnostic instruments.[26]

By the first decades of the twentieth century, education in scientific medicine had coalesced around a curriculum that included two years of instruction, with the first year devoted to the basic sciences, anatomy, physiology, and biochemistry, and the second year to pathology, bacteriology, and pharmacology. Classroom instruction was paired with hospital experience, replacing apprenticeships with something more

systematic and standardized.[27] The AMA encouraged this process of educational reform, stipulating an ideal course of study and its duration,
and conducting evaluations of medical colleges, which it reported in its
journal. In response, medical schools merged, reorganized, and closed.[28]
The Flexner Report, a 1910 survey of medical education in America by
the Carnegie Foundation for the Advancement of Teaching, further gal-
vanized the AMA's mission to standardize a science-based medical curriculum. Abraham Flexner, a secondary school educator, accompanied
by the AMA's secretary for the Council on Medical Education, inspected
and scored 155 American and Canadian medical schools, both regular
and irregular. Flexner focused his observations on the facilities, requirements, and resources, including number of faculty. Influenced by the
AMA, Flexner started from the premise that medical education should
cultivate excellent scientific researchers with a strong foundation in basic science taught in laboratories and clinics.[29] Flexner's survey reserved
its most scathing criticisms for eclectic, homeopathic, and osteopathic
institutions.[30] The AMA's Council on Medical Education reinforced
the findings of the Flexner Report by publishing at regular intervals its
ranking and grading of medical schools. By 1930, the Federation of State
Medical Boards affirmed the council's role as the "standardizing agency
. . . for all matters of premedical education, course of study, and educational requirements for the degree of Doctor of Medicine."[31]

    In the same period, members of the AMA energetically supported
the passage of the Pure Food and Drug Act of 1906, the first national legislation to restrict the proprietary medicine industry. The act reflected
the concerns of multiple reform groups promoting worker's rights, sanitation and hygiene, and health. The AMA lobbied for the passage of the
bill not only because it was consistent with principles of bacteriology
but also because it placed constraints on proprietary medicines and the
promises they made. The organization initiated its own investigations
into fraudulent drug claims through a new Council on Pharmacy and
Chemistry. In 1911, the AMA helped Congress pass an amendment to
the Pure Food and Drug Act prohibiting false statements on food and
drug labels. In concert with those efforts, the *Journal of the American
Medical Association* (*JAMA*), the nation's leading compendium of scientific medical thought, refused to print advertisements for patent med-

icines and inaugurated a regular column exposing quackery and other examples of medical fraud.[32]

The composition of state medical boards and boards of health also favored the consolidation of power among practitioners of scientific medicine. In this regard, the case of California is illustrative of national trends. In 1878, the state revised its "Anti-Quackery Act" to organize three separate boards with examiners appointed by the State Medical Society, the Homeopathic Medical Society, and the Eclectic Medical Society.[33] After 1901, California consolidated its three boards into one with nine examiners: five elected by regular physicians, two by homeopaths, and two by eclecticists. In 1907, the Medical Practice Act was amended yet again to include two representatives from the State Osteopathic Society.[34] This kind of organization—offering numerical superiority to regular physicians but including members of other medical sects—was common for state medical boards across the country.

Scientific and technological advancements alone did not account for the rise of regular medicine in the Progressive Era. Standardized education, federal and state regulations, and numerical dominance on state boards of medicine and health were the basis from which scientific medicine built its social authority. Enforcement of new laws was thus critical to the success of the entire endeavor. In the Progressive Era, regular physicians enthusiastically supported and often directly participated in campaigns to drive their unlicensed rivals—including the Chinese—out of business.

"Yellow Quacks"

Regular physicians recognized Chinese doctors as competitors as early as 1870. A newspaper article on Chinese medicine noted, "In San Francisco, the regular physicians complain bitterly of the inroads made upon their incomes by the Chinese doctors, and they will make an effort to keep the healing business entirely in their own hands."[35] In the decades that followed, Chinese doctors often became part of an undifferentiated assault on irregular medicine. Dr. George Lee Eaton, a president of the San Francisco Board of Health, declared, "The psychological effect of these fakers, whether they are beauty doctors, so-called specialists, or Chinese herb doctors . . . cannot be estimated. One and all they are of the same stripe. They prey on the ignorant and the morbid."[36] There were a few instances in which legislators proposed bills that specifically targeted Chinese medicine, but more commonly Chinese doctors were arrested under state legislation or municipal ordinances restricting general "quackery."[37] Chinese physicians selling prescriptions through the mail also found themselves in violation of postal statutes passed by Congress in 1872. Although the original intention had been to prevent fraudulent financial schemes from circulating via the mail, the postmaster general began to apply the statutes to "quack medicines" around the turn of the twentieth century. The postal statutes worked in concert with the 1906 Pure Food and Drug Act, overseen by another federal agency, the Bureau of Chemistry. Because the postal statutes adopted a wider definition of fraud, the Postal Service could pursue cases outside the jurisdiction of the bureau.[38]

Local medical societies sometimes threw their support behind regulatory schemes that promised to sweep up Chinese competitors. In 1891, the regular physicians of Butte, Montana, lobbied for a public health ordinance "for the suppression of quacks," which required all practicing physicians to show a certificate from the state medical board. A newspaper article quoted various doctors supporting the ordinance including Dr. R. L. Gillespie, who claimed it would "stop the practicing of the Chinese doctors, whose only certificate is heredity," and Dr. G. W. Monroe, who agreed that "it would shut out Chinese doctors and their tomfoolery. People should be protected against these Chinese doctors."[39] A judge in El Paso, Texas, appointed a board of medical examiners in 1887 and tasked them with "coppering the many Chinese doctors practicing there."[40] In Oregon, too, Multnomah County physicians organized a special committee to hire lawyers to prosecute complaints against "the quacks and charlatans now preying on the public in [Portland]" by practicing without a license, among them Wing Lee, who was convicted and fined seventy-five dollars.[41] Professional pharmacists also joined the push to restrict Chinese physicians. As early as 1893, a New Mexico newspaper reported, "The druggists of Las Vegas are persecuting a Chinese doctor under the provisions of the pharmacy act."[42] In 1907, the California State Board of Pharmacy identified the Chinese as the "most flagrant violators" of state medical laws and vowed to "pay particular attention" to them.[43] The Los Angeles branch of the American Pharmaceutical Association devoted time at their meetings to discuss the popularity and dangers of Chinese drugs circulating in the city: "A great many of the drugs from Japan, China, and the Philippines are adulterated and mislabeled . . . It is an astounding fact, but nevertheless true, that Chinese pharmacists and physicians practice without legal restriction on the coast."[44] Such anti-Asian rhetoric called on a prevalent nativism. As historian Alan M. Kraut has argued, American nativists wielded scientific medicine as a "weapon" against non-Anglo-Saxon immigrants.[45] In the case of anti-quackery campaigns, medical scientists deployed nativism to advance their own objective of marketplace dominance.

Regular physicians and pharmacists engaged in play-acting when they helped gather evidence against Chinese doctors. Doing their part to suppress the illegal Chinese herb trade, members of the California State Pharmacy Board acted out a frontier vigilante fantasy in San Bernardino in 1914. Three inspectors, disguised "in rough attire," swept into town to entrap unregistered druggists. The Los Angeles Times reported that the sting secured the arrest of seven sellers of morphine, a black woman in possession of opium, and three Chinese herbalists.[46] Sting-operations were not always so elaborately staged. In 1883, a member of the San Francisco Medical Society, F. A. Kelly, caught Joe Gong practicing medicine without a license. Pretending to be ill, Kelly went to Gong's office on Waverly Place to ask for treatment. When Gong could not show his license, a San Francisco police offer was at the ready to arrest him.[47]

Between 1914 and 1942, the California Board of Medical Examiners recorded 516 violations of the state's Medical Practice Act by Chinese physicians (table 4). The board recorded 230 guilty verdicts, among which 161 were sentenced to pay a fine (table 5). In 24 cases, the judge offered a choice: either a fine or a short jail term. In all instances, the violator chose to pay the fine, which was typically one hundred dollars but occasionally as high as six hundred.[48] Many physicians were

Table 4: Disposition of cases against Chinese physicians for violating the California Medical Practice Act, 1914–1942

Disposition	Number of cases
Guilty	230
Not guilty/dismissed	149
Pending	117
Not recorded	16
Mistrial, hung jury, moved	4

Source: Annual Reports of the Board of Medical Examiners, *Appendix to the Journals of the Senate and Assembly* (Sacramento, Calif.: State Printing, 1914–1942).

Table 5: Sentences for Chinese Physicians convicted of violating the California Medical Practice Act, 1914–1942

Sentences	Number convicted
Fine, fine + jail time (including suspended jail time), fine + probation	161
Probation	18
Suspended fine	11
Jail time	7
Fugitive	4
Discontinue advertising to suspend sentence	2

Source: Annual Reports of the Board of Medical Examiners, *Appendix to the Journals of the Senate and Assembly* (Sacramento, Calif.: State Printing, 1914–1942).

brought up on charges multiple times over the course of their career. Between 1914 and 1942, forty-seven Chinese physicians were accused of committing three or more violations. One herbalist, Wah Quack, was arrested twice within twenty-four hours for violating anti-quackery laws in 1919.[49]

When local officials were slow to act, individual doctors took matters into their own hands. In Hanford, a town nestled in California's San Joaquin Valley, Dr. J. A. Crawshaw wrote to Charles Tisdale to report on the activities of his Chinese and Japanese competitors:

> One L. T. Sue, a Chinese doctor, has been operating in
> Hanford, and has no credentials or authority to do so. Also
> Dr. Muriami, a Japanese, who operates under the wing of a
> M. D. here in Hanford. I have learned that this man writes
> prescriptions for patients, signs his name under the name of
> a regular licensed physician. These prescriptions are filled at
> the various drug stores in Hanford. This work has existed for
> one or more years. If you wish me to be of any service to you,
> I will be glad to collect any proof you ask me to.[50]

Tisdale responded dismissively, so Crawshaw filed a complaint against Sue in his own name and subpoenaed Tisdale. Although Tisdale repeatedly failed to answer the summons, the court heard the case in December 1909 and convicted Sue of practicing without a license. Sue paid a fine of one hundred dollars and went back to work.[51] Crawshaw fought on, but the Board of Examiners shuffled his correspondence among its various officials.

In frustration, Crawshaw consulted his local district attorney, who advised him to make his own case against Sue: "With [the district attorney's] advice I procured the service of three young men to call on the Chinaman and take treatment from him. This they did and swore to as many complaints."[52] By February, Sue was back in jail. The *Los Angeles Times* jokingly called him "the most arrested man in the [San Joaquin] valley."[53] This time, a representative from the State Board of Medical Examiners deigned to appear at trial but with little effect; Sue was acquitted. Crawshaw remained undeterred and exhorted his colleagues to show some backbone in a tortured metaphor that only a highly trained medical professional would appreciate: "Our spinal columns are composed of the hardest compact bony tissue, and not the flexible cartilaginous substance, that will readily bend or mold to the layman's idea of what constitutes the practice of medicine."[54] Showing bony spinal tissue in his own way, Sue continued to practice in Hanford until 1920 when he retired, enjoyed a grand tour of Europe, and then returned to live out his days in his native Canton.[55]

Compliance, Circumvention, Resistance

At first, Chinese physicians attempted to comply with the new statutes to protect their businesses. In the 1880s, state boards of health adopted a registration system for physicians, which typically required only a diploma from a medical college. Under this system, some Chinese doctors successfully secured their right to practice medicine, although often with the understanding that they would only treat members of their own race.[56] States and municipalities initially accepted diplomas from Chinese medical colleges but dealt differently with the problem of translating them. When Dr. Lou See On of Buffalo, New York, presented a degree signed by the Chinese emperor in 1880, the county clerk agreed to register the physician, stipulating only that a copy of his diploma would need to remain on file, perhaps in the off-chance that a skilled interpreter would pass through town to verify its contents.[57] In Sacramento, a clerk took on the unenviable task of copying a Chinese diploma, measuring a foot and a half square, by hand. He described the document as consisting of a "mass of Chinese hieroglyphics" as well as "fifty course outline sketches of the human figure, each being full of similar characters."[58] Other states required diplomas to be authenticated by Chinese officials in the United States. In 1887, the Louisiana Board of Health unanimously voted to approve the request of New Orleans doctor Kwai Ding Kwai to treat his fellow Chinese immigrants. As part of the registration process, Kwai had his diploma certified by the Chinese foreign minister in Washington and the Chinese consul in New York. States might also enlist translators to verify Chinese diplomas. Leavenworth doctor Ah Sam battled with the Kansas State Board of Health over its refusal to accept his degree from a medical college in Canton. Sam had emigrated from Canton to San Francisco as a twenty-one-year-old in 1879. In 1894, he moved to Leavenworth, where he established a practice that catered to some of the city's wealthiest white families. The county medical society arranged for him to be repeatedly and regularly arrested for practicing without a license. In response, he presented his diploma from a medical college in Canton to the State Board of Health, which sent the document on to Washington, D.C., for translation. Sam then continued to practice until 1902, when a new statute required him to resubmit his qualifications for inspection. Because of his good local reputation, the board agreed to issue him a license without sending his diploma out for another review.[59]

Don Sang of Crown Point, Indiana, faced greater scrutiny when he applied for a license with the Indiana State Board of Medical Examination and Registration in 1897. Dr. Sang—as he was known to his English-speaking patients—purportedly immigrated to the United States in 1849 to prospect for gold and, in 1892, made his way to Indiana via Illinois with his wife, children, and a nephew who worked as an assistant in his shop.[60] In 1897, Sang went before the Indiana State Board and claimed to be a graduate of a medical college in Canton operated by his family and established in 1407. As proof, he produced a diploma from that institution. The board then hired a Chinese student of theology at nearby DePauw University to serve as an interpreter. The student examined the diploma, translated it for the record, and gave his opinion that it was fraudulent. As evidence, he pointed to a blank seal that should have had some signifying markers. The board also engaged an expert witness who erroneously testified that there were no medical colleges in China except those operated by medical missionaries.[61] That mistake notwithstanding, in all likelihood Sang's diploma was a fake. He was probably trained to practice medicine within a family business, as many doctors of his socioeconomic class would have been, but it is not clear that the state board understood or cared about the nuances of medical education in China. After some deliberation, Sang was refused a license, but he appealed the decision, suing the board in federal court and demanding that he be allowed to sit for examination by a Crown Point physician who would determine his qualifications to practice medicine.[62] In the end, Don lost his appeal. By 1900, he had relocated his family to Chicago, where he ran a Chinese curio shop until his death in 1903.[63]

Idaho's most famous Chinese physician, C. K. Ah Fong, received a license to practice medicine around the turn of the twentieth century. In 1887, when the state passed its first licensing statute, it required doctors to present a diploma from a medical college or demonstrate that they had been practicing medicine before the passage of the law. Ah Fong, who had been working as a doctor in Idaho since 1875 and who claimed to be a graduate of the Kung Guh Medical College in Canton, fulfilled both criteria and received a license.[64] In 1899, however, the Idaho legislature added a new requirement that licensed doctors be American citizens or eligible for naturalization, which Chinese exclusion prohibited. Thus, in 1899, when Ah Fong went to renew his license, he was denied and ordered to stop practicing. In response, he went to court, charging the Board of Health with discrimination. After losing in the district court, he appealed and won his case in the state supreme court. On February 21, 1901, he became a fully licensed physician and surgeon in the state of Idaho.[65]

In these early decades of regulation, accommodations for Chinese doctors were not the product of their talents but rather a reflection of the fact that state boards of health and medical examiners were still insecure about their jurisdiction. They were therefore prone to adopting the most liberal interpretations of regulatory statutes. When the Louisiana Board of Health allowed Kwai Ding Kwai to practice medicine among his Chinese brethren in 1887, a member of the Committee on Registering Physicians justified the decision by asserting that the "board [of health] had no power to restrict any physician in his practice" so long as he had a "properly-authenticated diploma."[66] In 1893, when Omaha doctor Chang Gee Wo appealed his conviction for practicing without a license and challenged the constitutionality of medical licensing, the Supreme Court of Nebraska denied his appeal but insisted that "the board . . . is not to use its power arbitrarily nor to refuse a certificate in a proper case, nor to attempt to build up any particular system."[67] Implicit in the language of the court's decision was a common fear that one medical sect would monopolize licensing, as regular physicians endeavored to do.[68] American courts tended to agree that the state should be responsible for protecting the public from harm but favored regulation that gave different systems of education equal consideration.

By the 1910s, however, federal courts had become more comfortable with differential licensing. In 1915, four San Francisco herbalists appealed their convictions for practicing without a license and filed writs of habeas corpus arguing that not only did licensing statutes unconstitutionally discriminate against certain medical sects but that they violated international treaties with China that guaranteed certain rights to Chinese immigrants. Lawyers for the complainants argued that "accredited practicing physicians from other countries . . . were permitted to practice without examination or license."[69] The federal court denied their appeal, insisting that the decision to issue licenses according to different standards was within the jurisdiction of California's State Board of Medical Examiners.[70]

When all else failed, Chinese physicians deployed extralegal strategies to circumvent discriminatory laws. They undoubtedly presented many fraudulent diplomas to licensing boards, as in the case of Don Sang. Chinese doctors also bribed officials to "overlook" the law. In 1908, Los Angeles's civil service commission charged Nick Harris, a sanitary inspector in the health department, with accepting bribes from the city's Chinese doctors. Tom She Bin testified that he had given Harris gifts of a phonograph and a clock as well as money, and in exchange, Harris had not prosecuted him for practicing medicine without a license.[71] Witnesses for the defense countered that Harris arrested Chinese doctors with impartiality and that the phonograph in question was old and useless, but the commission dismissed him nonetheless.[72] In 1919, Lowe Bin was caught in a sting operation after attempting to bribe Frank M. Smith, a special agent of the State Board of Medical Examiners, with seventy-five dollars in exchange for immunity from prosecution for three Chinese doctors practicing without a license in Oakland.[73]

Some Chinese doctors partnered with licensed practitioners, effectively using them as a legal cover for the illegal operations. Upon the death of Pang Suey, it came to light that he had hired a registered physician named Robert Swift to work out of his office two days a week. Swift consulted with patients, diagnosed them, and then allowed Pang or his assistant to write and fill their prescriptions.[74] Los Angeles–area physician S. P. Lee relied on his family members. One of his sons was a licensed chiropractor and the other a licensed osteopath. Both worked out of the family's herb shops.[75] The cover of licensed medical practitioners allowed Chinese doctors to keep up the pretense that they were simply selling herbs.

Occasionally, Chinese doctors lobbied for new laws. In 1902, Leavenworth doctor Ah Sam and his colleague in Topeka, Andrew Wa, appealed to the Board of Health and requested that it exempt Chinese medicine from regulation because it was so different from "American" medicine. The Kansas State Board did not move forward with that request.[76] In California in the 1920s, Louise Leung Larson recalled her father, Tom Leung's attempts to lobby for state legislation licensing Chinese physicians alongside chiropractors. When that failed, he removed the word "doctor" from his advertisements and continued his work as an herbalist.[77]

Across the country in Boston, Pang Suey crusaded for licensing as a Chinese doctor and found some allies among Massachusetts legislators. Beginning in 1897, Pang had been a partner in the Los Angeles–based herb company Foo and Wing, managed by Li Wing and Tom Foo Yuen. Pang had a $1,200 stake in the firm and worked primarily as a druggist and sometimes as a salesman.[78] In 1909, he left Los Angeles for Boston although his motivations remain unclear. Tom Foo Yuen had opened a branch of Foo and Wing in Boston's South End in March 1904, possibly because he had a son attending college nearby. Fortuitously, the city's other two Chinese doctors died that same spring, shortly after the Boston branch opened its doors. The relative absence of competition may have created a business opportunity for Pang to start his own Boston office on Dartmouth Street in the Back Bay, where he sold medicines as well as rice and tea with the assistance of a Chinese American apprentice.[79] Foo later claimed to have loaned Pang $3,300 for just that purpose, but it was never proven to be true.[80] By 1912, Pang's apothecary and practice had achieved some local notoriety and became the subject of travel narratives published in northeastern newspaper articles.[81]

The law of the Commonwealth of Massachusetts required physicians to pass a written examination before the Board of Registration in Medicine. The exam was administered in English and centered on Western-style scientific medicine. The law did exempt certain categories of physicians, including army and navy doctors and psychologists, and Pang argued that it should not apply to him as a "dispenser of herbs" who offered free medical advice. Around 1914, Pang began to mobilize his white supporters to press for legislation that would protect his business, and in 1916, Representative Harold L. Perrin introduced a bill that would offer an exemption from registration for all "pharmacists or persons dealing in natural herbs in prescribing gratuitously."[82] Over two thousand individuals signed a petition supporting the bill, colloquially known as the Pang Suey bill. Prominent Bostonians including politicians, a professor at Boston University, and a rabbi appeared at the statehouse to testify on Pang's behalf before the Legislative Committee on Public Health.[83] The bill went forward but fizzled in the House by a vote of 129 to 94.[84]

The following year, Pang's supporters again introduced a bill, this time offering exemptions from licensing exams to graduates of foreign medical colleges. Opponents of the new bill cast aspersions on Pang's credentials. Dr. Walter P. Bowers, a member of the State Board of Registration in Medicine, claimed that he had investigated Pang's diploma and could not locate the Chinese college from which Pang had claimed to graduate. Pang's patients—including many women—packed the assembly room and "hissed their disapproval" of Bowers, and when Representative Joseph B. McGrath, who supported the bill, accused Bowers of lying, the two men almost came to blows.[85] The bill died in committee.

In April 1917, Pang succumbed to heart failure, leaving nearly $200,000 in cash squirreled away around his home in Boston. His wife and sixteen-year-old son, both in China, were named as heirs.[86] Yet Pang's true legacy may have been the loyalty and admiration that he inspired among his non-Chinese patients. In 1920, three years after his death, the Legislative Committee on Public Health again took up the question of exempting foreign doctors from examination. The *Boston Globe* reported that dozens of Pang's patients testified to their "restoration to health by either Pang Suey or his successor," Gouy Shang (Shong), who had trained under Pang's supervision.[87]

In California, Chinese physicians and herb companies also organized and sought the help of white allies to protest discriminatory
legislation and taxation. On January 21, 1925, California State Assembly
representative Edward J. Smith proposed a bill "to regulate the manufacture, sale, and use of herbs, roots, or other nature products used in
the administering of sickness or treating disease of a human being." The
bill required practitioners of Chinese medicine to receive approval from
the State Board of Health before prescribing or selling herbal remedies.
Believing that the bill would cripple their businesses, Chinese doctors organized the Herb Dealers' Protective Association of California with the
support of several Chinese American institutions including the Chinese
American Citizens Alliance, the San Francisco Chinese Consolidated
Benevolent Association, the Chinese Chamber of Commerce, and various Chinese churches and newspapers. Members of these organizations
as well as white allies spoke out against the bill in Sacramento or sent
letters to their representatives. They distributed pamphlets in Western-
style medical clinics and hospitals that extolled the health benefits of
Chinese herbs and asked for signatures on a petition opposing the bill.
They also collected funds to lobby state legislators, treating them to ban-
quets in San Francisco and deliveries of fresh flowers. Some lobbying
efforts may have verged into bribery, with Oakland doctor Fong Wan
and Sacramento doctor T. Wah Hing both implicated in a conspiracy to
pay various assemblymen, including Smith himself, to drop the bill.[88] In
the end, California's Committee on Medical and Dental Laws refused to
advance the bill, and it was withdrawn.[89]

"The Expense of Doing Business"

Despite all their pains to comply, circumvent, or change the laws, being arrested for practicing medicine without a license was a common
experience for Chinese doctors working in the early twentieth-century
United States. Chinese doctors learned to be on watch for police and
their informants seeking to gather evidence against them. According to
Louise Leung Larson, "The police, at times, used stool pigeons—people
pretending to be patients—and would arrest Papa after the usual consultation."[90] Larson recalled that when the Los Angeles police arrested

her father, "Papa was unflappable, even the time when he was hauled off in a patrol wagon. He had set up a routine for these crises." Tom Leung's secretary knew immediately to call his banker, A. C. Way, to pay for bail and his attorneys, Thomas White and Paul Schenck, to plead his case. Tom rarely spent a lot of time in lockup. Over the course of a thirty-year career, his family estimated that he was arrested over one hundred times and paid about five thousand dollars in fines.[91]

In rare instances, prosecution convinced Chinese physicians to leave the business. In 1920, an article for the *San Francisco Chronicle* reported that a series of arrests had compelled the departure of W. S. Ling from the Sierra foothill town of Oroville in which he had practiced medicine for twenty-five years. He became a porter in a San Francisco hotel, where he was far less likely to run afoul of the law.[92] For the most part, however, Chinese doctors simply accepted arrests as inevitable. The *California State Journal of Medicine,* which reported on violations of the Medical Practice Act, noted the frequency of repeat offenders. In 1920, when Wong Ting, Hong Wong, and P. S. Hsu were convicted and fined, the journal described them as a "Chinese triumvirate that specializes in breaking the Medical Practice Act . . . They mostly plead guilty, pay the fine, and hasten back to distribute the short dried herbs and gather in the long green."[93] That same year, when Los Angeles business partners G. S. Chan and H. T. Chan were convicted of the same violation, the journal recorded that they paid $250 and $100 respectively: "A few hundred dollars means only a few more herbs, and the weeds are full of them."[94] The penalties seemed inconsequential compared to what the Chinese doctor could earn. Thomas W. Wing, whose father, N. S. Sue, was repeatedly arrested for practicing medicine without a license in Modesto, California, recalled, "My father felt this was part of the expense of doing business, so he would go to jail, pay the fine, and happily stop by the grocery store on the way home to buy oranges and things for the family."[95]

Ironically, arrests, fines, and even short-term imprisonment in some cases might have been good for business. Tom Leung's family recalled, "The more he was arrested, the more business he got."[96] Thomas W. Wing speculated, "The publicity more than made up in new patients what it cost him [his father] to fight the [law]."[97] Newspaper

reports of arrests and trials could attract patients who remained un-
convinced of the merits of a state license. Oakland doctor Fong Wan
repeatedly used tales of his arrests and trials in his English-language advertising. In the 1930s, Fong became the target of an entrapment scheme
through his mail-order business. The postal inspector aimed to catch
Fong using the mail to defraud patients, and the office submitted sixteen
letters under various aliases.[98] After he was acquitted in 1932, Fong ran
an advertisement in the *San Francisco Chronicle* that emphasized "there
was no evidence that Fong Wan had used the mails to defraud" and insisted "there is no better proof of the curative properties of the Chinese
Herbs than" the not-guilty verdict.[99] In 1939, the Federal Trade Commission sued Fong for false advertising in his cross-state mail-order business. At the trial, his patients came to his defense and testified to their
miraculous recoveries thanks to his herbal remedies. Fong then paid to
reprint the entire court transcript—spanning a dozen pages of small
type—in both the *San Francisco Chronicle* and the *Oakland Tribune*.
Along the bottom of the first page, the business ran a banner that read,
"It pays to go to Oakland to see Fong Wan."[100]

After being arrested for practicing without a license, Chinese
doctors found ways to use the law to their advantage. This strategy depended on knowledge of the legal system and may have grown out of
Chinese immigrants' experience navigating complex exclusionary statutes. As historian Erika Lee and others have shown, the Chinese of all
social classes protested immigration laws and their enforcement by engaging the services of lawyers, filing appeals, and overturning denials of
entry.[101] During the 1900 outbreak of bubonic plague in San Francisco,
Chinese community leaders effectively used the court system to protest
mandatory vaccination and the quarantine of Chinatown that violated
their right to due process.[102] Similarly, Chinese physicians arrested for
practicing medicine without a license hired lawyers to fight and appeal
convictions.

Chinese doctors most frequently invoked a defense that rested on
the assertion that they only sold herbs and dispensed medical advice at
no cost.[103] The distinction was important on two levels: During the era of
Chinese exclusion, selling herbs allowed doctors to claim merchant status and thus an exemption from immigration restrictions. The "herbs-

only" defense also allowed Chinese physicians to claim exemptions from medical licensing statutes, which did not extend to purveyors of food and drugs. One of the earliest examples of this defense was deployed in 1879 when Sacramento doctor Loy Fook Wan was charged with practicing medicine without a license. Loy owned a drugstore on I Street, and the prosecution could not prove that he did anything more than compound and sell medicines.[104] In 1886, when Lee Wah was arrested for violating the California Medical Practice Act, which required physicians to take out a certificate with the State Board of Health, the prosecution called as witnesses two women who had purchased herbs from Lee at his shop in San Jose over a period of several weeks. The women testified to the fact that they had paid for herbs, but they insisted that Lee had provided diagnosis gratis. Lee was eventually exonerated.[105]

After repeated arrests for practicing medicine without a license, Utah doctor Yee Foo Lun developed a similar strategy for working within the confines of the law. In early May 1913, Yee Foo Lun made the move from Denver to Salt Lake City, where he opened an office above Hirschman's Shoe Store at 118 South Main Street.[106] Not two weeks later, he was arrested for practicing medicine without a license. The court charged him with violating the law of 1911 that required doctors to hold a certificate from the Utah State Board of Health before they offered medical advice or services. At his 1915 trial, he testified that he allowed customers in his herb shop to name their own ailments. Yee insisted that he did no diagnosis "because I always try to get away from doing anything against the law. I have been in court so much I know just what I have to do, and so I don't try to do that at all."[107] Well into the 1920s and 1930s, Chinese doctors were still claiming exemption from medical licensing statutes on the grounds that they only sold herbs, not advice.[108]

The defense in Yee's case also rested on the equivalence between Chinese herbs and an American tradition of self-care asserted in English-language advertising. At trial, his lawyers argued that Yee was exempt from the law as a seller of "domestic family medicines." Such exemptions were common in licensing statutes, but the definition of "domestic family medicine" was nebulous. Generally, such medicine was assumed to encompass curative substances that required no special training to administer. These treatments tended to be medicinal plants and minerals readily available in the home: Epsom salts, castor oil, camphor, quinine, and various spirits, for example. In some states, domestic family medicine was believed to be so obvious as to need no explanation. At Dr. Yee's trial, the Utah judge left it to the jury to decide the meaning of "domestic family medicine" and whether or not the herbs entered into evidence against Yee counted as such.[109] For his part, in the *Salt Lake Tribune*, Yee described what he sold as only "herbs and roots."[110]

Yee lost his case. In the 1915 appeal, the Supreme Court of Utah hired a chemist who found that Yee's prescriptions were a mixture of ginseng, cinnamon, licorice, sarsaparilla, "free from alcohol, chloroform, narcotic or alkaloidal drugs, and probably harmless." Harmless was not the same thing as effective, and the court argued that Chinese herbs were not "domestic family medicine." In fact, they were not medicine at all. "Instead of calling it a domestic family remedy, it is better," the decision read, "to call it by its right name—a subterfuge to deceive the credulous and the afflicted."[111] The language of the decision mirrored the negative portrayals of Chinese medicine that circulated in the academic and popular press: Chinese doctors were charlatans, and their patients were dupes.

The herbs-only defense Yee's lawyers deployed was a necessary fiction to protect Chinese doctors from discriminatory medical licensing, but it also contributed to the perpetuation of an Orientalist stereotype of Chinese medicine as primitive and unscientific. It reduced the practice to the simple act of selling herbal remedies and said nothing of the complex therapeutic principles that defined traditional Chinese medicine. As one of the many legal and extralegal defensive strategies deployed by Chinese doctors in the United States, the herbs-only defense obscured and minimized the diverse ways in which they served their patients and their communities.

Conclusion

In laboratories, clinics, and legislative halls, practitioners of scientific medicine laid the foundations for their social authority in the late nineteenth and early twentieth centuries. The enforcement of new licensing statutes was an important tactic in securing the market and political power they had struggled long and hard to achieve. Regular physicians who competed with Chinese doctors made them targets for surveillance, entrapment, and repeated arrests, fines, and sometimes imprisonment. Denied licenses and subject to arrests alongside other practitioners deemed "irregular," Chinese doctors learned to endure and navigate a new regulatory regime. The capacity of Chinese doctors to resist such legal persecution is evidence of the limited success of the Progressive Era movement to regularize medicine. However, enforcement was not the only weapon in the regular physician's arsenal. As the next chapter details, practitioners of scientific medicine simultaneously engaged in a rhetorical campaign against Chinese doctors that was just as relentless as their legal campaign.

F · I · V · E

Oriental Healers

I n not quite fifteen years since the passage of California's Medical Practice Act, the challenges of enforcement were plain to see. Fines and imprisonment did not sufficiently deter unlicensed practitioners of Chinese medicine. In some cases, legal persecution seemed to have the reverse effect, driving business to Chinese herbalists instead of driving Chinese herbalists out of business. C. B. Pinkham, the secretary of the Board of Medical Examiners, reflected on the failures of medical regulation in his state: "As far back as runneth the mind of man has the Chinese 'herb doctor' been a problem in California. We do not believe that there is a remote possibility of passing any legislation that either will effectively stop these Chinese herbalists from operating or put an end to their advertising, unless there be an unbelievable change of attitude in public opinion."[1] Scientific medicine had a public relations problem.

In the Progressive Era, regular physicians and their allies simultaneously waged a legal campaign and a rhetorical campaign against their Chinese competitors. Through a war of words, regular physicians aimed to demystify scientific medicine by debunking Chinese medicine. Depictions of Chinese medicine in the academic and popular press allowed regular physicians to elevate the status of Western-style medical science in terms that the public could understand and value. Chinese medicine and its practitioners were particularly useful to regular physicians and their allies because they were so obviously other. A long tradition of Orientalism had taught European American patients to perceive the Chinese as exotic and antimodern. Regular physicians and their allies overlaid that prevalent cultural discourse with one of their own. They made Chinese medicine the foil to Western-style scientific medicine, just as the Orient was the foil to the Occident, but they could not have anticipated how their Chinese competitors would respond.

Chinese doctors accepted that Orientalism conditioned American expectations of their practice, and they embraced it. Beginning in the late nineteenth century, as Chinese doctors entered the American medical marketplace, they found creative ways to reappropriate the Orientalist stereotypes deployed by regular physicians to discredit their practices. By self-Orientalizing, Chinese doctors claimed an innate, racial expertise in matters of human health that was difficult to dispute. To their non-Chinese patients, they delivered a safely exotic, comfortably strange experience that patients distrustful of regular medicine found appealing. Selling Chinese medicine as "natural medicine" did not necessarily come naturally to its practitioners. Rather, it reflected Chinese doctors' understanding of American medical cultures and their determination to compete in the American medical marketplace.

Natural Medicine

While nineteenth- and early twentieth-century advances in clinics and laboratories, medical education reform, and licensing did much to consolidate the meaning of the "science" of human health for academics, regular physicians still had a rather spotty record of success. Synthetic drug manufacturing remained a small segment of the drug trade, and surgical techniques were improving but still dangerous. For many patients, unschooled in the scientific method, the differences between irregular medicine and regular medicine were not obvious. There was no common consensus that scientific medicine was in fact superior to other systems of medical knowledge. In the spring of 1920, Mrs. F. C. Johnson of Somerville, Massachusetts, took her ailing daughter to see Pang Suey. "I didn't understand the Chinese doctor any more than I did the American ones I brought the child to," she explained to a reporter for the *Boston Globe*.[2] The ailing continued to seek out a broad array of healers and therapies as they always had.[3]

In the popular press, Chinese doctors could find themselves in the contradictory position of serving as both a critique and defense of scientific medicine. In 1895, a minister in Butte, Montana, delivered a sermon encouraging his parishioners to adopt the health and hygiene practices of the Chinese, which included—in his estimation—abstaining from alcohol, politics, and American medicine: "He isn't dosed with as much medicine as the white man, and he doesn't have as many physicians to bother with him. The Chinese doctor gives him some harmless stuff . . . [They] don't try to convince their patrons that they are sick in order to get a fee out of them."[4] A 1907 *Los Angeles Times* article ostensibly about "queer Chinese medicines" made space to poke fun at regular physicians' tendency to use Latin names to exalt themselves: "The Chinese doctor does not know Latin, and therefore does not deceive his patient by writing prescriptions in a dead language."[5] Another *Los Angeles Times* article satirized "hapless white physicians" outcompeted by their Chinese counterparts. In a mock interview, a "white doctor" explained that Chinese physicians "manage to get on in most cases by a great deal of bluff and shrewd guess work," but "when we white doctors don't know, we tell the patient his liver is out of order. I suppose they carry the bluff out a little further—and don't charge so much."[6] In that journalist's estimation, both Chinese and white physicians were charlatans. Descriptions of Chinese medicine in newspapers and magazines became a means to ridicule regular medicine and its pretensions.

A basic distrust of the elitism embodied by medical scientists went hand in hand with popular ambivalence toward not just modern medical science but modernity more broadly writ. As many scholars have argued, industrialization was both socially and psychologically unsettling for nineteenth-century Americans. In a classic work of American literary analysis, *The Machine in the Garden,* Leo Marx wrote, "Within the lifetime of a single generation, a rustic and in large part wild landscape was transformed into the site of the world's most productive industrial machine. It would be difficult to imagine more profound contradictions of value or meaning than those made manifest by this circumstance."[7]

New industries transformed landscapes and communities; new organizations recombined populations; new technologies—like the railroad and telegraph—seemed to alter space and time itself. By the Gilded Age, the material and cultural changes wrought by large-scale industrialization were pervasive. In art and literature, in strikes and protest, and in politics and reform, Americans expressed their discontent, their fears, and their hopes for a modern era. As historian T. J. Jackson Lears has argued, "Antimodernism . . . was ambivalent, often coexisting with enthusiasm for material progress."[8] The 1879 bestseller *Progress and Poverty* by Henry George captured that ambivalence:

> But just as such a community realizes the conditions which all civilized communities are striving for, and advances in the scale of material progress—just as closer settlement and a more intimate connection with the rest of the world, and greater utilization of labor-saving machinery, make possible greater economies in production and exchange, and wealth in consequence increases, not merely in the aggregate, but in proportion to population—so does poverty take a darker aspect. Some get an infinitely better and easier living, but others find it hard to get a living at all. The "tramp" comes with the locomotive, and almshouses and prisons are as surely the marks of "material progress" as are costly dwellings, rich warehouses, and magnificent churches.[9]

The success of *Progress and Poverty* in its time reflected the widespread resonance of its author's central concern: the benefits of modernization were great but not equally distributed.[10]

Scientific medicine seemed consistent with that disturbing pattern. As medical knowledge became more specialized and technical, care took place less frequently under the supervision of the family than under that of a private practitioner or hospital. Drugs were synthesized in the laboratory, not grown in the garden. These changes tended to improve health outcomes, but they were often prohibitively expensive to all but the most affluent.[11] Progressive Era patients remained understandably skeptical of what regular doctors seemed to represent: the elite, exclusive, and modern, all the things that their irregular competitors were not.

Over many decades, irregular physicians had capitalized on patient skepticism and worked hard to cast their regular rivals as enemies of nature itself. The discourse of natural medicine developed in the early nineteenth century as a critique of formally educated, primarily white and male physicians, who tended to prescribe mineral-based drugs and "heroic" interventions. Their rivals, who included self-taught or informally trained health care practitioners, women, and people of color, defined nature as something essential, universal, and democratic, and they extolled the benefits of medical knowledge systems that emphasized self-care (self-diagnosis, self-dosing); noninvasive procedures; and nonsynthetic, plant or animal-based drugs.[12] The term "nature cures" and its association with irregular sects like Thomsonianism became common parlance by the mid-nineteenth century, and in the Progressive Era, irregular physicians continued to deploy the discourse of natural medicine as a way to distance themselves from scientific medicine.[13]

Naturopathy is a prime example of the discourse of natural medicine in action. As a distinct school of medicine, naturopathy coalesced in the 1890s around the principles of herbalism, hydrotherapies, nutrition, and other practices that emphasized stimulating healing through close contact with sun, fresh air, and other natural elements. Epistemologically, naturopathy was remarkably inclusive, blending elements of a dozen or more medical sects from Thomsonianism and homeopathy to hypnotism and electro-therapy, but its adherents universally rejected Western-style scientific medicine. Their opposition targeted not only the American Medical Association's efforts to monopolize and standardize health care but also the scientific advances it championed, including vaccination. Naturopaths viewed vaccination as unnecessarily interventionist and incompatible with their beliefs in the body's ability to heal itself.[14]

For their part, AMA physicians saw their research and therapies as equally rooted in the natural world. Indeed if "nature's remedies" were characterized by their use of organic compounds, Western-style scientific medicine was no less dependent on nature than irregular medicine. Regular physicians relied on medicinal botanicals including belladonna, cannabis, opium (and its alkaloid, morphine), and emetine, and, to a lesser extent, animal byproducts.[15] While the historical record makes it difficult to state with any certainty the relative frequency with which regular physicians prescribed mineral versus botanical or zoological drugs, major medical compendia can gesture toward the possibilities.[16] In the 1910 United States National Pharmacopoeia, compiled decennially by the American Pharmacists Association and widely accepted as the mainstream authority on medicinal ingredients, nearly 57 percent of entries were botanical, which was proportionally similar to the classical Chinese formulary, the *Bencao gangmu,* dating from the late sixteenth century, which derived 51 percent of its ingredients from botanical sources. Zoological medicines accounted for another 6.5 percent of the American pharmacopoeia whereas the *Bencao gangmu* drew proportionally more of its *materia medica* from animal and human byproducts—29.5 percent.[17] At the very least, then, regular physicians had a large arsenal of organic drugs at their disposal.

The speeches and academic papers published in the *Journal of the American Medical Association* (*JAMA*) around the turn of the twentieth century reflect a prevalent feeling that regular medicine was the study of nature's laws of human health. In an 1895 address to the medical section of the AMA, Julius Kohl, a member of the State Board of Health of Illinois, described regular physicians as "students of nature" sworn to "point the way to obedience to those natural laws by which mankind must ever be governed."[18] In 1899, J. C. Wilson gave an oration in the same spirit in which he celebrated "the most wonderful century of the world's history" and the advances made in Western-style medical sciences: "The old was an art . . . relying largely on so-called specifics and not altogether scornful of charms and magic. The new is an art based on a group of correlated sciences and deriving its power from the forces of nature."[19] The desire to reclaim a connection between regular medicine and nature penetrated the popular press as well. In 1894, a *Los Angeles Times* article entitled "Chinese Doctors" took up the subject of the "Healing Power of Nature" and received the "warm indorsement of several prominent Los Angeles physicians," which the newspaper reported as an indication that "our modern school of American doctors is not so bigoted as some people would have us believe."[20] Perhaps the endorsement was an effort to rehabilitate the public image of regular medicine as divorced from nature. Regular physicians certainly recognized the problem they faced and discussed in their meetings how to publicize the natural basis of their practices. In 1904, *JAMA* exhorted its readers to withhold public criticism of "nature healers" and to "impress upon the public the fact that the [regular] medical profession is versed in the so-called 'nature' methods." Failing to do so threatened to undermine "the confidence of the public in the profession."[21]

Articles published in *JAMA* documented regular physicians' efforts to observe, understand, and assist natural processes. An 1896 eulogy for the esteemed British physician Edward Jenner described him as an "ideal country doctor" with a "passionate love for nature and a marked manhood and courage to investigate." His eulogist, William B. Dewees, praised Jenner's research: "He had the physicianhood and fortitude to search nature by following her and to honestly reveal the light he saw."[22] Wilhelm Hotz's 1897 article on hygiene applied a similar point more broadly: "What the physician *does* and the only thing he *can* do for the sick is certainly to assist nature in its efforts to restore health, and, as far as the symptoms indicate the need of the system, the physician has to be only a true student of nature in order to be also a successful physician."[23] In 1900, while calling for higher standards for basic science in medical college curricula, H. J. Herrick pondered the connection between medicine and nature: "Medicines modify functions; Nature heals. The doctor adjusts the broken bones and keeps the fragments at rest; Nature unites them. He provides the conditions; Nature is the benevolent healer."[24] This rhetoric continued unabated in the first decade of the twentieth century. "We are the servants of Nature," J. A. Work insisted in a 1908 article. "We should not dictate to Nature and say, 'Follow me.' Nature dictates to us and we must follow."[25] These examples are representative of a prevalent theme: an abiding curiosity and respect for nature animated the AMA's movement to standardize professional medicine.

In their quest to narrow the meanings of science and scientific authority, regular physicians did not reject all earlier or competing healing traditions but rather modified and incorporated them into new epistemologies and frameworks.[26] In 1884, James F. Hibbed wrote "A Plea for Greater Simplicity in Practical Medicine," in which he declared that the "guiding motto of every medical practitioner should be, 'All disease should be trusted to nature when art cannot declare an assured benefit by intervening."[27] In 1899, E. P. Hurd, president of the Medical Alumni Association for the University of Michigan, exhorted his fellow physicians to "avoid the danger of looking wholly at the material side of vital phenomena. Human life . . . cannot be explained satisfactorily from a consideration of its constitutional atoms."[28] Other physicians and surgeons publishing in *JAMA* argued pointedly against invasive procedures and for "nature cures." In a paper presented on nonsurgical treatments of an ophthalmological condition colloquially called "cross-eye" or "wall-eye," Edwin J. Gardiner "protest[ed] against hasty operative interference when Nature, properly assisted by science, can and does accomplish the result."[29] Similarly, Laurence Turnbull, an aural surgeon, recommended an antiseptic cleaning of a perforated eardrum so that "the healing process will commence, and 'Dame Nature' will complete the cure."[30] In the Progressive Era, papers and lectures published in *JAMA* tended to portray medical and surgical interventions as support for the body's natural capacity for self-healing.

Yet regular physicians also expressed an ambition to transcend the limitations of nature. Inaction ("letting nature take its course," so to speak) was akin to withholding the physician's power to heal and a violation of professional ethics.[31] In an 1883 paper on tracheotomies, surgeon W. H. Myer declared, "To trust to so called *vis medicatrix naturae* . . . is to forsake the path of duty to leave and to chance that which falls within the domain of reason." Myer placed no faith in nature's ability or desire to cure human ailments: "Nature pursues her ways with men regardless of their infirmities." He recalled for his audience the words of "Professor Houghton of Dublin" who scoffed at the notion of a "nature cure" for cholera by saying, "I will tell you what nature wants. She wants to put the man in his coffin, and that's what she succeeds in doing for the most part."[32] When obstetrician J. O. Malsberry offered his advice to new mothers, he touched briefly on abnormal presentations: "There are a few cases . . . in which nature throws up her hands, and mechanical assistance must be had, or the life of the mother or child or both will be sacrificed."[33] In the first decade of the twentieth century, the theme of assisting nature remained common. A 1910 article on diet in typhoid fever cautioned physicians, "Nature's method . . . should receive our encouragement and not our opposition . . . We could not interfere with the natural measures taken by the patient's metabolism itself to get rid of his infection. Neither should we leave it all to Nature's doubtful processes."[34] In the pages of *JAMA*, late nineteenth- and early twentieth-century physicians expressed ardent faith in their ability to make sense of nature and, in doing so, to improve upon it or overcome it.

Irregular physicians interpreted that faith as hubris. One early twentieth-century homeopath mocked the arrogance of regular physicians in a pamphlet on medical freedom: "'Tis nature that does it—but what right has she to be round curing people without a degree?"[35] That satirical portrayal was not too far from some of the actual sentiments expressed in *JAMA*. In a lecture on medical ethics, E. H. Bowman declared, "Our profession is the highest and holiest of any on earth . . . As our sphere is man in his entire nature, and we are thus brought necessarily into intimate connection and knowledge of the laws of his being, our profession is inevitably destined to take precedence of all other professions and lead in the van of the grand army of human progress."[36] Regular physicians, reveling in their elite status, did not endear themselves to the public.

Debunking Chinese Medicine

At the end of the nineteenth century, regular physicians confronted a set of entangled challenges. Their medical authority was derived from an extensive education in basic sciences and training in the use of new diagnostic technologies and clinical methods. Their patients were relatively less educated. Thus, regular physicians not only had to prove the therapeutic superiority of their science but they also had to teach consumers of medicine how to evaluate claims of authority: who to trust and how to identify quacks and charlatans. With the help of their allies in the press, regular physicians adapted the genre of the Chinatown travelogue to expose what they perceived as the false science of Chinese medicine. While travel accounts of American Chinatowns typically emphasized the traveler's encounter with the exotic, science writers covering Chinese medicine devoted more care and attention to explaining the principles and practices behind what they observed in the apothecary.

Science writers would have had various sources of information about Chinese medicine. In the late nineteenth and early twentieth centuries, medical missionaries in China continued to disseminate information about Chinese medical practices. Missionaries' studies of Chinese *materia medica* and healing practices continued as a byproduct of their educational initiatives and patient care at missionary hospitals. They published their observations of Chinese healing practices in new periodicals, including the *Chinese Recorder* and the *China Medical Missionary Journal*, as well as in longer monographs.[37] The Opium Wars between Britain and China (1839–1842 and 1856–1860) and "unequal treaties" with the British, French, and United States allowed missionaries to penetrate new territories through coastal and inland "treaty-port" cities where foreign powers asserted extraterritorial rights. It was difficult to maintain a supply of Western drugs in remote, inland areas, and interest in finding local substitutes surged. Publishers began to produce English-language guides to Chinese drugs, including F. Porter Smith's *Contributions towards the Materia Medica and Natural History of China; for the Use of Medical Missionaries and Native Medical Students* (1871) and G. A. Stuart's revision and three-volume update in 1911, *Chinese Materia Medica; Vegetable Kingdom.* Comparable compendia also existed for medicinal minerals.[38]

Unlike an earlier generation of texts by medical missionaries, late nineteenth- and early twentieth-century publications did not paint China as a vacuum of medical knowledge. They universally acknowledged the thousands of years of accumulated traditions, experiments, and even wisdom that constituted Chinese medicine. Yet at the same time, they affirmed the superiority of Western-style medical science and the necessary, redemptive role that it played in China. In 1869 and 1870, John Dudgeon, the physician to the British legation in Peking (Beijing), published a series of articles on "Chinese Healing Arts" for the *Chinese Recorder and Missionary Journal,* a periodical that communicated Chinese news and commentaries for English-speaking missionaries. Dudgeon's work was based on translations of Chinese medical texts that he did with the help of his students at the Imperial Medical Academy, where he was a professor of anatomy and physiology.[39] Dudgeon's primary interest was the use of magic, divination, and spirit worship in Chinese medical practices. He paid scant attention to systems of correspondence, *yinyang,* and the five phases. Even the brief discussion of *materia medica* concerned Chinese "simples" only inasmuch as they were conveyances for healing charms.[40] The emphasis on the magical allowed Dudgeon to paint Chinese medicine as a superstition-bound tradition, ignorant of modern science: "Belief in [magic and charms] was very natural at a time when the phenomena of nature which surrounded man[,] often sudden, august, and stupendous, such as eclipses, comets, earthquakes, famine, pestilence, etc., were imperfectly or not at all understood."[41] The persistence of magical and religious healing among the Chinese in the nineteenth century was, for Dudgeon, an indication of their primitivism and, perhaps, their turpitude: "Much that would not, in Europe, be considered morally wrong, in China forms an integral part of their religious systems . . . Both Emperor and people are alike addicted [to the use of charms]."[42] In this way, Dudgeon affirmed the moral and intellectual superiority of European American civilizations and, by extension, their right to exercise power over China.

Throughout the series, Dudgeon drew comparisons between the Chinese and the ancient civilizations of the Mediterranean. Such links helped make Chinese healing practices more comprehensible to European and American readers by drawing out cultural congruencies, but they also underlined the distinction between Chinese antiquity and European American modernity: "Like [Galen], the Chinese are diligent observers of the phenomena of disease; and they might become first class physicians, if their predilections and reverence for the theories of their ancestors did not warp and bias their judgement." Dudgeon used the series as an opportunity to endorse the advances that European medical science had made: "Not more than 150 years ago astrology and physic were practiced together in England and France. Some of the popular beliefs regarding healing are, in the present scientific age, almost incredible. By the largest majority, they are reckoned 'old wives' fables' or ignorant superstitious notions."[43] Later studies would echo Dudgeon's assessment that ancient Chinese traditions were falling out of favor among modern Chinese patients. In 1921, Harold Balme, dean of the School of Medicine at Shantung Christian University, wrote a history of medical missions in China in which the "vital forces of natural science, with its insistent demand for truth" swept aside the "queer fantastic notions of the Chinese physician."[44] As evidence of success, Balme pointed to the expansion of Western-style hospitals in the place of temples of medicine and healing shrines.[45]

Chinese students trained in missionary hospitals and Western medical colleges often assimilated that progressive narrative even when they ostensibly sought to complicate or correct it. In 1933, K. Chimin Wong, a high-ranking medical official in Hong Kong, published a history of Chinese medicine in which he argued that the Chinese had a long tradition of empiricism shaping their medical traditions, which prepared the Chinese people to receive and appreciate Western-style medical science. The example of smallpox vaccination served his point: "Since the Chinese were familiar with the feasibility of smallpox prevention, no better method than Jenner's inoculation could have been selected in order to gain a permanent foothold for western medical practice early in the nineteenth century."[46] Nevertheless, the book largely followed the contours of the narrative set out by Balme and others. Wong celebrated medical missionaries and Western-style scientific medicine as laying a critical foundation for modern China: "With its roots deeply embedded in the soil of four milleniums of empiricism, [Chinese medicine] only began to extend into the atmosphere of constructive effort when there was grafted onto it the vital principles of observation, experimentation, and coordination so characteristic of modern scientific medicine."[47] American medical scientists, reading such accounts, could take pride in their practices and dismiss Chinese medicine as retrograde.

In the nineteenth century, American research journals had offered scant but regular coverage of Chinese medicine, mostly translating and reprinting the treatises of European physicians on herbalism, acupuncture, and moxibustion. (Apotropaic healing, that is, healing with charms or talismans, was not considered sufficiently scientific to warrant study.)[48] But such coverage began to wane by the turn of the twentieth century. The consolidation of scientific medicine in the late nineteenth century discouraged new scholarship on Chinese therapies. Articles in *JAMA* from this period tended to treat Chinese medicine as a relic of a less enlightened time.[49] Yet there is evidence that interest in herbalism did persist in less visible ways. Some pharmacists continued to consult with local Chinese doctors in the analysis of traditional remedies.[50] At the local level, societies for physicians and surgeons kept discussion of Chinese medicine alive as part of efforts to eliminate "Oriental quackery." At a meeting in 1903, the Los Angeles County Medical Association invited as a speaker Yamei Kin, the first Chinese woman to receive a degree from a medical college in the United States. Born in Ningpo in 1864, Kin was the daughter of a Chinese pastor but was raised by American medical missionaries after the death of her family from a cholera epidemic. She spent most of her childhood in Shanghai and Japan, where her adopted father, Divie Bethune McCartee, was part of the Chinese legation until 1881. She eventually moved with her adopted parents to New York, where she attended the Woman's Medical College. After graduation, Kin worked as a physician in various hospitals in Philadelphia, New York, and Washington, D.C., including a rotation at the Chinese Asylum at Mount Vernon. She developed a reputation as a talented microphotographer and published an academic paper in the *New York Medical Journal* on the subject.[51] In 1888, Kin returned to Asia as a medical missionary first in Amoy (Xiamen), China, and then—while recovering from malaria—in Kobe, Japan. Between 1894 and 1904, she had a brief and unhappy marriage to a Spanish-Portuguese musician with whom she had a son. Together they toured the United States, where Kin would recount her life story while her husband performed Chinese music.[52] After her divorce, she returned to China, taking up residence in Szechwan, where she eventually received a grant from the Viceroy Yuan Shi-k'ai to open a Western-style nursing school for women in Tientsin (Tianjin) in northern China. In 1915, while she continued her work at the Tientsin hospital, she returned to the United States as a "publicity agent," touring the country to give lectures on various Chinese customs and practices, including nutrition and medicine, to audiences of physicians, society ladies, and other interested groups, including local branches of the AMA.[53] The minutes from the Los Angeles County chapter meeting reported that Kin "gave a very entertaining talk." She explained the tradition of medical education by apprenticeship in China and gave an overview of Chinese pharmacology. She also described the status of surgical procedures. We cannot know how the audience members responded. The minutes reported only that "there was no discussion" following Kin's presentation.[54]

Meanwhile, popular interest in Chinese medicine continued unabated. Regular physicians laid equal blame for the popularity of Chinese medicine on patients' inability to differentiate pseudo-science from science. An article printed in a New York newspaper noted, "The Chinese doctors are clever, and they do effect some cures in spite of their medicine. Lay it, perhaps, to the mental effect—the subtle influence of an alien personality combined with an awe of learning outrunning the oldest in America by so many hundreds of centuries."[55] Articles questioning the scientific basis of Chinese medicine aimed to correct such misplaced trust in so-called ancient learning. In 1894, the *Los Angeles Times* identified the Chinese medicine business on the West Coast as an example of the challenges that regular physicians faced serving patients possessed of "unreasonable" hopes for care and a dismaying pleasure in being "humbugged." The article concluded by calling for greater regulation of "Chinese quacks" and encouraging its readers "who are tempted to ignore the many excellent and conscientious physicians of all schools with which Los Angeles abounds in favor of the Chinese doctor should at least inform themselves a little in regard to the practice of the Chinese school of medicine."[56] Science writers hoped that a better understanding of Chinese therapeutic practices and principles might lead to more respect and trust in the authority of modern medical science.

Articles in the popular press about the "science" of Chinese medicine may have aimed to instruct the reader without formal scientific education in how to differentiate scientific medicine from pseudo-sciences like Chinese medicine, but they tended to do so by reinforcing racist assumptions about Chinese immigrants. In 1869, the *Overland Monthly* published "Medical Art in the Chinese Quarter" by Reverend A. W. Loomis, a former missionary to China and frequent contributor to the magazine on matters related to Chinese immigrant life and culture in

San Francisco. Like Dudgeon, Loomis described Chinese medicine as based more in mysticism than scientific evidence:

> So much study by so many learned men on one subject; so many thousands—yea, millions—of life-times spent in this study since the days of Noah until now, it might reasonably be supposed ought to have brought this science in China to a high state of perfection; but such is not the fact . . . There still remains a higher veneration for ancient than for modern discoveries, and the more smoky, thumb-worn, and worm-eaten a doctor's library appears, the more reverence, other things being equal, will usually be accorded to his opinions.[57]

According to Loomis, superstition prevented Chinese doctors from acquiring knowledge of anatomy or chemistry. Internal organs, nerves, and vessels, the author claimed, were "*terra incognita*" to doctors whose veneration for the intact human body prevented them from dissecting even postmortem.[58]

Loomis described the Chinese theory of anatomical correspondences and channels well enough to explain the basis of pulsology, but he summarily dismissed the practice as insufficient for diagnosis: "None but quacks . . . pretend to trust entirely to the pulse." Disparaging pulsology provided an opportunity for Loomis to educate readers on modern medical diagnosis: "The regular faculty speak of four methods by which the diagnosis must be obtain, viz.: 1st. By observation . . . 2d. By hearing . . . 3d. By questions . . . and 4th. The pulse."[59] The purported preference of Chinese patients for Western-style medicine became another standard feature of the genre. Loomis concluded his exposé of Chinese medical arts by cautioning his readers against forsaking "the new theories and freshly discovered medicines of the young nations of the West, for the theories which wise men of the East in the ages long ago invented."[60] Even Chinese immigrants to San Francisco, he claimed, once introduced to the "American" science of medicine, preferred regular doctors for treatment.

Across the country in Pittsburgh, the local newspaper recruited J. C. Thoms, a Chinese-born graduate of an American medical college, to explain Chinese medicine to its readers in 1889. Thoms had attended the Long Island College of Medicine, and soon after the publication of his *Pittsburgh Dispatch* article became the Chinese superintendent of the Chinese Hospital in Brooklyn.[61] The article combined a critique of Chinese medicine with a bildungsroman. Both parts served to exalt modern medical science. The discussion of Chinese therapeutic principles and practices reiterated common tropes of Chinese backwardness. Like Loomis, Thoms portrayed the Chinese physician as untrained; ignorant of anatomy, physiology, and pharmacology; and possessed of bizarre superstitions. Thoms restated Loomis's assertion that Chinese people preferred Western-style scientific medicine: "The more intelligent part of my countrymen freely confess this fact, and are now willing to employ the practitioners of the modern school in preference to the followers of the ancient Chinese methods."[62]

Thoms used his own intellectual biography to defend modern medical science. He portrayed himself as initially skeptical. "At first," he wrote, "I did not enjoy my studies, and the operations in the dissecting room were particularly distasteful to me, but I got used to them after a while . . . At first, I found it difficult to understand the English language and the long medical terms in Latin were hard to remember, but by diligent study and much practice I have succeeded in mastering the language."[63] Thoms's stated aversion to dissection may have recalled for readers the popular stereotype of Chinese doctors' opposition to autopsy or surgery, but his ability to overcome that limitation and discover, in his words, that he was "especially fond of the theoretical study of anatomy" provided an example of modern rationality overcoming primitive irrationality.

The ancient origin of Chinese medical principles and practices rehearsed Orientalist stereotypes of a civilization frozen in the distant past, and over the decades that theme featured prominently and consistently in science writing about Chinese medicine. An 1894 article in the *Los Angeles Times* claimed, "The standard medical works in China were compiled nearly four thousand years ago . . . and from the rules and precepts there laid down, no Chinese doctor must vary a hair's breadth, under penalty of [death] . . . Chinese medicine has, therefore, not taken a step forward for forty centuries."[64] A portrait of Boston doctor Pang

Suey published in the *New York Sun* in 1912 likened his practices to those of ancient Persian physicians "who treated their patients by means of an examination of a hand thrust through a curtain," and challenged its readers to "imagine a physician who asks no questions. Consider a doctor who holds your hand for a mere three minutes, then tells you what's the matter with you and proceeds to try to cure you . . . Here in this modern city appears a healer who asks only to lay his fingers on your pulse—and there you are, all pigeon-holed, tabulated, and diagnosed."[65] By underlining the incongruity of an ancient practice flourishing in a modern city, articles like this one encouraged their readers to be skeptical of Chinese medicine and to seek out modern healing practices more compatible with their culture and values.

Acupuncture, less commonly practiced in the United States than herbalism and pulsology, received special scrutiny as a prime example of Oriental barbarity.[66] While herbalism was very much a part of American folk medicine, and pulsology bore some superficial similarity to diagnosis by stethoscope or sphygmomanometer, acupuncture may have seemed comparatively more alien and, perhaps, menacing. Unlike the modern filiform needles developed in Japan and used in the late twentieth century, nineteenth- and early twentieth-century acupuncture needles were larger, with scalpel-like blades and retractor-like hooks, making acupuncture in some ways similar to minor surgical procedures. Indeed, the trained acupuncturist might encourage a little blood to flow to free the body's energy, or *qi*.[67] In San Francisco in 1887, the *Daily Alta California* reported that a Chinese physician had treated a woman with pneumonia by "piercing a row of portholes in her abdomen. The perforated patient died, though the doctor says this old treatment of pneumonia was discovered in China 250 years ago."[68] A death from blood poisoning in 1893 resurfaced public interest in acupuncture. Mrs. T. B. Jackson had been seeing Dr. J. E. Renken, a non-Chinese practitioner of the "needle-cure" in Oakland. The editors of San Francisco's *Daily Call* interviewed several regular physicians to ask, "Is needle-pricking from head to foot a cure for anything?" The unanimous answer was no. The newspaper article quoted a Dr. Staliard as describing acupuncture as "nothing but a piece of damnable quackery and humbug . . . It is impossible to keep the needles clean, and when people are punctured, eruptions arise, blood-poisoning sets in, and very often death follows." His colleague, a Dr. Lovelace, concurred, calling acupuncture "not only exceedingly cruel but supremely ridiculous."[69]

Articles on Chinese therapeutic principles and practices might discuss the systems of correspondence, doctrine of *yinyang,* diagnosis by pulse, and pharmacology with a reasonable degree of accuracy and neutrality, but acupuncture played the role of comic relief. In 1897, the *New York Sun* published an article by an American physician who claimed that "the Chinese practitioners seem to have a fondness for puncturing their patients . . . They seem to regard the human body as a great pin cushion, with which they have a great deal of fun."[70] A photograph of a doll pierced with dozens of acupuncture needles appeared in a 1919 issue of Klamath Fall, Oregon's *Evening Herald* accompanied by the question, "How would you like to go to consult a needle doctor in China?" The short article explained that doctors used the needles to "punch holes" in their patients' heads and bodies so that "little devils" might escape. It went on to solicit donations for a medical mission to China by Oregon Methodists, presumably aimed at modernizing Chinese medical practices.[71] By these means, acupuncture could speak to different aspects of Orientalist discourse: fears of Chinese savagery and ridicule of Chinese superstitions.

Science writers tended to attribute the backwardness of Chinese medicine to religion and superstitions, an explanation that reflected and reinforced a stereotype of Oriental irrationality. In 1880, the *San Francisco Chronicle* interviewed American physicians and sent one of its reporters undercover to expose "celestial" quackery in the city: "The principle cause of the backwardness of the Chinese medical practice is their religion. They are spiritualists and fatalists. They have neither a very deep fear of death nor do they believe the can die in any way but as ordained by fate."[72] Decades later, popular newspapers and academic medical journals alike were still rehashing the same themes. The *Sunday Oregonian* reflected on the persistence of "magic healing" in 1900 by interviewing two recently returned tourists to China, where they had observed an example of demonic healing, or exorcism. The writer then consulted with two Chinese physicians who informed him that "this has always been done in China and probably always will be because Chinamen do not change their ways of life."[73] In 1908, the *Los Angeles Times* reprinted an article from the *Medical Record,* a national journal of regular medicine and surgery, also describing the Chinese tradition of demonic healing: "After going through the usual examination . . . Dr. Wong-Yik Chee will diagnose the case and treat it, unless a devil happens to jump down the patient's throat. If this has happened the doctor can do the patient no good until he promises to set off 100 firecrackers to drive the devil away from his body and make a daily visit to a joss house."[74]

Beneath that sensationalism was an incomplete truth: Chinese medicine in the early twentieth century continued to encompass a wide variety of therapies, including magical and religious healing but also surgical interventions and drug therapies. The same was also true for American medicine of that era. The patent medicine industry thrived on its consumers' equal faith in science and magic.[75] The Christian Science movement, inspired by Mary Baker Eddy's 1875 publication *Science and Health,* attracted thousands of students to its Massachusetts Metaphysical College, and the Seventh-Day Adventists promoted a blend of spiritual and material therapies at their Health Reform Institute at Battle Creek, Michigan, from 1876.[76] Caricatures of "unscientific" Chinese medicine, however, allowed regular physicians and their allies to construct a convenient fiction about American medicine that erased its heterogeneity and asserted the supremacy of Western-style scientific medicine.

It was common for popular science writing to reduce Chinese doctor's qualifications to a matter of heredity alone. In 1891, a profile of New York doctor Choy Yeu Chong described Chinese medicine as "6,700 years old" and attributed his expertise to the fact that "his father was a doctor before him and his father's father treated the sick and collected his bills from his patient's executors . . . Yellower and dirtier and more furrowed than the diploma of the oldest living American graduate in medicine, Dr. Chong has his office at No. 26 Pell Street."[77] The reader could not have missed the satire implicit in the mention of the mortality rate among Dr. Chong's grandfather's patients and the equivalence between the "yellow and dirty" Chinese doctor and the "yellow and dirty" American medical diploma.

Representations of medical education in China and its deficiencies also reflected that same tendency to ignore the historical and contemporary realities of medical education in the United States. When Chinese doctors advertised their training in Chinese medical colleges and presented their diplomas before state medical boards, delegitimizing Chinese credentials in the public eye became all the more important. A widely respected volume entitled *Diseases of China* by medical missionaries W. Hamilton Jefferys and James L. Maxwell claimed, "To become a physician, a Chinese states to his friends and neighbours, 'I am a physician.' This is the limit of required preparation although it is usually a development from a former apprenticeship. His diploma is the more or less handsome signboard which announces his determination to the neighborhood."[78] Indeed, public licensure did not exist in China until 1909, and in 1910, when Jefferys and Maxwell published their seven-hundred-plus-paged tome, there were only a handful of schools of Western medicine in treaty-port cities in addition to the ancient and venerated Imperial Medical Academy. Thus, Jefferys and Maxwell correctly observed that most medical education in China took place through apprenticeships rather than through medical colleges. Of course, they might have said the same of the United States just forty years earlier.

Magical, Ancient, and Natural

When attacks on Chinese doctors in American scholarly and popular media ridiculed their therapies as antimodern or unscientific, their own advertising made that characterization a source of strength. In 1902, Wong-San of Bakersfield, California, invited patients to partake of "Oriental Medical Secrets that have been hidden from the eyes of the white man for untold centuries" in an advertisement that highlighted Chinese medicine's simultaneous exoticism, antiquity, and superiority. "Why not try the Oriental Methods?" he asked. "They save human life where the white doctor fails."[79] Such a strategy was well suited to attract non-Chinese patients who were both already conversant in the vocabulary of American Orientalism as well as skeptical of modern medical science.

With relative ease, Chinese doctors could capitalize on Orientalist notions of Asian luxury and decadence. As chapter 3 details, middle-class and affluent patients were attracted to waiting rooms adorned with silk scrolls, teak furniture, and other Orientalia. Orientalist notions of barbarity, on the other hand, were more difficult—but not impossi-ble—to rewrite. Chinese doctors creatively presented consumers of Chinese medicine with an opportunity to rethink the merits of Asian barbarism. Foo and Wing's *The Science of Oriental Medicine* claimed that Chinese backwardness and barbarism were in fact beneficial to the scientific process of discovery. According to its author (probably Foo and Wing employee Burton C. Platt), the "science" of *The Science of Oriental Medicine* was based on ancient and inhumane practices.[80] The book's discussion of anatomical knowledge was one example of this rhetorical strategy. Counter to prevailing myths that the Chinese did not understand how the human body worked, *The Science of Oriental Medicine* insisted that their anatomical knowledge was in fact superior to that of regular, American doctors because Chinese doctors dissected live humans, not cadavers:

> When the Chinese commenced to study medicine they went at once to the root of different questions involved by prac-ticing vivisection. Thousands of condemned criminals were taken and cut to pieces for the benefit of the living. In this way the functions of the vital organs such as the kidneys, the liver, the stomach, the spleen, and the heart were stud-ied in the living person. The intensely important questions involved in the digestion of foods were determined as well as the effects of different drugs. These investigations, made while the man was still alive, were a thousand times more thorough and reliable than the guesswork which civilized physicians have practiced for many years by cutting up the bodies of dead men, when heat, motion, and life are gone and death has destroyed every function.[81]

Foo and Wing claimed Chinese doctors, supposedly racially inclined toward barbarity, had used their unsavory predilection for the advancement of medical science. They could therefore comprehend what civility and morality prevented regular, white doctors from comprehending: how medications actually worked on the living body. In reality, Chinese doctors probably did not perform vivisections on condemned criminals or anyone else; early Chinese medical texts, like non-Chinese medical texts of the same era, relied on postmortem analysis of internal organs.[82] Nevertheless, the effect of such an anecdote might have been both shocking and comforting for potential white patients. By highlighting the unexpected benefits of barbarism, Tom Foo Yuen and Li Wing made Orientalism work for themselves.

Self-Orientalizing doctors emphasized the deep history of their medical knowledge. The depiction of Chinese medicine as an ancient healing art distinguished it from the new medical sciences. When Seattle doctor May You Ben was arrested in 1914 for practicing medicine without a license, he invoked what seemed like a bizarre argument in his defense: he testified that the prescription he wrote was in fact written by another doctor, Hee Wo, who had lived in China nearly two thousand years ago.[83] The newspaper covering the trial played the testimony for laughs, but it is worth considering what May might have meant by prescribing an ancient remedy to a modern patient. Such images corresponded to the Orientalist construction of China as an ancient and static civilization, but they also pointed toward a historical record of success that regular medicine did not have. Advertising mail-order medicines to readers of a newspaper in Bisbee, Arizona, San Francisco doctor Chin Mai Fong similarly linked his practices with antiquity, claiming not only that the "Chinese were medical experts before the white race was civilized" but that Julius Caesar himself had employed Chinese physicians when he fell ill.[84]

Chinese doctors contrasted the comforting constancy of old Chinese therapies with the unsettling dynamism of scientific medicine. In 1903, Foo and Wing began to run a lengthy advertisement in the *Los Angeles Times* promising "Medicines that Cure" and cautioning patient-consumers that "new ideas" were "not always improvements. Our ancient system [is] still the best." Foo and Wing characterized regular doctors as dangerously faddish and confused: "The result of all this shifting about and uncertainty and disagreement among doctors is that the

common people are constantly looking for remedies that they can understand, something that is not hidden in obscure chemical processes,
or set forth with a long name, something that was known to be good
years ago and is known to be good today." Foo and Wing promised that
their "Oriental system of medicine" was the safe and stable alternative
that the "common people" had been seeking: "Strangely enough that
system of medicine, which is easiest to understand, which involves no
hidden mysteries . . . is the oldest system of medicine in the world."[85]
When Tom Foo Yuen went into business with his nephew Tom Chong,
their half-page advertisement in the *San Francisco Chronicle* criticized
Americans for "looking constantly for something new in medicine . . .
The Chinese, on the contrary, keep the best of what has come to them
through the ages."[86] Oakland herbalist Fong Wan made a similar claim
in his 1936 advertising book, *Herb Lore,* when he promised, "One takes
no chances in using Chinese Herbs . . . Having been used by billions
of human beings with beneficial effects for approximately 5,000 years,
Chinese Herbs have long since passed the experimental stage." In this
statement, Fong asked his readers to trust in the longevity of Chinese
medicine over the novelty of scientific medicine.[87]

A reputation for dispensing "nature's remedies" became another
way for Chinese doctors to highlight the dissimilarity between their
practice and modern medical science. Chinese doctors often described
themselves as uniquely attuned to "nature" and their therapies as "nature's remedies." The coupling of ancient knowledge and organic drugs
was one of the most common and oldest marketing strategies deployed
by Chinese doctors in the United States. It dated all the way back to John
Howard's 1799 advertisement for "herbs and roots only" in Harrisburg,
Pennsylvania.[88] Chinese doctors' invocation of "nature's remedies" reflected the convergence of two compatible and contemporaneous cultural languages: American Orientalism and the discourse of natural
medicine. English-language advertisements for Chinese medicine in the
late nineteenth and early twentieth centuries borrowed from both of
those cultural languages. They rehearsed an image of Chinese medicine
that was based on "pure" and "growing things," not the "minerals,"
"chemicals," "poisons," "drugs," or surgeries associated with Western-
style medical science.

Although Chinese immigrant doctors were advertising their services to English- and Spanish-speaking patients as early as the 1850s, the language of natural medicine did not appear in print until 1877, when "Dr. Offo" promised "no poisonous medicines" to his Oakland clientele.[89] This timing coincided with a new wave of state legislation mandating public exams and licensure for health care providers, a movement largely supported by regular doctors.[90] References to nature became more prevalent in English-language advertisements for Chinese medicine after 1890, as Chinese exclusion diminished the number of co-ethnic customers, and non-Chinese patients became a larger part of their practice. Between 1890 and 1894, Chang Gee Wo ran ads in various Midwestern newspapers touting his "wonderful, marvelous, miraculous" cures, which were, in fact, "nature's remedies . . . tested for thousands of years in China."[91] Some thirty years later, having moved to Portland, Oregon, Chang continued to base his marketing on an appeal to nature, insisting that his prescriptions were "nature's own remedies, and contain no poisonous minerals or drugs."[92] In the 1890s and 1900s, an advertisement in the *Idaho Statesman* for Chin Man Sui promised that he used "nothing but the best quality Chinese herbs. Nature's own Remedy."[93] In the same decades, Chinese doctors advertising in California, Arizona, Washington, and Kansas made the language of natural medicine central to their value proposition.[94] In its 1902 edition of *The Science of Oriental Medicine,* Foo and Wing claimed that herbal remedies were "founded upon a complete understanding of Nature's laws. Americans carry their theories of science to extremes and get too far away from the simple, fundamental facts upon which health depends."[95]

Chinese doctors well understood that patients viewed Western-style medical drugs with trepidation. While historians have documented the declining use of mineral cathartics by American regular physicians by the 1860s, patient testimonials and articles in the popular press show that even in the early twentieth century, the public still associated regular doctors with harsh emetics and purgatives.[96] In 1928, Tom Leung declared to his Los Angeles patients that "the Chinese is a better physician than the American because of his familiarity with nature, a branch of curative science that . . . has been neglected in this country."[97] A "familiarity" with nature's remedies meant that Chinese physicians did not

prescribe mineral-based drugs or other botanical or zoological medicines that produced a dramatic, potentially toxic effect on the human
body: "For centuries the use of all minerals and of all poisonous herbs
or other substances has been forbidden by law in the Flowery Kingdom."[98] In contrast to the simple cultivation of medicinal herb gardens,
the use of medicinal minerals and metals might have seemed strange and
dangerous to patients. Chin Mai Fong criticized this tendency of regular medicine and invited patients to "compare the medicines obtained
from the mild, soothing, health-giving plants, provided by nature, used
by the Chinese, with the strong drugs used by many of the American
doctors."[99] A 1922 advertisement for the Oakland branch of the franchise Chan and Kong explained "how to get well and keep well" through
"remedies [that] consist of nature: barks, roots, herbs, and compounds
and not the chemical works or drugs."[100] Similarly, a pamphlet from
the 1920s for the Long Beach, California, apothecary S. P. Lee and Sons
entitled *Health Herbs: Nature's Great Gift to All* insisted, "God prepared
these natural herbs to aid the human sufferer. They are harmless. *Not
drugs;* but pure, natural remedies."[101]

Mentions of nature continued to appear regularly in advertisements for Chinese medicine up through the 1930s and 1940s.[102] In a
1936 advertising book for his Oakland apothecary, Fong Wan patiently
laid out the differences between drugs and herbs. While "each consists
of four letters," the similarities ended there. Fong insisted that an herb
"has life and it supplies nourishment for the building up and strength-
ening of the body." In contrast, drugs were "usually of mineral origin"
or "derived from vegetables or herbs, but only through a chemical process," thus "it has no life and has a deadening or killing effect" on the
human body.[103] While Chinese herbs were not raw but minimally processed to prevent spoilage in shipping, their naturalistic appearance may
have been reassuring for patients dubious of medicines synthesized in
a laboratory.

Chinese physicians used long-form advertising to equate their
practices with traditions of American folk medicine and its pastoral
connotations. In *Things Chinese,* a hundred-page book that publicized
Chang Gee Wo's office and herb shop in downtown Portland, Chang
described his ingredients as "roots, bark, herbs, vegetables, and flow-

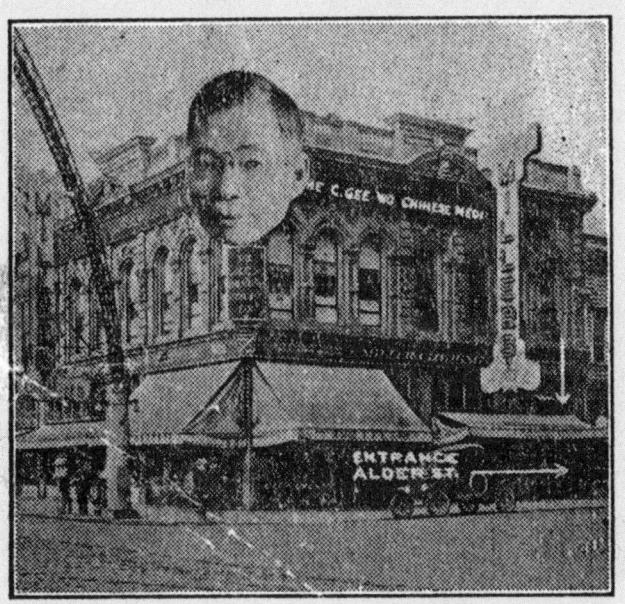

Cover of Chang Gee Wo's *Things Chinese,* 1930s. Courtesy of
the Oregon Historical Society.

ers" and explained how Chinese herbs were harvested wild and then
tended in farmyards "in the same manner as a gardener tends to his
choicest flowers."[104] Garding Lui, an herbalist who immigrated to the
United States in the 1920s, published several English-language books
and articles on Chinese medicine, including a lengthy piece in the *Los
Angeles Times* in which he explained the nature of medical education
in China:

> The Chinese physician takes his premedical course in the herb
> store or apothecary shop. He begins by learning to grind and
> mix the powders and herbal compounds that he must pre-
> scribe when he has become a full-fledged doctor. Some of the
> prescriptions he learns to fill are as beautiful as a poem, call-
> ing for orange and honeysuckle leaves or for the white bloom
> of the chrysanthemum. The Chinese apothecary's shop bears
> little resemblance to that of the American pharmacy. Such
> oriental stores still can be seen in Chinatown—with embryo
> doctors who seem to be rowing boats but are, in reality, roll-
> ing herbs into powders to alleviate their people's distress.[105]

Such pastoral and humane images worked against images of apothecaries
packed with desiccated animal and human body parts. In 1943, Lui published the work he would be best remembered for, a short book entitled
Secrets of Chinese Physicians. An introduction, written by Jesse Forest
Silver, an American doctor and self-styled poet, encouraged readers—
also presumed to be American—to suspend their prejudice against the
Chinese by reflecting on their own traditions of folk medicine: "We talk
about the superstitions of the Chinese people. Are we immune? . . . We
have resorted to the use of crafty psychology and hypnotic therapy in
the healing of the sick . . . We go and get goat and monkey glands to
make us young again."[106] Put so plainly, American medical practices did
not seem so dissimilar from those of the Chinese. Practitioners of traditional Chinese therapies embraced contradictions. In the American
medical marketplace, their medicine was both irredeemably other and
comfortingly familiar.

    Chinese doctors were aware that modernization and industrializa-
tion in the late nineteenth century had changed the meanings of nature
for many Americans, although not in entirely predictable or coherent
ways. Nature in Progressive Era America could simultaneously signify
the antimodern and the modern. The preservationist desire to commune
with a pristine "Nature" was founded on an antimodern impulse, but
the principles of conservation were undoubtedly products of a modernizing state and science, which was equally characteristic of the time.[107]
Advertisements for Chinese medicine frequently played on the seem-

ingly contradictory valences of nature to depict a practice and philosophy that was both "modern" (based on science) and "old-fashioned"
(based on ancient folkways).

The coupling of ancient medicine with modern science, its presumed opposite, was not as common as the language of natural medicine but it did appear in short- and long-form advertisements beginning around the turn of the twentieth century. In 1897, Dr. Wong Him
alerted his customers that he was moving to "more modern premises"
with an illustration that showed a Chinese man's bust (presumably his)
adorned in an old-fashioned Oriental cap.[108] A 1909 advertisement for
Yee and York, a pair of Chinese doctors practicing in Walla Walla, Washington, identified them as "great scientific men of China."[109] Longer advertisements were sometimes, but not always, better suited to explain
the subtleties of the relationship between Chinese medicine and science.
An 1896 letter in the *Los Angeles Times* from Li Wing Fawn and his business manager, Burton C. Platt (shortly before he joined Foo and Wing),
combined the language of science with the traditions of Chinese medicine. They described their commitment at the Flowery Kingdom Herb
Company to educate the "American people in the merits of a truly rational system of medicine." The system was herbal, and it was not static,
but dynamic and adaptive. The occasion prompting the letter to the *Los
Angeles Times* was the store's addition of a surgical department, which
would "offer advice and remedies for the cure of all difficulties that under American methods, would be supposed to require operations." Li
and Platt probably added the service to their roster to compete with
regular physicians. Their announcement begged further explanation
given Chinese medicine's reputation for noninvasive procedures. The
letter explained that the approach to surgery depended on the "either
internal or external" application of herbal remedies. Where American
surgeons deployed scalpels and forceps, "the Chinese surgeon accom-
plishes astonishing results without the use of instruments, apparatus, or
mechanical contrivances of any kind."[110] Li and Platt conjured an image
of the magical capabilities of the Chinese surgeon but kept the details of
the procedures deliberately vague.

Some herbalists appropriated the language of science and its most
recognizable conventions to describe their "ancient" practice. In 1902,

Jung Hong seemed to reference the germ theory of disease in an advertisement for his Los Angeles shop: "Chinese Herbs will wash your blood the same as you wash your hands."[111] In the 1924 edition of *Things Chinese*, Chang Gee Wo explained that he moved his business to a building that could house his "modern equipment" and "laboratory."[112] In the same decade, Tom Leung's *Chinese Herbal Science*, featured testimonials from European American patients including C. M. Melick, who declared—with a liberal use of capitalization for emphasis—that Leung was "MORE thoroughly and SCIENTIFICALLY EDUCATED" than the regular, American physicians he had consulted for his tuberculosis and cancer. Melick explained, "I was IGNORANT of the thorough and scientific education of the CHINESE HERBALISTS, and because of the PREJUDICE and EGOTISM WE AMERICANS have against any other than the white race."[113] For American patients, references to scientific methods or a formal education in science helped make Chinese healing practices seem sensible and safe without undermining the antimodern concepts that distinguished them in the medical marketplace. According to *Chinese Herbal Science*, "T. Leung has mingled Oriental splendor with American modernism until he has now succeeded in establishing one of the most model herb dispensatories to be found anywhere in the United States."[114] Chinese medicine promised the best of both the ancient and modern worlds to European American patients.

    Nutritional advice also became a means by which Chinese doctors could characterize their work as simultaneously embedded in antimodern and modern environmental understandings. *The Science of Oriental Medicine* cited "an exhaustive study" from a chemistry professor at the University of California, Berkeley, Walter C. Blasdale, on the medicinal benefits of Chinese vegetables: "He believes that many of these will ultimately become of general use and of great value to American and European nations." *The Science of Oriental Medicine* asserted that the knowledge of these healing vegetables was "ancient" but also confirmed by a modern scientist, in this case a chemist.[115] Chang Gee Wo's *Things Chinese* played up the "scientific" aspects of his practice. The fifth edition included an article by a white doctor on the medicinal value of vitamins, a recent discovery in 1924: "Our grandmothers had 'herb teas' that shamed the apothecary's art. The Indians' 'roots and herbs' were the Puritans' delight. The Chinese have a remarkable faculty for choosing matchless herbal remedies. At Portland, Oregon the well-known C. Gee Wo Chinese Medicine Company has the acme of reputation for giving out the very best of such preparations, and best because they are rich in remedial vitamins."[116] Pairing references to grandmothers, Indians, and Puritans with vitamins simultaneously underscored the deep, historical roots of Chinese herbal remedies and connected them to Americans' emergent understanding of diet and nutrition.

Like herbal remedies, Asian foodstuffs also became part of American conceptions of Chinese health practices and their inherent harmony with the natural world. Explaining the science of Chinese food to American consumers became a cornerstone of the career of Yamei Kin. In the 1910s, she helped popularize soy food products in the United States. In 1917, the U.S. Department of Agriculture commissioned a report by Kin on the uses of the soybean in China and methods of its cultivation.[117] Kin's description recalled much of the language used to promote herbal remedies: the Chinese, Kin reported, had been eating soybean food products for four thousand years, and this ancient custom stemmed from principles of conservation familiar to her modern audiences: "The word is in need of tissue-building foods . . . and cannot grow animals in order to obtain the necessary percentage of protein."[118] In her exultation of the soybean, Kin relied on an implicit understanding of resource scarcity and efficient land management that were the hallmarks of early twentieth-century conservationists like Gifford Pinchot.[119] The cultivation of soybeans reflected a Chinese version of American conservationism: "The Chinese do not know what worn out soil is. Some places are so fertile and are cultivated with so much care and skill that three or four crops are regularly gathered." Kin explained that soy products such as *natto,* tofu, miso, *yuba,* and *shoyu* allowed people to "live cheaply in China and yet produce for that nation a man power so tremendous that this country must pass an exclusion act against them." Kin promised that the soybean would increase the productivity of American farms and, by extension, the vitality of the American people.[120]

Asserting an equivalence between Chinese drugs and foods did not always serve the interests of Chinese herbalists. That fact became apparent in the 1940 case *Oy Wo Tong, et al. v. United States* when San

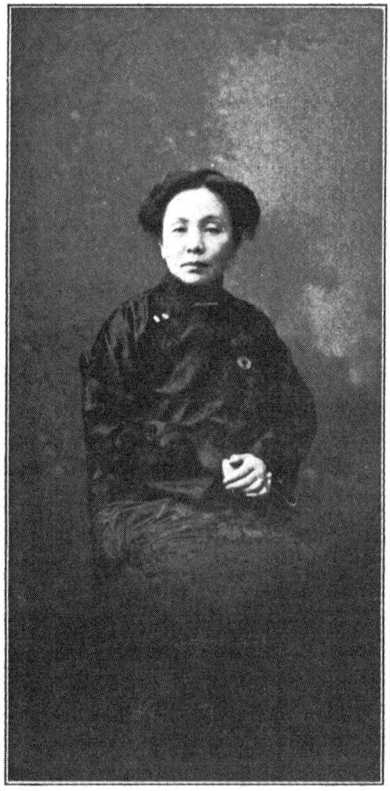

Yamei Kin, the first Chinese woman
to graduate from an American
medical college and an early
promoter of soybeans in the United
States, 1915. Wikimedia Commons.

Francisco importers found their shipments of herbal medicine taxed as
processed foods. In 1940, the San Francisco herb import companies—
Oy Wo Tong, Tin Bow Tong, and Ton Chong Gauk—filed a complaint
with the U.S. Customs Court after a collector at the Port of San Francisco assessed a duty on a variety of traditional herbal remedies. The
San Francisco customs agent insisted that they were, in fact, prepared
foods and therefore subject to a tariff.[121] The companies insisted that
the assessment was illegally collected because the customs officer should

have classified their imports as "crude" drugs that were "included on the free list." Other Chinese importers had filed similar complaints with the court for the same herbs: *hoi pak lien* (lotus nuts or seeds), *bak hop* (various parts of the lily, including its petals, bulbs, and bulb scales), *sui sit* (another kind of flowering lily), *yuen yuk* (longan fruit), and *sar sam* (the root of a bellflower plant).[122] A 1920 case before the Treasury Department had found that canned lotus nuts had lost their germinating potential and had to be considered prepared food.[123] Thus, the decision in the *Oy Wo Tong Co.* case would hinge on proving the "edibility" of imported medicinal plants or the lack thereof. Both the defendants and the plaintiffs in the case submitted seeds, fruits, lily bulb scales, and other vegetal matter in question. The court sent the plaintiffs' samples out for chemical analysis by Bella Kahn, a chemist at the U.S. appraiser's laboratory in New York. The results were not helpful. Kahn could not isolate any alkaloidal or cathartic drugs in the samples, but the court determined that Kahn's finding was insufficient "to show that such commodities do not have medicinal or therapeutic properties."[124]

In the absence of empirical data to classify the Chinese herbs as food or drug, the court called on cultural knowledge. The defense introduced four witnesses to testify to the fact that the imported herbs had no medicinal value or customary use as medicine among Chinese people. The first two witnesses were credentialed American scientists: Archibald Wallace Dunn, an American doctor who had practiced medicine in China, and Walter C. Blasdale, the Berkeley chemist who had been quoted extensively in the advertising materials for Foo and Wing. The other two witnesses called on behalf of the United States were not scientists but rather individuals of Chinese descent: Harry Lewis, a customs inspector identified by the courts as "an American of Chinese parentage," and his wife, a China-born woman raised primarily in New York City. Both testified that Chinese American communities used the commodities as both food and drugs. Mrs. Lewis (as she was called in court documents) claimed that she was "familiar with *luk mei*, a soup or broth which is made from six ingredients: *wai san, sar sum, bak hop, yuen yuk,* and two more." Consuming medicinal ingredients in a soup did not confirm or deny their status as foodstuffs as it was customary to reconstitute dried medicines in boiling water, but Mrs. Lewis's next statement seemed to offer more definitive support for the government's classification. She testified "that she buys all of these ingredients in grocery stores, not drug stores."[125] Yet Mrs. Lewis's distinction between a grocery store and a drugstore was misleading, perhaps deliberately so. In the Chinese American community, herbalists imported both medicines and assorted dry goods, their shops simultaneously serving as apothecary and grocery store.[126]

For the plaintiffs, eleven Chinese witnesses, all involved in the herb business as importers, sellers, or doctors, testified that the samples had no food use and were strictly employed in medicinal applications. The court's decision privileged their testimony: "We think the testimony of these witnesses is entitled to great weight inasmuch as they are the ones who purchase the commodities and consume them, in accordance with the medical customs of their race."[127] Thus, the court determined that the commodities in question were indeed drugs, not food, and it surmised that the drying, slicing, and other light processing was most likely in service of preventing damage to the items during shipping. The herb companies won their case and recovered the illegally collected assessment.[128] What was at stake for the plaintiffs was arguably more than the 10 percent tax. By protesting the categorization of their imports as "advanced in value" by processing, Oy Wo Tong, Tin Bow Tong, and Ton Chong Gauk reinforced a popular understanding of Chinese medicine as close to its original state in nature. The lack of processing or synthesizing was the essence of Chinese medicine and its value proposition to American patients.

Lost in Translation

The meanings of nature in traditional Chinese medicine were not directly translatable into European American categories. Traditional Chinese medicine, as a compilation of doctrines and practices, did not conceive of nature as the opposite of science or modernity. Nor were herbs more natural than minerals by virtue of being organic instead of inorganic. Chinese practitioners believed that health relied on a harmonious balance of complementary (or corresponding) elements, which were both magical and material. In this way, Chinese therapeutic principles and practices had elements that resembled both premodern and modern sensibilities about the body and its physical environment. Linda Nash, in her book, *Inescapable Ecologies,* argues that the expanding acceptance of the germ theory of disease in the late nineteenth- and early twentieth-century United States led to a reconceptualization of the body from one embedded in a particular environment ("the ecological body") to one independent of the environment ("the modern body"). Whereas the ecological body existed in a constant state of exchange with its environment, and wellness reflected a sustainable balance between the two, the germ theory of disease taught physicians that pathogenic agents (germs, bacteria) caused sickness and that human health depended on protecting the modern body from those agents. To borrow Linda Nash's categories, the body in traditional Chinese medicine was both modern and ecological.[129] Chinese doctors considered the physical environment in their diagnoses and prescriptions, but it was not necessarily determinative of wellness or disease. Ill health might just as likely be the consequence of a pathogenic agent, emotional turmoil, inherited conditions, or an evil spirit. Good diagnosis examined the interdependencies of the body, mind, and physical environment.[130]

Over the centuries, Chinese physicians had of course absorbed new discoveries about human physiology, etiology, and pharmacology into an ancient framework of complementary, counterbalancing forces. A wave of epidemic diseases in the seventeenth century led Chinese scholars to postulate that infectious agents causing tuberculosis and smallpox might be transmitted through unclean environments ("impure *qi*") passed to individuals through the nose and mouth. In this regard, seventeenth-century scholars blended the preexisting concept of *qi* with a rudimentary understanding of contagion emanating from material conditions like stagnant water, rotting food, or other decay.[131] When Chinese doctors began immigrating to the United States during the late nineteenth and early twentieth centuries, principles of environmental health were undergoing reconsideration by scholar-physicians in southern China. Between the 1850s and 1870s, southern scholars concerned with how regional climate affected diseases accompanied by high fevers developed a consensus that the treatment must depend on local *qi,* that is, endemic conditions of the patient's physical environment. According to historian Marta Hanson, "In the minds of Chinese physicians them-selves, specific geographic locales required distinct therapeutic inter-ventions."[132] Hanson argues that, by the end of the nineteenth century, this theory of localized medical knowledge had successfully penetrated the medical canon and received wide acceptance.[133] Although doctors who immigrated to the United States were not typically part of the elite, scholarly class that engaged in such debates, they were likely aware of major epistemological shifts and may have incorporated theories of lo-cal *qi* into their clinical work.

The majority of immigrant doctors received their training not in universities but in family businesses, and changes in that stratum of the Chinese medical profession would have had the most direct bearing on their work in the United States. In the late nineteenth century, family medicine was also rethinking its approach to drug therapy. Historian Volker Scheid has argued that the medical families of Menghe, a transport hub between the cities of Shanghai and Nanjing in the late Qing period, were particularly influential among clinicians of their social class. The descendants of Menghe physician Fei Boxiong promoted drug thera-pies that emphasized "harmonization and moderation" (*hehuan*, 和缓). Disciples of this therapeutic method from the 1880s into the early twen-tieth century aimed to prescribe "bland" or "light" drugs that worked in concert with one another over a long period to restore balance to the body.[134] According to Scheid, adopting this therapeutic method was a way for family doctors to distinguish their services from competitors of a lesser social rank, specifically folk healers, who tended to peddle powerful emetics and purgatives.[135] In its gentle, non-heroic approach to drug therapy, the principle of *hehuan* bore some similarity to the dis-course of natural medicine circulating in the United States, but its logic was not rooted in a concept of antimodern nature. Chinese physicians had to borrow the dichotomies of American "nature cures" to sell their non-dichotomous therapeutic principles to American patients.

A comparative consideration of Chinese-language advertisements in the United States suggests that Chinese doctors marketing their ser-vices to a co-ethnic clientele did not employ the language of natural medicine. In the pages of *Chung Sai Yat Po* (世界日報), a Chinese-language newspaper published out of San Francisco, health care providers—including two women—and drugstores advertised Chinese, Japanese, and Western medicine for sale in San Francisco, Chicago, and Los Angeles. In 1900, Ng Poon Chew, an immigrant from Canton, established the four-page daily to cater to his fellow Cantonese-speaking immigrants.[136] A sample of ninety-three health-related advertisements between 1900 and 1911, while far from conclusive, suggests several recurring themes in the marketing of Chinese medicine to Chinese patients.[137] The sample included no references *hehuan*, local *qi*, nor to other terms that might be linked to harmony, moderation, or balance. Instead, advertisements in *Chung Sai Yat Po* tended to emphasize the expertise of the practitioner and his or her reputation for curing diseases where other doctors had failed.[138] In eight advertisements in the sample, doctors employed the term *miao* (妙), describing their treatments as marvelous or miraculous.[139] Chinese-language advertisements also frequently remarked on the superior ingredients employed in the shop. The Tai Wo Company, a Chicago-based apothecary, maintained that is proprietary eye medicine was made from "high-quality material" (上品名藥).[140] San Francisco practitioners similarly ran advertisements between 1901 and 1904 that described their imported medicines as high-quality (上藥) or expensive (貴重之藥).[141] References to "miraculous" and other superlative language did not distinguish Chinese doctors from their American counterparts.

In the case of Tom She Bin, a physician with offices in San Francisco and Los Angeles, it is possible to compare his advertisements across Chinese, English, and Spanish. As early as 1889, Tom was promoting his services outside his Chinese community in the pages of the *Los Angeles Times* and later the *Los Angeles Herald, San Francisco Chronicle,* and *Sacramento Record-Union.*[142] He also reached out to patients in *Chung Sai Yat Po*, where he promised that his special, proprietary medicine would provide an instant and amazing effect (立服立止) for patients suffering from coughs and stomach ailments.[143] For the most part, his English- and Spanish-language advertisements played on similar themes, especially the ability of his tonics and other treatments to effect a cure where other doctors had failed. "He is a Medical Wonder!" an advertisement in the *Los Angeles Times* declared beneath an illustration of "Dr. Tom," dressed in the robes of a Mandarin scholar, taking the pulse of an elegantly attired woman.[144] In at least two English-language advertisements, however, Tom used the discourse of natural medicine to characterize his prescriptions. An 1898 advertisement in the *Sacramento Record-Union* explained Tom's exclusive use of "remedies, which are extracted from roots, bark, and herbs." Tom promised, "No minerals are used by us, we thus avoid the dire effects of poisons left in the system so often by the use of mineral remedies."[145] In a 1907 advertisement

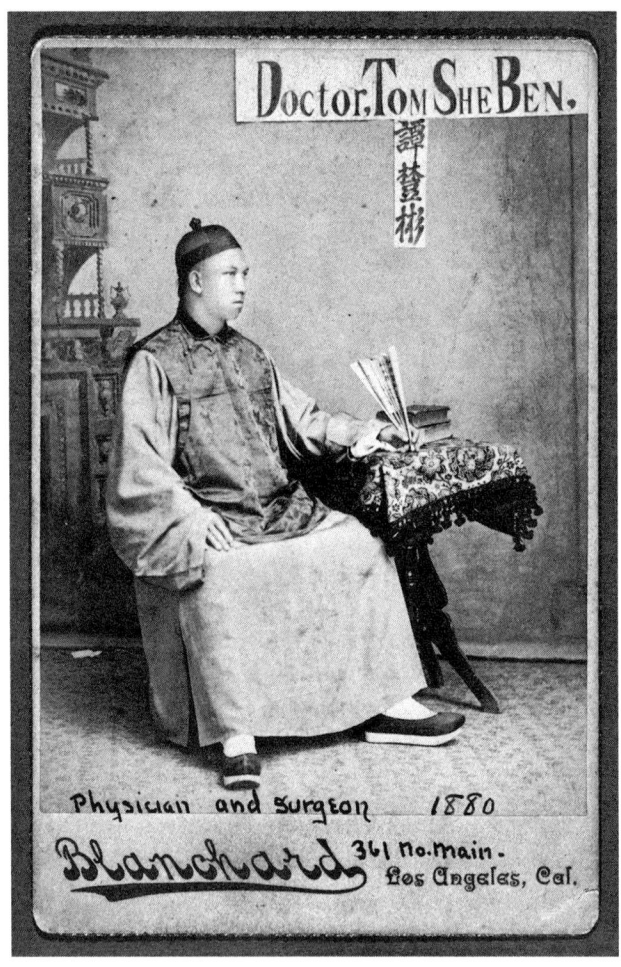

Tom She Bin trade card, 1880. Courtesy of the Huntington Library, San Marino, California, Hazard-Dyson Collection.

printed in the *Los Angeles Times*, Tom listed the many afflictions "readily cured through the natural medium of our 600 herbs and teas."[146]
The absence of the discourse of natural medicine in Chinese-language
advertisements suggests that Chinese doctors did not see *hehuan*, local
qi, or other principles related to environmental health as major selling
points for a co-ethnic clientele more interested in efficacy and quality.
Nature's frequent appearance in English-language advertisements, on
the other hand, suggests that Chinese doctors understood they were targeting a patient population with a very different set of cultural associations with nature and its relationship with irregular medicine. Although
non-Chinese patients in the late nineteenth- and early twentieth-century
United States may have interpreted Tom She Bin's "natural remedies" as
a translation of an exotic and ancient Chinese natural philosophy, it was
more likely an adoption of an American medical vernacular.

Conclusion

During the Progressive Era, concepts of nature, modernity, and Orientalism became entangled, and Chinese health practices and therapeutic
systems thrived in the spaces where medical scientists failed to assert
their authority. Efforts to discredit Chinese herbalists with the negative
tropes of Orientalism did not just fall short of their mark; they seem to
have had the ironic effect of deepening public interest in Chinese medicine. Chinese doctors crafted an image of Chinese medicine for American patient-consumers. It was an "ancient" science, boasting herbal
remedies that were simultaneously familiar and exotic, natural and
strange. Whether it was a form of capitulation or defensive strategy, that
approach enabled unlicensed Chinese physicians to distinguish themselves from their regular counterparts and appeal to patients distrustful
of state-sanctioned, "modern" medical science. In the coming decades,
new local and global challenges only reinforced the contradictions of
selling Chinese medicine in the American medical marketplace.

Decline

In 1971, a wrecking ball leveled eight blocks of squat wooden buildings in downtown Boise and with them Chinatown. A window recovered from the rubble reads, "Gerald H. Ah Fong, Chinese Remedies and Herbs," and it hangs in the Idaho State Historical Museum as part of an exhibit honoring Gerald's grandfather, C. K. Ah Fong.[1] From 1892 on, Ah Fong and subsequently his sons and grandson diagnosed illnesses and compounded herbs in two locations in Boise's Chinatown, which radiated from the corner of Capital Boulevard and Idaho Street. By the time Gerald etched his name on the window, Chinatown was fading. During the mining boom of the late nineteenth century, there had been several thousand Chinese moving about Idaho, but their numbers had declined to just over eight hundred in 1910 and then—after the Great Depression—roughly two hundred, concentrated in major urban centers like Boise and Coeur d'Alene. By 1970, Idaho's Chinese population had rebounded somewhat, with 498 Chinese men and women living in the state, and 116 in the Boise metropolitan area alone.[2]

Meanwhile, the overall population of Boise City was growing tremendously but unevenly. Between 1960 and 1970, the city more than doubled in size, but its new inhabitants gravitated toward the less-developed edges, stripping the urban core of its vitality and necessity.[3]

A writer for *Harper's Magazine* and a native Boisean noted that "downtown Boise gives the impression that it has recently been visited by an exceedingly tidy bombing raid conducted by planes that cleaned up after themselves." The neighborhood merchants, he acknowledged, put up a "brave show of doing business . . . but no one seems to be paying much attention."[4] Downtown Boise seemed ripe for redevelopment.

In the 1960s, federal programs offered funds for "urban renewal." It was a capacious term, and Boise's planners adopted a scorched earth interpretation of it. Their "renewal" involved razing retail shops, laundries, and restaurants and replacing them with an indoor shopping mall, spanning 800,000 square feet and orbited by a nebula of "satellite" parking lots with space for more than 4,000 cars. Downtown merchants and residents scattered. In the end, only Billy Fong held out. An eighty-four-year-old cook who worked at a local Chinese restaurant, the Golden Wok, Fong refused to leave until the rumbling of the approaching demolition trucks drove him, literally waving a white flag, from his home.[5] By that point, Gerald Ah Fong was long gone. He had retired to sunnier climes in California in 1964. There was no one to witness the destruction of his grandfather's legacy and the remnants of the community he had served.[6]

In a work of fiction, the razing of Boise Chinatown, and with it C. K. Ah Fong's herb shop, might seem like an overwrought and all-too-obvious symbol for the end of Chinese medicine in the United States. With a shopping mall of planetary proportions rising from the wreckage, a novelist might spin a tragic tale of traditional herbalism eclipsed by mass consumerism in the post–World War II era. Indeed, Chinese herbalists struggled mightily in the middle decades of the twentieth century. They fought through the lean years of the Great Depression only to face a spate of wars in Asia that severed supply lines across the Pacific and made it difficult, if not impossible, for them to restock apothecary shelves. Consequently, as historian Haiming Liu has argued, the American Chinese herb business "shrank rapidly" in this period.[7] Global economic and political crises were not the only threats to the livelihood of Chinese herbalists in the United States. Early to mid-twentieth-century innovations in science and marketing heralded the dawn of a "Golden Age" of biomedicine, which made it more difficult for Chinese herbalists to compete in the American medical marketplace.[8] At the same time, World War II and the Cold War expanded opportunities for Chinese immigrants and American-born Chinese to pursue careers in licensed medical professions, which diminished the status of Chinese herbalists within their communities.

The Chinese American Herb Business in Depression and War

Between 1930 and 1970, Chinese herbalists continued treating a mixed-race clientele with herbalism, pulsology, and other traditional Chinese therapies, and their advertising pitch remained unchanged.[9] English-language advertisements from the 1940s reflect that Chinese herbalists still marketed to non-Chinese patients with the well-rehearsed themes of ancient, miraculous, and natural remedies. Dr. Wing's Herbs encouraged readers of the *Los Angeles Times* to learn how to "regain health naturally" by writing away for a free booklet or visiting his office on South Vermont Street for a free consultation. "Why suffer when natural Chinese herbs may be able to help you?" the advertisements asked. "Let the wisdom gathered through the ages relieve you in a simple, natural way."[10] Direct appeals to women also persisted with promises of special attention to their health concerns. A 1943 advertisement for Los Angeles doctor T. B. Chew included a testimonial from Eunice Tedford, who "report[ed] amazing recovery from female trouble!"[11] The promise of the "free consultation" allowed Chinese herbalists to circumvent medical practice laws by concealing the diagnosis behind the sale of unregulated herbal remedies.[12]

Yet, in some ways, the middle decades of the twentieth century also seemed like an end to an era. First-generation Chinese doctors had come to the United States as young men in the late nineteenth century. By 1940, they were either quite elderly or dead. C. K. Ah Fong died in 1927.[13] Tom Leung of Los Angeles passed away in 1931.[14] His cousin and mentor Tom Foo Yuen outlived him by sixteen years.[15] Yitang Chang died in 1952.[16] In eastern Oregon, Ing Hay survived until 1952 (his business partner Lung On died in 1940), but the herbalist was nearly blind and too infirm in the final decade of his life to practice medicine.[17] N. S.

Sue, the Modesto physician memorialized by his son Thomas W. Wing in the memoir *Son of South Mountain and Dust,* retired in the 1930s and went to live out his days in Los Angeles.[18]

In many cases, relatives—mostly sons, grandsons, and nephews, or occasionally widows—inherited the herb businesses after deaths or retirements, but world events conspired against these second-generation Chinese doctors. The Great Depression affected Chinese herb shops as it did any other business. Tom Leung's widow, Bing Woo, and his son Taft tried and failed to make their mail-order business offset the loss of foot traffic to their two shops in Los Angeles. They eventually gave up their lease on one space and laid off their one nonfamilial employee (who moved to Pomona to open his own herb shop).[19] For a few years thereafter, Bing Woo and Taft ran a reduced clinic and apothecary out of their home with the mother compounding prescriptions in the kitchen and her American-born, English-speaking son receiving patients in the front parlor.[20]

If the Great Depression delivered the initial blow, the series of midcentury wars in East Asia was the knockout punch for many Chinese apothecaries. The Sino-Japanese War that began in 1937 rolled into the global conflagration of World War II. The conflict disrupted trade between wholesalers in China and shops in the United States. As it became increasingly difficult to import traditional remedies from China, some herbalists exited the health care profession altogether. Taft Leung found alternate work as an accountant for Chinatown merchants, and he and his mother closed down the family herb business.[21] When World War II made it impossible to stock his Tucson apothecary, Chan Doo Sung, the roving herbalist who had opened and closed a series of Chan and Kong Herb Stores across the Far West, abandoned medicine and became a cashier at a local restaurant.[22] The end of World War II did not restore the supply chain between China and the United States. After the Communist takeover of China in 1949, the United States imposed a ban on Chinese imports that later escalated into a formal suspension of trade between the countries during the Korean War. That embargo remained in place until the Nixon administration normalized relations with China in 1971.[23] As a result, scarce imported medicines became even scarcer.[24]

The Chinese herb business in the United States undoubtedly struggled and probably did diminish in the middle decades of the twentieth century, but it is difficult to quantify the decline. While English-language directories fail to capture the practitioners who advertised only in Chinese-language media or by word of mouth, comparisons across the years for Los Angeles and San Francisco—the American cities with the largest Chinese populations—can at least suggest the direction and magnitude of change that the herb business experienced. In 1940, the Los Angeles Directory Company included thirty-seven Chinese herbalists; six years later, the Western Directory Company named a few more, with forty-five listings for herbalists in the city.[25] These numbers generally accord with Los Angeles herbalist Garding Lui's estimate that there were about 120 practitioners of traditional Chinese medicine working in California, with about 40 in Los Angeles in 1948.[26] Seven years into the U.S. trade embargo on China in 1956, the Pacific Telephone and Telegraph Company Directory listed only twelve Los Angeles herbalists, nearly a 75 percent decline over a decade. It is possible that the other herbalists moved out of Los Angeles to a lower-rent city or that they removed themselves from the city directory, but their absence may also reflect a precipitous decline in the herb business. In San Francisco, the city directories show a less dramatic but earlier drop off that the embargo cannot explain. In 1940, the Polk's Crocker Langley Directory listed forty-six Chinese herb companies and herbalists in San Francisco, but only thirty-two in 1948 and the same number in the 1955–1956 edition.[27] These data suggest that while Chinese herb companies in the United States may not have thrived or expanded in this period, many did survive. How did they do it?

Chinese herbalists pursued legal and extralegal strategies to cope with the various setbacks of the mid-twentieth century. As supplies of imported herbs dwindled and prices soared, foresighted herbalists stockpiled a reserve.[28] Others found viable substitutions. Yitang Chang shifted his business to Japanese wholesalers who moved their product through the British-held Hong Kong instead of Canton.[29] In some cases, domestic sourcing was possible. In New York City, a Chinese restauranteur, Sou Chan, reached out to a supplier of snakes and wildcats in Brownsville, Texas, who sold the medicinal animals for fifty cents

a pound plus the cost of shipping.[30] In Los Angeles, Garding Lui remarked on the "abundant production" of medicinal herbs in the United
States, Mexico, and Canada although he conceded that even "with all
that, it was exceedingly hard [for Chinese doctors] to get anything desired."[31] In John Day, Oregon, Ing Hay's nephew Bob Wah, an herbalist
who came from Idaho to take over Kam Wah Chung from his elderly
uncle around 1940, used local plants and animals but only reluctantly.
He complained that they were weaker, so much so that each prescription seemed to require a greater quantity of the ingredient to be effective.[32] Nonetheless, by these means, Wah kept his uncle's business going
until 1948.[33]

Smuggling herbs was another solution to the supply chain problem.
In the early years of the embargo, the *San Francisco Examiner* reported
that the Oy Wo Tong Company had been raided for illegally smuggling
herbs from China.[34] In 1959, federal marshals arrested ten men—seven
Chinese and three Canadians—who transported Chinese herbs across
the Canadian border to Chicago and Memphis for distribution across
the country. By these means, the ring had brought more than a million
dollars' worth of contraband into the country in just a few years.[35]

In addition to making do with the limited medicine that managed
to cross the Pacific, Chinese herbalists diversified their skillset by studying other areas of medicine. During the Depression and war, Garding
Lui counted twelve of the city's forty or so herbalists who had become
licensed chiropractors.[36] Advertisements from the 1940s for Los Angeles herbalist G. S. Wong emphasized his experience in both Chinese
herbalism and "American" physical therapy. By so doing, he promised
his patients the best of both the "ancient and new."[37] From a business
perspective, diversification presented some clear, practical advantages.
Becoming a licensed chiropractor or physical therapist offered protection from arrests and fines for unlicensed herbalists, but perhaps more
importantly for this era, it reduced their dependence on a dwindling
supply of imported medicines.

While training in other therapeutic systems may have been a common strategy among Chinese herbalists, it is not obvious how it transformed the practice of Chinese medicine in the United States. Scholars
including Paul D. Buell, Linda L. Barnes, and Sarah Christine Heffner

have studied how Chinese doctors adapted their therapeutic practices in the United States, but more work is necessary to understand the full extent of the changes, particularly for practitioners who sought out formal credentialing in other medical systems.[38] The case of Los Angeles herbalist Tseung Bowquong Chew suggests that such training altered neither the image nor the primary offerings of Chinese herbalists in the medical marketplace. During World War II, self-described "Famous Herb Specialist, T. B. Chew" enrolled in a three-year course of study at the Southern California College of Chiropractic.[39] Becoming a chiropractor might have opened up new opportunities for his business, but he never seems to have practiced what he learned.[40]

Trained as a traditional herbalist in Canton, Chew immigrated to the United States in 1915, just two years after the birth of his second child and namesake. He initially settled in San Francisco, with his wife, daughter, and son soon joining him in 1920, and the reunited family opened an herb shop on Clay Street in the heart of Chinatown. By 1924, Chew had another daughter—Mary—and his wife had died. These tumultuous life changes may have prompted him to relocate to Los Angeles, where he opened one store in the city's Chinatown and another in Santa Monica. Chew quickly remarried and had two more sons, and they all squeezed in to the back quarters of Chew's Santa Monica office. Years later, his eldest son would recall that "ninety-nine percent" of his father's patients were American.[41] In 1940, the U.S. Census Bureau found "Thomas" B. Chew still living in Santa Monica (although no longer in the back of his herb shop). His oldest daughter was married to a Chinatown dentist, and his sons were off studying in China. Only his American-born daughter, eighteen-year-old Mary, remained at home.[42] The Great Depression and World War II were hard on the business. During that time, Chew embarked on a new phase of his career as a licensed chiropractor. It did not last long. In 1947, Chew retired to China.[43]

If Chew's training as a chiropractor materially changed his practice, it was not apparent in his advertisements or his legacy. Throughout the 1930s and 1940s, his business continued to run the same advertisements promising cures for a wide spectrum of ailments using traditional herbs ("nature's way to a healthy life") and made no mention of chiropractic therapies.[44] After his retirement, he left the practice to his eldest son, also a licensed chiropractor, who carried it on at least until 1972, when a reporter for the *Los Angeles Times* profiled the business. As the reporter flipped through the testimonial scrapbooks in the office waiting room, he noted, "The letters are not about the chiropractic methods [Chew] is licensed to use. They are from people who have been treated with Chinese herbal medicine."[45] Despite the myriad difficulties they faced, for Chew and his son, herbalism remained the core of the business and the basis of their reputation among patients.

Biomedicine's Golden Age

Through adaptation and substitution, smuggling, and sheer grit and determination, Chinese doctors pushed through the difficult middle decades of the twentieth century. For these small business owners, the global crises that disrupted herbal supply lines and affected the bottom line were obvious setbacks to overcome, but they faced more nebulous challenges as well. In both the United States and China, biomedical scientists were successfully consolidating their social authority. The outbreak of World War I propelled new discoveries in health science. From the late nineteenth century, the industrial giant Germany had led the world in pharmaceutical development. As the Allied powers mobilized for war, their governments vigorously invested in their domestic drug industries to keep soldiers healthy and reduce their dependence on the Germans.[46] Pharmaceutical innovation—particularly the discovery of antimicrobial compounds called sulfonamides—flourished in the 1930s. The interlocking interests of government, academic medicine, and pharmaceutical corporations created research partnerships that produced a multitude of "wonder drugs" in the 1930s and 1940s, most famously penicillin, which had been discovered in 1928 but was not mass-produced until 1942.

In the United States, biomedical scientists—who commanded state boards and major medical colleges—were in a prime position to take advantage of new federal funds flowing to research institutions and hospitals. In 1938, the Food, Drug, and Cosmetic Act (FDCA) a revision to the old, toothless Pure Food and Drug Act, raised the barriers of entry in the pharmaceutical industry, and new patent laws protecting proprietary remedies made it more profitable to be in the business of making drugs. During World War II, antibiotics, synthesized in laboratories and produced in factories, saved tens of thousands of people who might have otherwise died from infections, and the American pharmaceutical industry surged ahead of its counterpart in war-torn Germany. In peacetime, the pace of innovation continued at an even more astounding rate. Alongside antibiotics, researchers discovered new classes of drugs like antidepressants and diuretics.[47] Military doctors and surgeons returned from the war to find that advances in drug therapy and federal research monies permitted them to apply their hard-won experience and make progress in other areas of health care like cardiology, cardio-thoracic surgery, and transplant surgery.[48] For Chinese herbalists who appealed to patient fears of drugs and surgery, the great leap forward for biomedicine in the mid-twentieth century dulled their competitive edge.

Across the Pacific, China was experiencing a parallel revolution in its medical institutions and cultures. Despite the efforts of British and American medical missionaries, Western-style scientific medicine was a negligible part of the Chinese medical marketplace up until the early twentieth century. The Qing government's reforms to its civil service examinations in 1905 created more opportunities for Chinese men and women to travel abroad to study medicine, particularly in Japan, where Meiji Era modernization had sidelined indigenous medical traditions and permitted a German-style system of education to flourish. With their freshly inked diplomas, Chinese students returned to their homeland to establish the country's first scientific medical professional organizations between 1907 and 1915.[49] Although Chinese patients largely continued to rely on traditional practices, Chinese medical scientists pressured government officials to emulate Japanese, European, and American models of medical regulation and education. A strong and "modern" state, they argued, rejected "superstitious" healing traditions.[50] In the late Qing and early Republican periods, their rhetorical efforts gained traction in public health initiatives that combated epidemic disease and expanded rural health care by drawing on the expertise of Western-style scientists.[51] When the Nationalists came to power in 1928, Western-style medical scientists wrested control of the newly established Ministry of Health and secured government funding for Western-style medical colleges.

Emboldened by the political support, Western-style doctors ramped up their efforts to push aside traditional Chinese medicine. They convened a national conference and unanimously passed a resolution entitled "Abolishing Old-Style Medicine in Order to Clear Away the Obstacles to Medicine and Public Health." Although practitioners of traditional Chinese medicine effectively thwarted the attempt to transform the resolution into policy, medical scientists managed to maintain a privileged position within the nascent national system of health care.[52]

Perhaps most importantly, in this era many traditional Chinese medicine doctors realized their political survival depended on making their practices consonant with scientific methods and epistemologies. Historian Volker Scheid has argued that the selective assimilation of Western medical knowledge into traditional practices dated back to the earliest contact with the system in the Ming Dynasty, but China's culture wars in the 1920s and 1930s elevated the stakes of remaking Chinese medicine. The state's campaign for modernization seemed to pivot on Western-style scientism. During the Republican period, Chinese reforms to traditional medical education and practice ranged from a wholesale purge of the mystical and the metaphysical to a subtler reimagining of therapeutic tenets to make them harmonize with Western-style theories of physiology, pathology, and pharmacology.[53] All but the most conservative doctors thus had to concede that Western-style empiricism should guide the integration of traditional Chinese practices into modern health care.[54] To reject science was to lose a seat at the political table.

The distance of an ocean, even one as vast as the Pacific, did not insulate overseas Chinese from changes to medical cultures back home. As described in chapter 2, Chinese immigrants to the United States had always experimented with European, American, and other non-Chinese healing practices. For specific problems like cataracts and trachoma as well as acute conditions including infections, fractures, and other traumas, the Chinese preferred Western-style medicine if given the choice.[55] Brothers Eugene and Harvey Leong, whose family ran an herb shop in Bakersfield, California, until 1945, recalled that their mother treated them with Chinese herbs except in two instances: once when their sister Ruth suffered an acute case of appendicitis, and again when Eugene required a tonsillectomy.[56]

Early twentieth-century advertisements in the *Chung Sai Yat Po* suggest a more general attraction to "scientific medicine" among immigrant patient-consumers. Some Chinese doctors advertising to a co-ethnic clientele emphasized their experience in American or European hospitals or training with "Western" doctors. In advertisements for his San Francisco dental practice, Charlie Fong described himself as a licensed practitioner trained by Westerners when he was young (少遊西學).[57] Lee Chai Leong's 1904 advertisement stated that he had special access to combinations of Western and Chinese medicine, capable of curing near-fatal diseases (西醫學堂).[58] References from Western patients might also have served as evidence of a Chinese practitioner's expertise and widely held esteem. An advertisement for Mack Q. Ying from 1901 offered testimony from prestigious Western patients, including mention of a gift of an inscribed plaque honoring his service from the Fresno Police Department (警局送區額).[59] While this marketing strategy may have been a manifestation of the pro-assimilationist politics of the newspaper's founder, Ng Poon Chew, it likely also reflected the growing popularity of Western-style scientific medicine among the Chinese.[60]

Western-style biomedical care gradually became more available to Chinese American communities over the second half of the twentieth century. In major cities, bilingual social workers organized Chinatown health teams to connect low-income immigrants with public health services. When UCLA ethnographer Alvin Yiu-Cheong So canvassed Los Angeles's Chinatown in the 1970s, he observed that the ethnic Chinese community (which included new arrivals from Hong Kong, Taiwan, and Vietnam) used Western-style biomedicine and traditional Chinese medicine almost interchangeably: "As soon as the Chinese patients think the Western medical treatment is ineffective, they will turn to Chinese traditional medicine for help."[61] A growing number of Chinese and Chinese American M.D.s opened private practice offices in Chinatowns and offered consultations in multiple Chinese dialects. So noted a marked decade over decade increase in the number of M.D.s, seeing fifty, sixty, or more ethnic Chinese patients each day.[62] Across the country, Chun-Wai Chan and Jade K. Chang studied the health practices of New York City's Chinese immigrants—primarily working-class men and women from Hong Kong—and found that the overwhelming majority exclusively saw M.D.s when seeking professional medical care. Chan and Chang summarized the sentiment among their respondents: "Going to traditional practitioners is cheaper, requiring less time and involving fewer painful procedures, but . . . Western doctors are actually more reliable and more accessible."[63]

Medicine and the Model Minority

The increased presence of Chinese and Chinese American M.D.s in the American medical marketplace was in large part a result of changing diplomatic relations between the United States and China during World War II and the Cold War. On December 17, 1943, the United States lifted the restrictions on Chinese immigration first established by the Exclusion Act of 1882. China was an ally of the United States in the war against Japan, and, in the words of President Franklin Roosevelt, the repeal of exclusion "represent[ed] a manifestation on the part of the American people of their affection and regard."[64]

In the same month, the *Ladies' Home Journal* published a glossy spread featuring three generations of James Hinquong Hall's Chinese American family, all smartly dressed in Western-style "sports shirts" and "frilly clothes" in their California home.[65] Hall was a doctor but not an herbalist. He had graduated from Stanford Medical School and completed an internship at San Francisco Hospital. After a year of postgraduate training at Peking Union Medical College, he returned to the United States to settle in Los Altos, not far from his alma mater. He then worked his way toward a position as the chief of staff at the Chinese Hospital on Jackson Street in San Francisco's Chinatown.[66] The circumstances of James Hall's life, admiringly portrayed in the pages of the *Ladies' Home Journal,* signaled a new chapter in the social history of Chinese immigrant doctors. Although there had been a few exceptional Chinese M.D.s in the late nineteenth and early twentieth centuries, Hall was at the forefront of a generational wave of Chinese men and women who received degrees from American medical colleges and who pursued careers in licensed medical professions in the United States.

In the mid-twentieth century, members of Hall's generation benefited from the United States' rapprochement with China. While the

Chinese Nationalist government had encouraged its citizens to seek out technical and scientific training in the United States as early as the 1920s and 1930s, cooperation between the governments in the area of international education deepened during and just after World War II. Initially, these technical and scientific exchanges were designed as a means to cultivate diplomatic relationships with future foreign leaders, but they evolved into efforts to meet the labor needs of American industries and military.[67]

American universities welcomed young Chinese men and women as "exemplary international students," particularly when they devoted themselves to courses of study in the sciences or engineering, fields with obvious utility for a country racing to out-modernize and out-compete its Communist rivals.[68] Widening opportunities in education first flowed to Chinese nationals taking up temporary residence in the United States, but they eventually trickled down to American-born Chinese as well.[69]

The Cold War created new incentives for the federal government to liberalize its immigration policies in ways that permitted the entry of scientifically and technically skilled workers, or knowledge-workers. All major immigration legislation from this era—the Displaced Persons Act of 1948, the McCarran-Walter Act of 1952, the Refugee Relief Act of 1953, and the Hart-Cellar Act of 1965, and other one-time measures— created special provisions for immigrants with economically or strategically useful training, including physicians, surgeons, nurses, and dentists.[70] A perceived doctor shortage in the United States that dated back to World War II seemed to grow more acute in the postwar decades and spurred the recruitment of foreign medical graduates, especially from Africa and Asia.[71] Among the Chinese in the United States, the wave of students and knowledge-workers admitted under such exemptions was a tiny fraction of the overall population. In 1960, they numbered just 5,000 out of 237,292 Chinese and Chinese Americans enumerated by the U.S. Census, but, as historian Madeline Hsu has argued, their professional visibility and success paved the way for American-born Chinese to step out of ethnic economic niches and into the "middle-class mainstream."[72] By 1960, the U.S. Bureau of the Census reported that the number of Chinese in professional and technical occupations had grown to 17 percent, compared to 2.5 percent in 1940. The Bureau of the Census also found that Chinese men and women had completed some years of college education at higher rates than white or black Americans.[73] By the 1980s, the Asian American model minority myth conveyed the stereotype of Asians as genetically and culturally predisposed to mathematical and scientific superiority.[74]

Rising expectations of aptitude helped open doors for Chinese American men and women at American medical colleges. Whereas herbalism might have been the only medical career open to their parents, Chinese American sons and daughters were becoming chiropractors, dentists, pharmacists, physical therapists, nurses, osteopaths, and biomedical doctors. Beginning as early as the 1930s but accelerating in the post–World War II period, graduation records from the American medical colleges nearest to San Francisco—the city with the largest Chinese American population—reflected a small but growing cohort of American-born Chinese M.D.s. Prior to 1930, only two Chinese Americans—Shin Tive Pond Mooar Jee and Carl Leslie Hong—had graduated from the University of California, San Francisco. The medical school at Stanford University did not admit its first American-born Chinese student—David Kiong Chang—until 1928. After 1930, however, both schools consistently graduated one or more Chinese American students each year, with gaps during and just after World War II.[75]

In the 1930s, mainstream medical professions threw up significant barriers before the children of Chinese immigrants, but they no longer seemed insurmountable. During the Great Depression, Thomas W. Wing, an American-born son of Modesto physician N. S. Sue, attended junior college in Los Angeles. He knew that he wanted to follow his father's footsteps into the medical field, but having observed the elderly herbalist's struggles with the Food and Drug Administration and state medical board, he was reluctant to pursue the study of Chinese medicine. Many years later, he recalled, "It was clear to me that the profession [of Chinese medicine] was fading fast." His memoirs reflect the ambivalence that the young Chinese American man felt as he weighed his career options. He worried that if he abandoned Chinese medicine, he would lose his patients' presumption of embodied authority: "I knew Americans wouldn't come to me if I were a chiropractor, but the license would protect me from arrest and medical harassment . . . If I became an M.D., I would learn modern diagnosis, the use of clinical and laboratory testing, and have no patients." Wing applied to the Southern California College of Chiropractic. He believed the therapy offered the best blend of traditional Chinese holism and Western-style biomedicine: "I had grown up in Chinese medicine learning about balancing the flow of energy throughout the body. I wanted to learn Western diagnosis and apply it to my knowledge in Chinese herbs. The chiropractic approach made sense to me. For me, it was the ideal way to go."[76]

First-generation Chinese doctors encouraged their children to pursue medical careers outside of traditional Chinese therapies. Second-generation Chinese health practitioners recall their parents pushing them toward biomedicine, pharmacy, and other licensed professions because of the security and status they held in American culture. Having endured more than twenty arrests, Oakland doctor Fong Wan understandably felt as though he were under constant siege by the state medical board. A career in herbalism was too insecure, so even though he employed his eldest sons, Richard and Edward, as apprentices in his shop, he forced them to apply to American medical colleges. Edward became a radiologist and did not look back, but Richard—a family practitioner—married Gracina Ding, the daughter of a San Francisco herbalist, and initially worked out of his father's Tenth Street apothecary. Even after he moved offices, Richard continued to prescribe herbal remedies to his patients. Fong's third child—a daughter, Evelyn—became a chiropractor and sublet office space in the family herb shop.[77]

American-born Arthur W. Chung descended from a family of Chinese herbalists. In Canton, his grandfather, three of his uncles, and one brother were in the herb business. His father, Yitang Chang, apprenticed in a Cantonese herb shop before immigrating to the United States and opening an apothecary at the corner of Seventh and Hill Streets in downtown Los Angeles. Arthur was born in the family home, just two blocks from the shop, in 1913. During the Depression, the herb business struggled, and Chung's father sent him back to China in hopes that the economy would improve while the young man was away. A decade later, Chung finally returned to Los Angeles with a degree in Western-style medicine from Shanghai Medical School. With some additional training at Harvard Medical School, New York's Bellevue Hospital, and the Los Angeles County Hospital, Chung became a pathologist. His father, the herbalist, was supportive of the decision. It seemed to both the elder and younger Chungs that it would be easier for a Chinese man to make it in America with a professional degree.[78]

Struggling to keep an herb business afloat during the Great Depression also convinced herbalist Tom J. Chong that his American-born son Paul should pursue a degree in Western-style medical science rather than take over the chain of apothecaries the family had established in the greater Los Angeles area. Unable to pay for medical school tuition, Paul Tom recalled, "pharmacy was the next best thing." In 1933, Tom became a licensed pharmacist, and with a handful of Chinese business partners, he opened the first Chinese-owned, Western-style drugstore in Los Angeles. Located on "the Plaza," the historic center of the city, Tom's drugstore sold makeup and ice cream alongside pharmaceuticals to a mix of Chicano and Chinese customers. Decades later, an interviewer asked Tom if he attempted to continue the tradition of Chinese herbalism in his career as a pharmacist, but Tom said no. He explained that his entire family used "western medicine and stopped believing in Chinese herbs."[79]

Chinese M.D.s often had conflicted feelings about traditional Chinese medicine. Margaret Jessie Chung, the first known American-born Chinese woman to receive an M.D. from an American medical college, encountered a challenging professional environment after she completed her studies at the University of Southern California in 1916. Chung intended to become a medical missionary to China, but after the Presbyterian missionary society rejected her application, she floundered. As her biographer, Judy Tzu-Chun Wu, has argued, Chung's circuitous career path stemmed from an ambivalent relationship with her heritage and with other members of the Chinese immigrant community. After graduation, Chung briefly accepted a nursing position before securing an internship and residency at a Chicago hospital, dabbled with the settlement house movement in Chicago, and then returned to Los Angeles to become a surgeon to musicians and movie stars. She famously performed a tonsillectomy on silent-film darling Mary Pickford.[80]

In 1920, Chung fulfilled her missionary dream of bringing "modern" medicine to the Chinese by opening a clinic in San Francisco's

Chinatown in the 1920s, but her open disdain for Chinese traditions—
including traditional medicine—and her limited Chinese-language skills
as well as, importantly, her gender made it difficult for Chung to integrate into the local medical community. She became a target for criticism
and even outright defamation among her colleagues, including James
Hinquong Hall, who was chief of surgery at the San Francisco Chinese
Hospital. Sexist suspicions of sexual promiscuity and homosexuality
circled around Chung and shrank her roster of Chinese patients. Increasingly, she provided services to European American health-tourists,
primarily middle-class men who found it thrilling and perhaps titillat-
ing to receive Western-style medical treatment from an Asian woman
in the distinctly "Oriental" setting of her Chinatown office. Even with a
degree and a license to practice medicine, Margaret Chung had to self-
Orientalize to compete in the American medical marketplace.[81]

For those who primarily worked with Chinese immigrant communities, traditional medicine could sometimes seem like a challenge
to overcome. When the medical staff at the San Francisco Chinese Hospital solicited brief autobiographies from its founding doctors, one of
them, D. K. Chang, who had received his M.D. from Stanford University, named the "many problems that I had to confront at the beginning
of my practice in 1928" with "the herbalist" near the top of the list. He
recalled that his patients' "strong belief in Chinese herbs" was an "ob-
stacle to meet and tackle," and lamented the loss of patients who refused surgeries and opted instead to self-medicate with traditional remedies.[82] Another early Chinese Hospital physician, Helen Tong Chinn,
a graduate of the medical college at the University of California, San
Francisco, mourned the death of children whose immigrant parents refused to vaccinate "because everyone was suspicious of strange [West-
ern] medications."[83]

Members of the American Chinese Medical Society (ACMS), a
professional club for Chinese biomedical scientists in the United States,
took pains to distance their professional identities from practitioners
of traditional Chinese medicine. First organized in New York in 1964,
the ACMS brought together Chinese biomedical scientists who had immigrated to the United States as refugees in the 1950s. Such professional
groups were common among foreign doctors, and indeed the ACMS

modeled its constitution and bylaws on the American Hungarian Medical Society. Like other organizations of its kind, the ACMS served as a social node for a community that shared a common language, national origin, and vocation, but for members of the ACMS, there was an added incentive: Chinese biomedical doctors needed to differentiate themselves from practitioners of traditional Chinese therapies like herbalism, pulsology, and—eventually—acupuncture.

The organization's bylaws quite deliberately excluded from full membership anyone without a degree from a medical, osteopathic, or dental college.[84] At the same time, the ACMS newsletter, printed four times per year and mostly in Chinese, translated scientific papers and journal articles authored by its members and announced awards and other achievements. In that way, the newsletter underscored the contributions of Chinese American M.D.s to the biomedical field. In 1973, the group raised funds for a scholarship to support young Chinese American men and women pursuing an M.D. or D.D.S. degree and an annual scientific award honoring a member for outstanding research in biomedicine. In 1985, the organization took the next step to differentiate its members from practitioners of traditional Chinese medicine by adopting a new name: the Chinese American Medical Society. Interposing "American" between "Chinese" and "Medicine" retained the expression of identity shared by its members but underscored their insistence that they "knew little to nothing" about traditional therapies.[85]

In the 1960s and 1970s, Chinese American social workers collaborated with biomedical professionals on publications that linked poverty in Chinatowns to Chinese immigrants' adherence to their traditional remedies.[86] In 1971, Frederick P. Li, an M.D. who had emigrated from Canton as a child and worked at the National Cancer Institute's field station in Boston, and Elaine Shiang, a medical student at Harvard, published a report of a case in *JAMA*. The report concerned Li and Shiang's observations of the Chinese immigrants in Boston and the dangers of their adherence to ancient medical practices. In the report, Li and Shiang described the case of a twenty-year-old male college student from Hong Kong who suffered severe gastro-intestinal distress over a period of seven months. Rather than submit to biomedical care, the student treated himself with Chinese herbs and acupuncture. Within a year, he had died of liver cancer. Li and Shiang stressed that the young man's death could have been avoided had he not delayed "proper therapy," meaning Western-style biomedical treatment.[87] The *JAMA* report reflected the difficult position that Chinese American M.D.s occupied in the American medical marketplace. Their heritage and language skills allowed them to work with Chinese immigrant communities in ways not always possible for their non-Chinese colleagues, but they resisted seeming too sympathetic to "unscientific" healing practices. Li and Shiang's rejection of Chinese herbalism and acupuncture signaled their belonging among biomedical scientists.

Conclusion

By the time that Ah Fong's apothecary met the wrecking ball in downtown Boise in 1971, Chinese herbalists had endured three decades of economic depression and wars. Survival in such a business environment required making do with local substitutes, smuggling illegal imports, or diversifying into new services. It could also lead to letting go of failing family businesses. The ascendance of biomedicine in the early twentieth century heightened competition for herbalists in the medical marketplace. At the same time, new opportunities in licensed medical professions for their children and grandchildren made traditional medicine less of a necessity within the Chinese American community. Many members of this generation had an ambivalent relationship with traditional Chinese medicine or even actively rejected it. The rising numbers of Chinese American men and women pursuing careers in biomedical professions might have spelled the demise of traditional Chinese therapies, particularly in the United States, where its roots were not so deep and its practitioners were relatively few. But it did not.

In the middle decades of the twentieth century, patient-consumer habits and the demographics of medical professionals were changing. The new landscape of American health care, monopolized by biomedical politics and institutions, might have seemed to diminish demand for traditional Chinese medicine, but it did quite the opposite: it created an opening for its resurgence.

Rediscovery

The decline of Chinese medicine in the United States laid the basis for its eventual rediscovery and revival in the 1970s. In 1971, the same year that Boise razed its Chinatown, a celebrated American journalist named James Reston underwent an emergency appendectomy in a Beijing hospital. Grumpy and gassy the following day, he acquiesced to a course of acupuncture for post-operative pain relief and broadcast his experience to the readers of the *New York Times*. Reston's article was a perfectly timed catalyst for a process already under way. New developments in American medical consumerism and the changing demographics of Chinese American communities explain the sudden surge of popularity of Chinese acupuncture in the early 1970s.[1] Dissatisfaction with the so-called Golden Age of American biomedicine primed a critical segment of affluent patient-consumers to seek out alternatives, including traditional Chinese medicine. At the same time, World War II and the Communist takeover of China in 1949 yielded an exodus of refugees, including trained acupuncturists. Thus, the metaphoric wrecking ball did not destroy Chinese medicine as the actual one did to Ah Fong's shop in downtown Boise. The middle decades of the twentieth century comprised an era of deaths, retirements, and disappearances, but in unexpected and unintended ways, these endings created new beginnings.

"An Experimental Porcupine"

On July 15, 1971, clad in a gray suit and blue tie fashionably coordinated with the podium and draperies, President Richard Nixon appeared in a live television broadcast from the White House to announce that he would travel to China in February of the following year. The historic visit was the culmination of National Security Advisor Henry Kissinger's efforts to accelerate the normalization of relations with China after two decades of estrangement. Nixon, with Kissinger's encouragement, hoped that restoring communication and trade with Communist China would earn the country's support as the United States pressured North Vietnam to negotiate an end to the Vietnam War.[2] One day after Nixon's announcement and over six thousand miles away in a Beijing hotel, the *New York Times* vice president and columnist James "Scotty" Reston doubled over with a sharp pain in his abdomen. Reston was one of a handful of elite journalists who received permission from the Chinese government, beginning in April 1971, to tour the country and reintroduce its culture and people to the American public in advance of Nixon's historic visit.[3] Eight days into a six-week tour, Reston suffered an acute case of appendicitis, underwent surgery at the Anti-Imperialist Hospital in Beijing, and then received acupuncture for postoperative pain from Li Chang-yuan, a thirty-six-year-old staff acupuncturist at the hospital.[4]

The presence of a staff acupuncturist at a state hospital was most proximately the result of Mao Zedong's medical policy, but the initial revival of the therapy dated back to China's Republican Era. During the nineteenth century, the Chinese elite had relegated acupuncture to the lower strata of health care, but in the 1930s, Dan'an Cheng, a scholar-physician, famously rehabilitated its image among his class by simplifying, secularizing, and effectively "scientizing" the ancient needle therapy. Cheng had studied both traditional Chinese medicine and Western-style medicine in Shanghai in the 1920s, but he first came to appreciate acupuncture as a patient, seeking relief from debilitating back pain. His successful course of treatment led him to found the first acupuncture correspondence college in Wuxi in 1930 and, three years later, the nation's first acupuncture journal. In 1934, Cheng went to

Japan to study the style of acupuncture that had evolved there. Japanese medical reformers had applied Western-style medical principles
of anatomy and physiology to the ancient Chinese concepts of channels and meridians. Cheng built on those foundations. He linked the
mechanism of acupuncture to the nerves and revised the placement and
number of acupoints—sites where a practitioner inserts the needles.
He recommended the use of very fine metal needles, which eliminated
the bloodletting once associated with the release of *qi*, and he discouraged burning moxa too close to the skin, which could cause scarring.
Significantly, he also rejected the use of astrology or divination, which
had historically determined the timing of treatment. Historians have argued that Cheng's "revisions" essentially reinvented acupuncture. His
work shaped the therapy's teaching and practice in postwar China and
its eventual dissemination to the rest of the world.[5]

Modernized and simplified, acupuncture became part of China's
national health care system. When the Communists, led by Chairman
Mao, came to power and established the People's Republic in 1949, they
inherited an enormous public health problem. More than a decade of
war had dismantled the nation's medical infrastructure, and there were
millions of poor, predominantly rural people without access to hospitals, trained doctors, vaccinations, or good sanitation. At the same time,
the Communists faced another challenge that was more political and
cultural. Mao's party had to foster unity. The Chinese had to see themselves as part of a common enterprise founded on not only a shared class
struggle but also a single, glorious heritage. Reviving traditional Chinese
medicine became a means to solve both material and political problems
of governance in Communist China. To deal with a shortage of qualified physicians, the Chinese government under Mao recruited 300,000
practitioners of traditional Chinese medicine to be part of the official
health care system. These men and women became the backbone of a
new medical infrastructure that administered vaccines and dispensed
advice about modern hygiene while at the same time practicing some
version of ancient therapies, including acupuncture.[6]

Mao called traditional Chinese medicine "a great treasure house,"
and he encouraged the Chinese people to take pride in it as an ancient, indigenous science. In state hospitals, Mao demanded that his

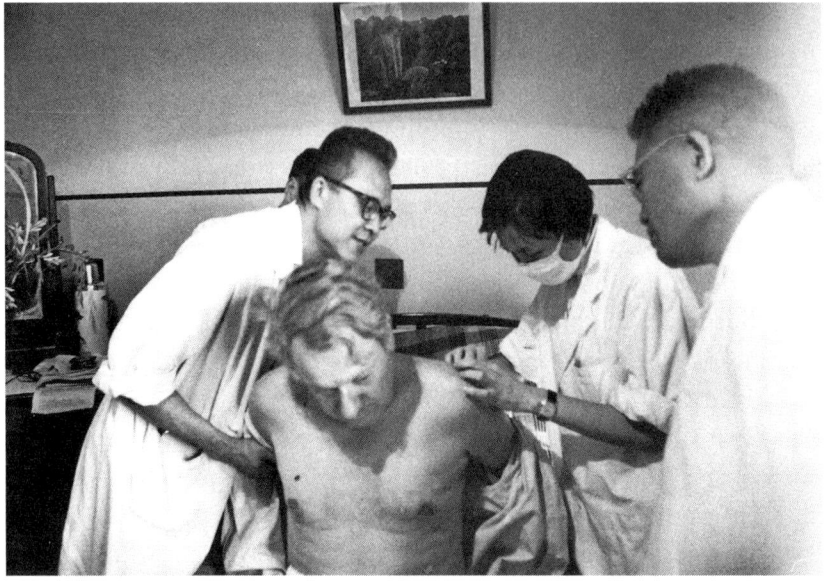

James Reston recovering from an appendectomy in Beijing, 1971. Courtesy of
the University of Illinois at Urbana-Champaign Archives, record series
number 26/20/121.

government "take Chinese medicine seriously." Continuing the efforts
undertaken by Western-style scientists in the Republican period, Chinese chemists worked hard to identify the active chemical compounds
in herbal medicine, and government scientists aimed to uncover physiological or psychological explanations for the efficacy of acupuncture.
Under Mao, an eclectic system of medicine became regularized. It
came into the laboratories, clinic exam rooms, and surgical theaters.
In Chinese state hospitals, herbalists, acupuncturists, and biomedical
scientists worked side by side. Consequently, when the Chinese government invited American journalists and physicians to visit China in the
early 1970s, they were able to observe—or in the case of James Reston,
receive—acupuncture firsthand.[7]

Reston filed a report of the experience for the readers of the *New
York Times*. While the acupuncture seemed to relieve his discomfort,
he groused, "It was a rather complicated way to get rid of gas on the
stomach." It was hardly a ringing endorsement. Reston's ambivalence

for his new status as "an experimental porcupine" did nothing to dampen the enthusiasm of the American public, however. Recovering at the hospital, Reston fielded numerous requests to confirm reports of "remarkable cures of blindness, paralysis, and mental disorders" and other "great new medical breakthroughs in the field of traditional Chinese needle and herbal medicine." Reston demurred: "I do not know whether this speculation is justified, and am not qualified to judge."[8] But his readership clamored for more. Curious and eager Americans wanted to know: How did it work? What could it cure? Was it all just a Communist hoax?

American patient-consumers were receptive to a "medical miracle" from China, but up until the 1970s, they had relatively few sources for information about acupuncture. The first generations of Chinese doctors who had immigrated to the United States were poorly equipped to educate their non-Chinese patients about the needle therapy. They had left China at a time when acupuncture had a reputation as a low-class surgery. As members of a merchant class, very few immigrant doctors had any training in acupuncture or moxibustion, a frequently paired modality.[9] The meager coverage of acupuncture in American popular media simply described it as one of the many "exotic" and puzzling therapies associated with China's ancient knowledge system. A 1947 *New York Times* column of fun facts about global ancient medicine simply described Chinese acupuncture as "the practice of *thrusting* hot steel needles into selected anatomical areas of the patient."[10] Other articles similarly made mention of the "pricking" without additional context or explanation.[11] Sensational accounts played on a prevalent squeamishness toward needles while offering no way to understand their utility.

Much like nineteenth-century Chinatown travelogues, mid-twentieth-century newspapers and magazines continued to treat Chinese medicine, including acupuncture, primarily as a curiosity, but increasingly in the 1950s and 1960s, a new Cold War–era rhetoric overlaid older Orientalist tropes. When American newspapers covered the development of "Traditional Chinese Medicine" under Chairman Mao, they tended to characterized Mao's medical policies as a reversal of progress made under the tutelage of Western-style biomedical scientists. Before the Communist takeover in 1949, the Rockefeller Foundation, the China

Medical Board, Yale University, and other philanthropic and religious organizations had made profound investments in building up biomedical education, facilities, and networks in China. According to the *New York Times,* Communism reversed that progress, leaving the country "isolated" with "too few modern hospitals and too few modern doctors."[12] Chinese biomedical scientists thus resorted to acupuncture and herbalism because they had no other options.

The American popular press painted a picture of China as a desperate and destitute society, resistant to change. In 1959, P. K. Padmanabhan, a correspondent for the *Los Angeles Times* Asian Bureau, reported that "in spite of relentless efforts by the [Chinese] government to whip them on modernity, millions of Chinese continue to take treatment only from herbal doctors."[13] The American press scoffed at Mao's program to biomedicalize traditional therapies and insisted that it had barely advanced Chinese society beyond base superstition. A *New York Times* article glibly noted that "in Communist China today, when it comes to treating the sick, witches are out but eels' blood is in."[14] Another *New York Times* article reported that Chinese biomedical scientists who refused to collaborate with acupuncturists and herbalists were publicly castigated for "being poisoned by bourgeois ideology."[15] In such coverage, China remained characterized by its inferiority, made manifest through its dependence on archaic and esoteric medical practices.

Elsewhere, the American press identified the revival of ancient therapies as a form of Communist indoctrination. Peggy Durdin, a freelance writer for the *New York Times,* described a meeting of the Chinese national congress where a practitioner of traditional Chinese medicine linked human longevity to the teachings of Marx, Lenin, and Mao. "No one in the audience, however highly trained in science, dared refrain from hearty applause," Durdin reported. She went on to lament the reduced status of China's biomedical scientists under Mao. Many of them had trained at American-sponsored institutions like Peking Union Medical College but found themselves compelled by Mao's medical policies to study and accept traditional Chinese therapies in their practice: "Traditional medicine is taking them away from their legitimate function of healing sickness and saving lives." According to Durdin, "no group today better illustrates than do China's doctors the

[Communist] party's almost paranoiac determination to break a man's independence and control his every attitude, belief, and thought."[16] It was not clear if China's innate backwardness or Maoism retarded the spread of Western-style biomedicine. Cold War Orientalism made Chinese civilizational deficiencies indistinguishable from the deleterious effects of Communist ideology.

The supposed lack of scientific evidence for acupuncture was a recurring theme in American media coverage. In reality, however, acupuncture and other traditional Chinese therapies had been the subject of continuous research in modern laboratories and clinics around the world. Only a combination of American provincialism and prejudice made it seem otherwise. In China, Western-style medical scientists had formally studied acupuncture since the 1930s, and under Mao's pressure to centralize authority in Beijing and standardize medical practices in the 1950s, clinical experiments with acupuncture and chemical analyses of Chinese *materia medica* multiplied in state hospitals and medical colleges.[17] When American physicians began to visit China in 1971, they praised the vibrant and innovative research programs at state hospitals.[18] The Chinese Medical Association made translations of Chinese research available in its English-language journal, which had gone through many iterations since its inception in the 1880s. By the 1950s, the *Chinese Medical Journal* was the leading English-language source for biomedical interpretations of traditional Chinese medicine, but Maoist officials suspended its publication in 1966 during the Cultural Revolution.[19]

Outside of China, Japan was the most important center for the study of acupuncture. The Japanese had practiced Chinese acupuncture since at least the sixth century and developed their own theories and variations.[20] Seventeenth-century European travelers made some of their earliest observations of the needle therapy there.[21] In the late nineteenth century, American newspapers were at least as likely to associate acupuncture and moxibustion with the indigenous medical practices of Japan as they were with those of China.[22] In the late twentieth century, Japanese researchers not only continued to translate ancient Chinese acupuncture texts but also produced new studies, including unique contributions to the understanding of moxibustion and its effects on the immune system.[23]

While the close relationship between China and the Soviet bloc during the Cold War expanded the region's interest in acupuncture, Western Europe had a longer and deeper history of academic inquiry in the area of traditional Chinese medicine.[24] France was the center for biomedical research into Chinese acupuncture. Through its colonies in Southeast Asia and its diplomatic forays into China, French imperial authorities had ample contact with ethnic Chinese doctors. From the 1930s to the 1950s, French doctors Charles Flandin and Paul Ferreyrolles energetically promoted the scientific study of acupuncture, having been introduced to it by George Soulié de Morant, the French consul to China. While stationed in Beijing, Soulié de Morant observed cholera treated with acupuncture. After leaving the diplomatic corps, he meticulously translated the work of Japanese scientist T. Nakayama on acupuncture and other Chinese therapies, and he enlisted Flandin and Ferreyrolles to share it with their colleagues.[25] Flandin and Ferreyrolles's publications—occasionally with other coauthors—highlighted the application of acupuncture in nerve, muscle, and skin disorders.[26] They inspired other French researchers in the fields of psychology, obesity, dentistry, veterinary science, and physiology.[27] Among them was the anatomist and surgeon Pierre Huard, who made the general study of classical Chinese medicine, along with its manifestations in Vietnam, Japan, and Korea, the centerpiece of his scholarship from the 1940s to the 1980s.[28]

In Paris, the Val-de-Grâce Hospital offered medical students and physicians theoretical and practical courses in acupuncture from 1934 (with only a brief interruption during World War II) and held an open clinic from ten o' clock to noon every Friday. The hospital published annual statistics from its clinical practice as evidence of "the scientific and logical basis" of the therapy, which seems to have been primarily applied in cases of chronic pain.[29] In 1943, French physicians—working under the guidance of Japanese and Vietnamese practitioners of classical Chinese medicine—organized the Société Internationale d'Acupuncture in Paris to disseminate the latest scientific studies on acupuncture to a global roster of members.[30] The evacuation of French physicians from Vietnam during the First Indochina War in the early 1950s swelled the ranks of the society with members who had closely observed acupuncture practiced by ethnic Chinese doctors.[31]

France's neighbors Germany and Great Britain also maintained an academic interest in traditional Chinese medicine. Throughout the mid-twentieth century, German and, to a lesser extent, British biomedical journals regularly published research on Chinese medical therapies—especially the use of acupuncture in pain management.[32] Like France, Germany established a biomedical organization, the Deutsche Zeitschrift für Akupunktur, in 1953 to share scientific research.[33] (An equivalent society did not form in Britain until 1980.)[34]

The United States lagged behind to say the least. A few individual scientists with unique ties to China did publish research prior to the 1970s. In 1924, clinical pharmacologist Ko Kuei Chen and his coauthor, Carl F. Schmidt, famously isolated the active alkaloid in *ma huang* (*Ephedra vulgaris* or *Ephedra sinica*), an herb used in traditional Chinese remedies for respiratory ailments.[35] An immigrant from Shanghai with an M.D. from Johns Hopkins University, Chen proved the effectiveness of ephedrine as a vasoconstrictor and convinced the pharmaceutical company Eli Lilly to manufacture a drug based on the stimulant for asthma and allergies. Chen went on to become the director of pharmacological research at Eli Lilly and dedicated a forty-year career to the study of Chinese *materia medica,* supported by his employer from 1929 to 1963, and later the medical college at Indiana University.[36] Chen's relationship with Eli Lilly and the success of ephedrine was unusual for its time. For the American pharmaceutical industry in general, herbal remedies were of little interest. They offered too little potential for producing patents and, thereby, profits.[37]

Lower-tier, regional medical journals offered some discussion of traditional Chinese medicine. In the late 1940s and 1950s, Albert Fields, a recently returned medical officer with the U.S. military in China and a professor of medicine at the University of Southern California, published a series of articles on Chinese therapies, particularly the aspects he found most relevant to his interests in physical therapy, in California-based biomedical journals.[38] Fields emphasized the congruencies between Chinese and biomedical epistemologies, likening the ancient *yinyang* doctrine to modern scientific dualities like hormone and anti-hormone, enzyme and anti-enzyme.[39] In his academic publications, Fields endeavored to balance his biomedical perspective with a tacit acknowledgment of its limitations: "Like many others who have seen them examine patients, I have repeatedly been amazed at their almost uncanny ability to determine the seat of disease from the pulse alone."[40] We might read his work on ancient Chinese therapies in the late 1940s and early 1950s as an early example of what the medical community now calls "integrative medicine." By looking to the past, Fields was ahead of his time. Perhaps consequently, his research does not seem to have risen beyond minor field journals.

Aside from Fields's work, coverage of traditional Chinese medicine in regional journals was sporadic and motivated foremost by anthropological curiosity. In 1951, the esteemed College of Physicians of Philadelphia invited William Cadbury, a medical missionary to Canton, to speak before its section on medical history. Cadbury offered a cursory explanation of the theories of *yinyang* and correspondences as well as pulsology and acupuncture. Throughout the lecture, the prevailing attitude was one of condescension. Cadbury scoffed at the Chinese physician's "ignorance" in the treatment of fractures. While he cursorily nodded toward some overlap between the Chinese and American pharmacopoeia, he savored each gory detail as he described the use of animal sacrifice in Chinese healing practices: "A remedy that I have not infrequently seen applied to a patient in extremis is as follows: a rooster is killed and the body cut in half, longitudinally, and the bleeding half is quickly applied to the skin of the patient's abdomen. If there is any possibility of a cure this is supposed to be infallible." Reading the reprint of the lecture, one can almost hear Cadbury pause for laughter. In his characterization of the typical Chinese doctor, Cadbury highlighted the attachment to "magic and astrology," which were inextricably bound in with the Chinese theory of the human "organism." Such anecdotes simultaneously entertained his audience and reassured them of their scientific supremacy.[41]

Less famous authorities copied Cadbury's approach. In 1958, Jerome D. Waye, a recent graduate from Boston University's School of Medicine, summarized half of a dozen English-language histories of Chinese medicine for the *Boston Medical Quarterly*. Calling its classical therapies "fanciful" and veiled in the "shrouds of mysticism," Waye criticized modern China for rejecting biomedicine: "They have undoubtedly been held back in this as in other spheres of knowledge by their extreme reverence for ancestral beliefs and customs."[42] The attachment to traditional therapies rehearsed an old Orientalist trope of Chinese backwardness and cemented a priori assumptions of the inferiority of Chinese medical knowledge systems.

For the most part, however, if scientists in the United States conducted serious research into acupuncture prior to the 1970s, their work went unnoticed by the most prestigious, national biomedical journals. In the middle decades of the twentieth century, the *Journal of the American Medical Association* (*JAMA*) published only one article on Chinese medicine, a survey of acupuncture by a University of Chicago professor, Ilza Veith, in 1962. The subtitle of her article implicitly posed the question of whether acupuncture was "verity or delusion" and came down squarely on the latter. She characterized the therapy as "bizarre" and "irrational." She predicted that acupuncture would not survive truly rigorous scientific inquiry. "Founded as it is upon fanciful ideas of anatomy and physiology," she wrote, "it can scarely [*sic*] be expected to survive as a form of rational and scientific therapy, despite its continuous popularity for over 2,500 years and its recent inclusion into some modern systems of treatment."[43]

Even after Reston's appendectomy and *New York Times* article, late twentieth-century portraits of acupuncture and its practitioners in the popular press rehashed many of the same Orientalist tropes that Progressive Era chroniclers had applied to herbalists. Journalists disparaged acupuncturists as hucksters and charlatans, peddling fantasies to gullible, often female patients. A profile of a Taipei clinic by John Saar, a Far East reporter for the magazine *Life*, held up the therapy for ridicule. "It seems less like a hospital than a visit to your friendly neighborhood sorcerer," Saar scoffed, describing its "grubby" exterior and "cluttered" and "dingy" waiting room. A photo of a patient wearing a crown of two-inch needles accompanied the article, a sight that Saar likened to "casualties from a flock of arrows loosed by Lilliputian archers."[44] A *Los Angeles Times* investigation into the city's acupuncture trade characterized the therapy as "more mystical than medical" and identified among its believers not just "cultists" but also "California housewives" and Hollywood ingénues seeking relief from injuries sustained in the frivolous pursuits of a privileged class: tennis, skiing, and horseback riding. With barely concealed contempt for his subjects, the journalist profiled a handful of female patients, including Joan Shumway, identified only as "the attractive wife of a prominent West Sider," who made regular visits to a West Hollywood acupuncturist for tennis-related knee and back pain. The article quoted Shumway as describing the clinic in terms that highlighted its alterity: "The place is very mysterious," she reported. "There is no sign on the door. His wife opens the peephole and says 'Come.'" Of her acupuncturist, she claimed, "He has these marvelous hands, as if they had eyes in them." Shumway's account reinforced a prevalent notion that acupuncture was part of both an underworld and another world.[45]

Academic skepticism filtered into the popular press. When *Newsweek* made acupuncture its cover story in August 1972, the headline asked if the needle therapy was "myth or miracle." Chinese hospitals, the magazine acknowledged, had published research documenting the efficacy of acupuncture in various treatments, but *Newsweek* cautioned its readers not to put too much faith in the findings: "Chinese doctors, for the most part, do not believe in the rigidly controlled studies comparing various modes of treatment that are standard in the West." It would be better, the article concluded, to await verification by American scientists.[46] But American patient-consumers were impatient. They did not want to wait for the deliberate speed of the scientific method.

In the early 1970s, Americans wrote to their congressional representatives, to the White House, and to the Department of Health, Education, and Welfare demanding to know more about the mysterious needle therapy.[47] Almost a year to the day after Reston's appendectomy, the United States' first clinic devoted to acupuncture opened on the Upper East Side of Manhattan. An internist, Arnold Benson, assisted by four Chinese acupuncturists, charged twenty dollars per visit. In its one week of operation before the New York State Health Department shut it down, the clinic saw three hundred patients and boasted three thousand more on its waitlist.[48] Around the same time, celebrity athletes like Los Angeles Rams quarterback Roman Gabriel, Kansas City Chiefs defensive lineman Ed Lothamer, and San Francisco Giants players Willie McCovey and Sam McDowell reported miraculous recoveries from injuries after a course of acupuncture.[49]

Popular magazines like *Life, Vogue,* and the *National Review* rushed to run articles on acupuncture in 1971 and 1972.[50] The frequency of mentions of the terms "acupuncture" or variations on "Chinese herbs" or "Chinese medicine" in the *New York Times* spiked dramatically after July 1971. Whereas these terms appeared in 95 unique records (including advertisements, editorials, and news articles) in the 1960s, they appeared in 724 records in the 1970s. Lillian Africano, the editor of *Acupuncture News Digest,* observed, "Acupuncture may have run second only to Watergate as a consumer of newsprint."[51] In the summer and fall of 1972, acupuncture began to appear on primetime television. NBC aired a documentary on acupuncture anesthesia narrated by an American surgeon who had toured China, and a nighttime soap opera, *The Bold Ones: The New Doctors,* had one of its main characters, played by Carl Reiner, experiment with acupuncture for pain relief in an episode entitled "A Nation of Human Pincushions."[52] Sensational representations of acupuncture also circulated in low-brow entertainment. A martial arts movie released in 1974 entitled *Golden Needles* capitalized on popular associations between the "Orient" and sexual licentiousness. The film depicted American actors racing through the streets of Hong Kong in pursuit of acupuncture needles with magical capabilities to enhance the user's sexual virility.[53] In New York, modern-day snake oil salesmen peddled therapeutic stainless-steel bracelets from the "Oriental Land of Acupuncture." They promised to cure the wearer's unspecified ailments with "magnetic rays."[54] In the public imagination, the opposing forces of attraction and revulsion that underlay American Orientalism continued to shape popular associations with Chinese medicine and, more specifically, acupuncture.

In many ways, changes in the American medical marketplace and its regulation in the mid-twentieth century invited the public frenzy for Chinese acupuncture. As Nancy Tomes has argued in *Remaking the American Patient,* America's "Golden Age of Medicine" ironically alienated the class of patient-consumers it most benefited.[55] Scientific advances in the first half of the century had several profound effects on the provisioning of health care: they cemented the social authority of biomedicine, encouraged specialization among its practitioners, and set its costs soaring. The financing of health care began to change as well, with salaried hospitalists and private managed care plans replacing the simple fee-for-service arrangements between individual doctors and patients that had prevailed before World War II. Biomedicine's trend toward greater sophistication and specialization made health knowledge impenetrably complex for the ordinary patient. New and expensive surgical procedures sparked a protracted public debate about "unnecessary surgeries" in the 1950s.[56] Meanwhile, the increased scrutiny of the FDCA did not eliminate concerns about pharmaceuticals. Terrifying reports about the misuse or overuse of prescription drugs circulated in the popular press.[57] Setting aside the dangers of unknown side effects and interactions, new drugs effectively contained infectious disease but could do little for chronic disorders like heart disease, cancer, and pain syndromes.[58]

The postwar economic boom afforded middle-class and affluent patient-consumers the freedom to devote time and energy to their health. This class of patient-consumers thus simultaneously experienced fewer freedoms and more entitlement. They bristled at the physician's professional authoritarianism, balked at the escalating costs of care, and lamented constraints on choosing therapies and providers imposed by insurance plans. Patient-consumers in the 1950s and 1960s sought out alternatives to biomedicine for the same reasons as their Progressive Era progenitors: an aversion to costly, potentially harmful drugs; fear of unnecessary surgeries; and desire for greater sovereignty over their own health care. In an era of increased specialization, practitioners of Chinese medicine may have seemed comfortingly general.[59] Herbalists who advertised in English-language newspapers commonly claimed to cure an astonishing array of ailments including "female troubles," gastro-intestinal distress, chronic pain, sleeplessness, respiratory infections, asthma, and headaches.[60] The Chinese apothecary was a one-stop shop.

New currents in medical culture flowed through a wider countercultural moment in American history. Counterculturalists represented overlapping and intersecting movements of feminists, civil rights activists, anti-colonialists, and anti-capitalists, groups that shared some

common traits. They were universally distrustful of traditional, patriarchal authority and often skeptical of science and industry. They
promoted consumer rights, multiculturalism, and the freedom of self-
determination. Asian religions, philosophies, and healing systems attracted counterculturalists' curiosity. They invited Indian gurus to pre-
side over public events; practiced yoga, transcendental meditation, and
Zen Buddhism; and identified Ayurvedic, Tibetan, and Chinse medicine as systems of "natural" healing.[61] In the 1970s, civil rights activist
and black nationalist Mutulu Shakur introduced Chinese acupuncture
at Lincoln Hospital in the Bronx as means of democratizing access to
health care among drug addicts, the poor, and the elderly.[62] In this way,
the diffusion of Chinese medicine to the United States played a part in
anticolonial politics, but its principal beneficiaries were initially middle-
and upper-class, mostly white Americans.

Countercultural ideologies of naturalism, holism, and vitalism became the primary frameworks through which such American patient-
consumers interpreted Chinese acupuncture and other traditional therapies. These ideologies had distinct historical trajectories, but they were
reasonably congruent with traditional Chinese therapeutic principles
and practices. At the heart of naturalism was a rejection of the idea that
modern science and technology could improve on the workings of nature. Naturalists had lived through the atomic age with its veneration
of science, and they emerged on the other side with a deeply seated fear
of what it could do. They worried about nuclear fallout—radioactive
isotopes in the groundwater, in the air, in the food that they ate. They
worried about chemical pesticides like DDT and their effect on ecological and human health. As a philosophy, then, naturalism promoted a
way of life presumed to be closer to nature. Its adherents recoiled from
what they perceived to be the overuse of pharmaceuticals. When they
sought out remedies, they gravitated toward those conceivably grown
in gardens.[63] Since at least the eighteenth century, American patient-
consumers had associated Chinese medicine with "nature's remedies,"
a shorthand for the prevalent use of organic, rather than inorganic, medicinal compounds.[64]

The Chinese propensity to seek psychosomatic explanations for illness registered with mind-body enthusiasts, and the Chinese philosophy

of balancing the body's vital forces through special diets and exercise would have felt familiar to the readers of J. J. Rodale's *Prevention* and other similar publications concerned with chronic diseases. Holism originated in models of ecology that considered not just the discrete organisms and inorganic factors present but also their interactions with one another. Holism entered medical discourse in the 1970s as a language with which to criticize biomedicine. In that context, it implied an approach to health care that took into account not only physiology but also psychology, social context, and spirituality. Holistic medicine, like traditional Chinese medicine, stressed the individuality of the patient and the multidimensional particularities of his or her condition. Two individuals presenting a similar set of symptoms might receive very different diagnoses.[65] Vitalism imagined a universe through which unseen forces of energy flowed. Balancing or unblocking that flow was the key to health and healing. Meditative exercises like t'ai chi or qigong attracted the curiosity of vitalists.[66] The intersection between counterculturalism and medical consumerism made Americans receptive to the key tenets of traditional Chinese medicine when they had an opportunity to reconnect with them in the 1970s.

"As Covert as It Is Chic . . ."

In the years just after Reston's appendectomy, American demand for the needle therapy far outstripped the supply. Charter busses transported the truly desperate across state lines in search of an acupuncturist. Thousands of patients lined up for treatment from practitioners with dubious qualifications.[67] There were probably between one and two hundred illegal practitioners scattered across American Chinatowns and just a dozen licensed physicians—mostly Chinese American—who included acupuncture in their practice.[68] In a 1972 article for the *Los Angeles Times,* a reporter documented his struggle to find an "expert needler" as he paged through the phonebook and roamed the streets of Los Angeles's and San Francisco's Chinatowns. "Acupuncture," he concluded, "is as covert as it is chic."[69]

Good acupuncturists were hard to find because they were, quite literally, hiding. It was illegal to practice medicine without a license, and

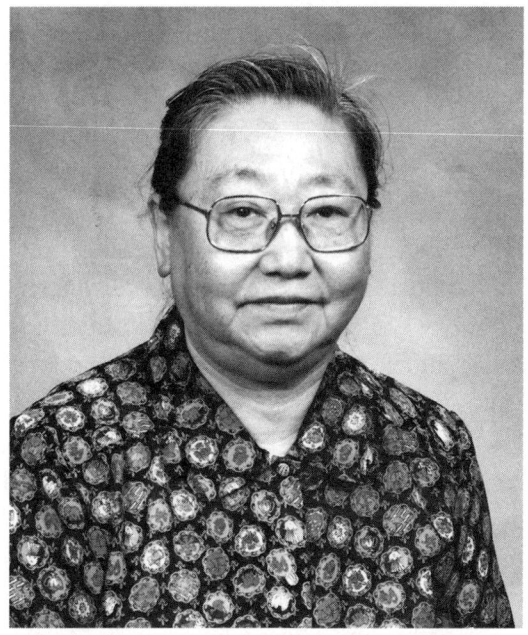

Miriam Lee, the "Mother of Acupuncture in
California." Courtesy of Frank He.

in nearly all states, procedures that pierced the skin counted as medicine.[70] In 1972, an elderly acupuncturist in Los Angeles practiced out
of a motel room at the Royal Pagoda Motel while a chiropractor maintained her anonymity by performing the needle therapy in the Beverly
Hills Hotel.[71] Kung Fu teacher George Long offered acupuncture to his
students at his studio in San Francisco.[72]

Miriam Lee, who eventually trained so many California acupuncturists that she would be remembered as the "Mother of Acupuncture
in California," began her practice out of her home.[73] A native of the
Shandong Province of China, Lee was a nurse, midwife, and acupuncturist before her family fled the country in the wake of the Communist
Revolution.[74] By 1969, she had settled in Palo Alto, California, and was
working on the assembly line at the Hewlett Packard plant. When her
coworkers complained of shoulder or neck pain, she treated them with
acupuncture in her off-hours.[75] Word of her services spread quickly. She

helped the Chinese American son of a fellow church member recover from spinal surgery, then a pair of American women with chronic pain. Soon she was operating an acupuncture clinic out of her home with patients sneaking up the back staircase. "At one point," Lee recalled, "there were so many people waiting on the stairs to get in the staircase broke."[76]

Some biomedical physicians in private practices offered space for unlicensed Chinese doctors. These clandestine arrangements typically became known only when exposed by the authorities. Fresno anesthesiologist Alice Lee allowed three acupuncturists—John Lee, Virginia Young, and Paul Sy—to practice in her office.[77] Similarly, Harry Oxenhandler, a Palo Alto M.D., began allowing Miriam Lee to see patients out of his offices between five o'clock in the morning and one o'clock in the afternoon. Business boomed. "For seven hours a day, five days a week, I saw between seventy-five and eighty patients," she reported. "I had four beds for those who had to lie down. People in wheelchairs were treated in the bathroom. Those who could sit I treated in the waiting room or on the foot of the treatment tables."[78] The success of Lee's operations alerted the authorities and led to her arrest in Oxenhandler's office for practicing medicine without a license on April 16, 1974 (the day after Governor Ronald Reagan vetoed a bill to legalize acupuncture in California). Police stormed the office at 6:45 in the morning while she was in the midst of treating ten patients. She removed the needles and went off to jail. At trial, Lee's patients—both Chinese and non-Chinese—flooded the courtroom, each one ready to testify to the efficacy of acupuncture and to defend her right to practice.[79]

As acupuncture-mania swept the nation, Chinese American M.D.s who had been secretly practicing traditional therapies alongside their regular biomedical practice enjoyed a moment in the spotlight. Dr. Sung J. Liao, a specialist in physical rehabilitation who held a degree from the Yale School of Medicine, found his services in high demand once it became public that he used acupuncture to treat chronic pain.[80] Dr. E. C. Wong, a Denver-based biomedical physician, toured the country lecturing on acupuncture and other traditional Chinese therapies and charging attendees $175 each. "Seven years ago, I was called an Oriental quack," he told a Chicago audience. "But now you are all so open to new methods."[81] Hong Kong doctors similarly cashed in on the new zeal for acupuncture by coming to the United States to offer correspondence courses, weekend-long seminars, and even "acupuncture cruises," where American M.D.s received training while enjoying a day at sea.[82] There were no schools of Chinese medicine in the United States. The People's Republic of China allowed a select few to train in the regularized and simplified form of acupuncture practiced in state hospitals, but anyone interested in learning more traditional therapeutic approaches had to study with master practitioners in Hong Kong, Taiwan, Western Europe, or British Columbia.[83]

Without legalization, acupuncture largely remained in the hidden corners of the American medical marketplace. In the early 1970s, most state legislatures had kicked around acupuncture licensing bills.[84] By 1973, Kansas was the only state to outright ban the needle therapy, but Arizona, Colorado, Delaware, Connecticut, and New York as well as various states of the upper Midwest all defined acupuncture as equivalent to the practice of medicine and therefore restricted its practice to state-licensed physicians. That legislation effectively excluded the majority of practitioners who did not hold a biomedical degree from an American school of medicine or dentistry.[85] The New York law shuttered the doors of the "nation's first acupuncture clinic."[86] Other states, including California, permitted nonlicensed physicians to participate in acupuncture research at state-approved universities and under the oversight of a licensed physician. It was up to the acupuncturist to find a biomedical doctor, osteopath, or dentist willing to do the supervision.[87] After her arrest and acquittal, Miriam Lee used the California exemption to continue to practice as part of experimental research conducted in the medical school at the University of California, San Francisco.[88]

With varying degrees of urgency, state chapters of the American Medical Association (AMA) opposed efforts to legalize acupuncture, but by 1974, the national organization had conceded support for compromise measures that restricted acupuncturists to practicing under supervision by licensed physicians.[89] State legislators found supervision appealing as it encouraged scientific study of acupuncture and left the door open to the possibility that, with a sufficient record of efficacy and safety, the states might license acupuncturists to practice independently at some point in the future. If the states hoped such compromise regulation would quiet some of the public clamor for more access to needle therapy, it did not. In a best-case scenario, licensed physicians and practitioners of Chinese medicine might work cooperatively, but as Ginger McRae noted in her review of acupuncture regulation in this period, supervisory relationships had "inherent possibilities of abuse," particularly for practitioners with limited English-language skills or insecure immigration status.[90] More obviously, supervised practice did little to expand the supply of qualified acupuncturists for patients in need. Practitioners of Chinese medicine, biomedical allies, and patients continued to lobby state legislatures to liberalize licensing statutes.

While lobbying efforts moved forward in fits and starts, acupuncturists and their supporters found creative ways to circumvent the law. Morton W. Barke opened the first chain of acupuncture clinics in California in the early 1970s. Barke was a young M.D. from the University of California, Irvine, where he specialized in obstetrics and gynecology. A self-described "medical maverick," Barke was (and remains) almost compulsively entrepreneurial. After school, he branched out into a number of medical fields, mostly unrelated to his original area of specialization. In 1971, Barke read the headlines about James Reston's miraculous appendectomy, and it piqued his interest. He rented an old real-estate office in the affluent Los Angeles enclave of Beverly Hills, purchased twenty chiropractic beds, and opened an acupuncture clinic. The fact that he knew nothing about acupuncture did not deter him.[91] Barke hired a team of three Korean acupuncturists—Jang Ho Kim, Joon Pil Lee, and Tae Eul Yun—asked them to bring along a translator, and started receiving patients.[92]

The clinics complied with California's law by guaranteeing that licensed physicians would insert the needles under the supervision of the Korean "master acupuncturists." In his public statements, Barke was careful not to overstep state regulations. "We don't do X-rays," Barke told a staff writer at the *Los Angeles Times*. "Every patient we treat must have a written diagnosis from his physician. We don't offer acupuncture instead of other treatment . . . We do not claim to cure anything."[93] Barke's clinics offered a treatment of last resort for patients for whom Western-style biomedical science had failed, most commonly chronic pain conditions like arthritis, migraines, or back pain. The Korean doctors marked red dots on the patients and licensed physicians placed the needles as instructed. The clinic was soon overflowing with patients. Within months, Barke had opened new clinics in San Francisco, Riverside, Santa Barbara, and Santa Ana.[94] Soon he was running ten acupuncture clinics spanning the state from San Diego in the south to San Francisco in the north.[95]

Despite his precautions, the Board of Medical Examiners still accused Barke of unprofessional conduct and won an injunction against him that prevented the acupuncturists from touching patients, even if only with a red pen. The entrepreneurial Barke had to improvise. He arranged for the Korean doctors to demonstrate the placement of the needles by marking up eighteen-inch-high plastic dolls instead of patients. They then passed the dolls to the licensed physicians, who placed the needles as indicated on the model. At the same time, Barke and two of his patients, A. Everett Leopold and Joyce Solomon, filed a class-action suit against the Board of Medical Examiners to challenge state's restrictions. They claimed that the law unduly and unfairly restricted access to the treatment. Only participants in acupuncture research could receive the therapy.[96] In the end, the attorneys negotiated a compromise in which Barke and his patients agreed to drop the civil suit and the California Board of Medical Examiners permitted the clinic to resume operations.[97] Decades later, Barke recalled that the judge was married to a Chinese woman, which he conjectured may have tipped the scales of justice in his favor. Meanwhile, Barke's clinics offered classes for biomedical doctors in acupuncture, with the idea that these licensed trainees would eventually replace the unlicensed Korean acupuncturists.[98] While Barke found a clever way to keep his business aboveboard, in California, the state with the largest population of Chinese residents by a factor of two, the practice of traditional Chinese medicine remained illegal.

Ultimately, it was not California but Nevada that became the first state to legalize Chinese medical therapies—including acupuncture and herbalism—in April 1973. While there had been Chinese doctors practicing herbalism in the state as early as 1870, a century later the state had a negligible Chinese population, most of whom worked in the entertainment industry.[99] The reasons that Nevada would become the first state to legalize acupuncture were not self-evident. The movement may have benefited from relatively little resistance by Nevada's biomedical scientists. The state suffered from a chronic shortage of physicians, and the legislature did not organize a college of medicine until 1969.[100] There was a local chapter of the AMA, and its members did campaign against the law, but the organization was in the throes of major leadership changes and preoccupied with more pressing concerns such as skyrocketing costs of malpractice insurance.[101] In such an environment, irregular physicians could enjoy a wider range of freedom.

The vote to recognize traditional Chinese medicine as a "learned profession" followed a public demonstration of acupuncture orchestrated by a Las Vegas real-estate developer named Arthur Steinberg. In 1972, Steinberg and his wife had toured Asia and encountered acupuncture while in Hong Kong. There are conflicting explanations of how Steinberg became the unlikely champion of acupuncture in America. Some say that Steinberg, who suffered hearing loss in his left ear, had flown to Hong Kong with the express purpose of seeking "needle therapy treatment" and returned with a successful restoration. Other reports imply that the couple had a chance encounter with acupuncturist Lok Yee Kung, who cured Steinberg's wife's migraines. Regardless, Arthur Steinberg returned to Nevada and founded the American Society of Acupuncture. Using his own money, he began to lobby the state legislature to allow acupuncturists and other practitioners of traditional Chinese medicine to practice without supervision by licensed physicians.[102]

Steinberg paid for Lok and his wife, Chien Ching, to fly from Hong Kong and set up a temporary free clinic in the Ormsby Hotel and Casino, located opposite the statehouse in Carson City. Over three weeks, Lok and his wife treated more than four hundred patients, including half of the state's sixty legislators.[103] *Time* magazine covered the event with some incredulity, and it did not pass up the opportunity to make a Las Vegas–themed joke: "It is refreshing to know that even legislators in Nevada check the deck before dealing."[104] The results of the treatment were convincing. Nevada lawmakers claimed to have been cured of a range of ailments from sinus trouble to chronic knee pain, and they

voted nearly unanimously to authorize the practice of Chinese medicine and establish a Board of Oriental Medicine on April 20, 1973, with
Senate Bill no. 448. The members of the state's chapter of the AMA registered their displeasure at Nevada's legislation by likening acupuncturists to a "two-armed bandit." (Manipulating the needles required both
hands, a *JAMA* article explained.)[105] Lok Yee Kung and Chien Ching
Lok remained in Nevada, eventually settling in Las Vegas and raising
their family, which included a son, Peter Pak Ming Lok, who went on to
earn an M.D.[106]

The road to licensure was longer for practitioners of Chinese
medicine in California. In memoirs and other recollections, many individuals take credit for the eventual legalization. In reality, its success was
the product of multiple contemporaneous initiatives among formally
trained and self-taught practitioners and their devotees, working in
semi-organized fashion to lobby state legislators as early as 1972. Some
acupuncturists, like Zion Yu, presided over lucrative and prominent
clinics. In 1967, Yu had moved to Los Angeles from Taipei with his wife,
Shiao Pin, who was an expert in skin care. The pair established a successful West Hollywood clinic that catered to celebrities with ailments ranging from chronic pain to allergies to aging skin.[107] Other participants in
the movement for legalization practiced more covertly. In 1971, Barbara
Bernie was an architecture and design consultant living just outside San
Francisco. Suffering from chronic fatigue syndrome and desperate for
relief, Bernie traveled to Vancouver to seek treatment from Kok Yuen
Leung, a famous acupuncturist. Leung referred Bernie to a San Francisco practitioner who worked secretly out of a condemned Chinatown
building. Her experience as a patient inspired her to study acupuncture
at a college of traditional Chinese medicine in Warwick, England. In
1973, she returned to the United States and began touring California
with her British mentor, J. R. Worsley, to promote acupuncture and
champion its legalization. On the lecture circuit, Bernie met Miriam
Lee. The women joined forces to lobby for the right to practice without
supervision.[108]

Meanwhile, Pedro Chan, a recent college graduate, was making a
name for himself as a promoter of acupuncture among non-Chinese
communities in Los Angeles and San Francisco. In 1967, Chan had

emigrated from Macao to the United States to study engineering, first
at Whittier College and then at California State University in Los Angeles. Back home, his father owned a chain of herb stores with locations
in Macao, Hong Kong, and Canton, and over time, Chan became acquainted with doctors in Los Angeles's Chinatown, just a bus ride away
from his dormitory. Chan knew the local practitioners of Chinese medicine spoke little to no English but nonetheless served a diverse clientele of Chinese and non-Chinese patients. The growing interest in acupuncture among non-Chinese patients gave Chan the idea to make the
most of his skillset: fluency in English and personal connections to the
Chinatown acupuncturists. In 1972, Chan self-published *Acupuncture,
Electro-Acupuncture, Anaesthesia: A Small Needle Works Wonders,* which
promised to "familiarize the English-speaking people with acupuncture
in order to arouse their interest and investigation."[109] It would be the
first of several short, English-language guides to acupuncture that Chan
sold in Chinatown herb shops in Los Angeles and San Francisco. Subsequently, he contracted with a few trade presses to put out two additional
short, inexpensive books: *Wonders of Chinese Acupuncture* and *Finger
Acupressure.* These works displayed the hallmarks of more professional
production, including endorsements by prominent biomedical physicians that praised Chan's ability to translate Chinese concepts into language that "Western" readers could understand.[110]

Chan's fluency in English and his relationships with Los Angeles
and San Francisco acupuncturists and herbalists equipped him to organize efforts for legalization in California. Chan raised funds among
practitioners and patients to hire a lobbyist, Art Krause, who pressured
Art Torres, Herschel Rosenthal, and George Moscone, the state assembly
members from Los Angeles and San Francisco, and Alfred H. Song, the
first Asian American elected to the California legislature. Krause worked
his magic. On July 12, 1975, almost four years to the day after Reston's appendectomy, the newly elected California governor Jerry Brown signed
a bill sponsored by Moscone and Song and coauthored by Gordon
Duffy that loosened restrictions on acupuncturists. The legislation created a licensing process for practitioners of Chinese medicine.[111] It established an Acupuncture Advisory Committee, which reported to the

state medical board and took responsibility for vetting applicants and administering a licensing exam. California acupuncturists and herbalists celebrated the victory and hailed Governor Brown as the "father of California acupuncture."[112]

But the law left in place a significant restriction: acupuncture patients had to present a referral from a licensed biomedical physician, chiropractor, dentist, or podiatrist. In 1978, Torres introduced an assembly bill that lifted the requirement and recognized acupuncturists as primary health care providers. In the same year, Jim Keysor, another state assemblyman from the greater Los Angeles area, sponsored a bill that authorized coverage for some acupuncture costs through Medi-Cal, the state's health insurance program for low-income residents.[113] For California practitioners of traditional Chinese medicine, this legislation not only expanded the pool of potential patients; it also put their therapies on par with other scientifically certified medical practices. Within just a decade, Hawaii, Rhode Island, and New Mexico had passed laws similar to those of Nevada and California, and nine other states had created licensing exams or certification provisions enabling non-physicians to practice acupuncture without supervision.[114] In 1980, a Supreme Court case, *Andrews v. Ballard,* opened up the possibility for Chinese herbalists and acupuncturists to practice independently and without fear of prosecution.[115] While it did not protect a fundamental right to practice for non-physicians, it did chip away at biomedical authoritarianism by privileging patient-consumers' access to the treatment of their choosing.[116]

The legalization of acupuncture created new business opportunities for Chinese American herb companies. In the late 1970s and 1980s, advertisements for acupuncture clinics often included nutritional recommendations and herb therapy on their lists of services.[117] As dedicated schools of Chinese or "Oriental" medicine began to proliferate in the United States in the 1980s, most required some courses in herbology even though they concentrated on acupuncture.[118] As of 2014, only six states—including California and Nevada—required exams in Chinese herbology, but twenty-nine defined acupuncture and its scope of practice to include recommendations for traditional Chinese remedies.[119]

This capacious definition indirectly extended the legal protections enjoyed by acupuncturists to herbalists.

Ambivalent Orientalism

Legalization allowed practitioners of acupuncture and other traditional therapies to advertise more freely in English-language newspapers. In the 1970s and 1980s, display advertisements were typically spare, perhaps reflecting a high cost of printing, but in the more elaborate examples, some themes from the Progressive Era did resurface. Late twentieth-century practitioners continued to define their value in opposition to biomedicine. They played on patients' anxieties about pharmaceuticals and surgery. Advertisements for San Diego acupuncturists declared, "Chinese Acupuncture is phenomenal, an alternative to medication and surgery."[120] Los Angeles acupuncturist Leona Yeh promised "safe effective results" for a panoply of ailments "without the harmful side effects of drugs or medications."[121] Across the country, a chain of acupuncture clinics promised "painless natural treatment" in New York City's Chinatown, Queens, and Long Island.[122]

Other practitioners drew comparisons with biomedicine more obliquely as they linked acupuncture to ideas associated with holism, energy healing, and homeopathy. The California Acupuncture College explained, "This time-revered practice has one of its fundamental concepts that man exists as a series of integrated energetic systems and that disease results from an imbalance between those systems. Further, man is viewed not as an isolated entity but as a whole person interacting with all aspects of his environment."[123] Meanwhile, D. E. Kendall's clinic outside of Los Angeles claimed that acupuncture "balances the flow of energy and rechannels it to or from the abnormal areas. The body's own healing processes take over from there."[124] These advertisements broadly gestured toward Chinese therapeutic principles, but they primarily served to make acupuncture seem similar to other American irregular sects and dissimilar from biomedical science.

Vocabulary and images associated with "the Orient" served as a reminder of the persistent compatibility between the discourse of natural medicine and Orientalism. The modern *yinyang* symbol—a simplified

version of a pattern that dated back to at least the eleventh century—
made frequent appearances in advertisements for Chinese acupuncture.
Los Angeles herbalist Wei-Ming Chung encouraged patients to "feel the
stress free feeling of being back in balance" with the *yinyang* symbol
graphically representing both "balance" and the "Orient" at the same
time.[125] In Cleveland, the North Coast Acupuncture Clinic described itself simply as a "wholistic practice" with a *yinyang* symbol pierced by an
incongruous and unexplained lightning bolt.[126] References to the "miraculous" and an emphasis on Chinese medicine's ancient origins were
also common. In 1979, Kyoung H. Kim insisted, "Pain Relief—A Miracle? Maybe So. Five thousand years of continuous practice should be
proof for you to try it."[127] Such English-language advertisements tended
to depict China as an ancient civilization, locked into premodern habits of magical thinking, but for patients skeptical of modern science,
that was not necessarily a bad thing. Among practitioners of traditional
Chinese medicine in the United States, professional sovereignty could
still rest on their capacity to embody American Orientalist stereotypes.
Ironically, Morton Barke, who opened Los Angeles's first legal acupuncture clinic in 1972, noticed that his business dropped off when Asian
practitioners became licensed: "People preferred the certain aura that
Asian people had," he recalled.[128]

For the Chinese doctor, the racialized shorthand of Orientalism
was useful but only up to a point. Historically, collaborating with licensed medical professionals had generated certain indirect legal protections, and borrowing their concepts helped demystify foreign medical concepts for American patient-consumers. After the passage of state
licensing laws, practitioners of Chinese medicine began to perceive new
advantages. In many states, acupuncturists could only work under the
supervision of licensed medical professions or required patient referrals from them. The language of Orientalism was useful insofar as it
highlighted the alterity of Chinese medicine, but it was a poor foundation for forging partnerships with biomedical scientists. Thus, for every
advertisement that distanced Chinese therapies from Western-style biomedicine, there was another making claims for obvious and "natural"
compatibilities between the knowledge systems. In 1974, the Center for
Health Education, an acupuncture clinic outside of Los Angeles, urged

the readers of the *Los Angeles Times* to seek out the needle therapy "when all else fails." Their advertisement promoted the clinic's affiliation with an "American M.D. Board Certified Anesthesiologist trained in Oriental Medicine as well as American Medicine." The Center for Health Education held out the promise of Chinese acupuncture "combined with Western medicine."[129]

Pedro Chan found creative ways to use biomedical vocabulary as he promoted Chinese acupuncture in his books. His first publication, *Acupuncture, Electro-Acupuncture, Anaesthesia,* sped through the history and philosophy of Chinese medicine in fewer than fifty pages—with a couple left blank at the end for notes. Chan offered a lengthier discourse on the apparatus of acupuncture, which partly reflected his education in biomedical engineering but also an inclination toward translating traditional therapeutic principles and practices into biomedical terms.[130] Subsequently, when promoting a new volume on acupressure, Chan's advertisements made multiple references to his partnerships with biomedical physicians and the White Memorial Medical Center, a major Los Angeles hospital, as well as to the seeming endorsement of *JAMA* for the techniques his book described. Perhaps most striking is Chan's explanation for acupressure's mechanism of efficacy: "There are small electrical currents in the body—currents that medical science can measure. When we feel pain, these currents convey messages to the brain. Now with Pedro Chan's amazing technique . . . you can lessen pain or even 'turn it off' just as you were turning an electric switch."[131] Without even passing reference to the classical Chinese theories of channels and meridians, Chan strategically applied the language of nerve conduction that would have been familiar to chiropractors, physical therapists, neurologists, and their patients.

In many ways, the translation work of acupuncturists recalled the tendency of earlier generations to link their ancient practices to modern science. In the first decades of the twentieth century, when Chang Gee Wo claimed to concoct herbal remedies in his "laboratory" in Portland or Tom Leung boasted of his "model herbal dispensatory" in the pages of *Chinese Herbal Science,* they were—however crudely—identifying their therapeutic practices and principles with those of scientific medicine. Early twentieth-century Chinese doctors like Chang and Leung understood that for some patient-consumers and regulatory agencies, the legitimacy of Chinese medicine in the United States, and consequently their freedom to practice it, rested on its compatibility with biomedical epistemologies. Chang's and Leung's counterparts in the late twentieth century approached that persistent problem at a different moment in American medical culture. Middle-class and affluent American patient-consumers had rushed ahead of biomedical science and its institutions. By the 1990s, their demand would pressure research institutes, insurance companies, and medical schools to reenvision irregular medicine as "complementary" to regular medicine. In the 1970s and 1980s, however, the concept of "Complementary and Alternative Medicine" or "integrative medicine" was as yet ill defined, but practitioners of traditional Chinese medicine—alongside chiropractors, naturopaths, and homeopaths—were in the process of inventing its possibilities.

Conclusion

In the decades after World War II, American biomedicine's trend toward specialization, skyrocketing costs, and the rise of managed care alienated some patients and sent them looking for alternatives that traditional Chinese medicine seemed to provide. News of James Reston's postoperative acupuncture in the summer of 1971 reached an audience of middle-class and affluent American patient-consumers eager and financially able to experiment. Practitioners of traditional Chinese medicine—particularly acupuncturists—seized on this moment. They made their therapies comprehensible within concepts familiar to American patient-consumers. As with earlier generations of herbalists, late twentieth-century practitioners continued to use "Oriental" difference as the basis of their value proposition and their professional authority, but they also borrowed freely from other irregular medical sects and even and especially biomedicine. The translation of ancient Chinese therapies into biomedical paradigms made it possible for practitioners to recast themselves as purveyors of medicine that was both alternative and complementary to biomedical science.

Epilogue

A New Medicine

The year 1971 was an inflection point in the long history of Chinese medicine in the United States, and it marked events with significance at global, local, and personal scales. While James Reston's post-appendectomy encounter with acupuncture captured the attention of a trans-Pacific audience, the destruction of Boise's Chinatown—and with it Ah Fong's abandoned apothecary—might have registered only in regional news. For one Chinese family, 1971 was momentous for entirely different reasons. As the dust settled over downtown Boise and Reston returned to the United States minus an appendix, a twenty-one-year-old foreign student from Hong Kong named Ka-Kit Hui was about to begin his first year of medical school at the University of California, Los Angeles (UCLA). Although incalculably more people took note of Reston's grumbling than Hui's achievement, the young scientist and others like him would go on to have a far greater impact on the trajectory of Chinese medicine in the United States.

Hui came from a medical family. His grandfather Hee Wan came from Guangdong (Canton) Province to the United States to study optometry and scientific medicine in San Francisco. Upon completion of his studies in 1910, Hee returned to China to practice Western-style medicine and set up clinics and optometry shops in Shanghai. In 1949, with China in the throes of the Communist Revolution, Hee fled the country with his family to Hong Kong. Ka-Kit Hui was born shortly thereafter.[1]

In 1968, Hui came to the United States to pursue a bachelor's degree in chemistry at UCLA and stayed on for medical school with the support of a Regent's Scholarship. In the months following Reston's appendectomy, Hui followed reports of Chinese acupuncture on television and radio. Growing up in Hong Kong, he remembered having some exposure to traditional therapies—herbalism, of course, as well as t'ai chi and massage, but not acupuncture. He voraciously consumed cheap paperback books on traditional Chinese therapies that his parents brought over on their visits to the United States. A trip home to Hong Kong in 1973 gave Hui an opportunity to take a course in acupuncture and other Chinese therapies with a master teacher. However, it was not clear how he could combine scientific medicine with traditional Chinese medicine. A career as an internist and a clinical pharmacologist seemed as reasonable a first step as any.[2]

As a professor of medicine at UCLA, he made incremental progress toward integrating Chinese medicine—particularly herbalism, but also acupuncture—into a biomedical career as he pursued sub-specializations in clinical pharmacology and drug development. He conducted studies of hypertension, heart failure, and receptor regulation, areas where he saw potential synergies with traditional Chinese therapeutic principles. "Going up for tenure," Hui recalled, "it seemed like I was all over the place."[3] But like a sailboat tacking into the wind, Hui eventually arrived at his intended destination. In 1994, with the support of his wife; his parents; his longtime mentor, Medical School dean emeritus Sherman Mellinkoff; and his department chair, Alan Fogelman, Hui founded the UCLA Center for East-West Medicine. Just a year earlier, David Eisenberg and colleagues at Harvard Medical School—who once trained under Hui's supervision—had published the results of a survey showing that in one year, Americans' total number of visits to practitioners of "alternative" medicine—defined as therapeutic systems not widely taught in major medical schools—exceeded the number of visits to conventional, biomedical doctors.[4] When the Center for East-West Medicine opened its doors, the popularity of a new category of care—Complementary

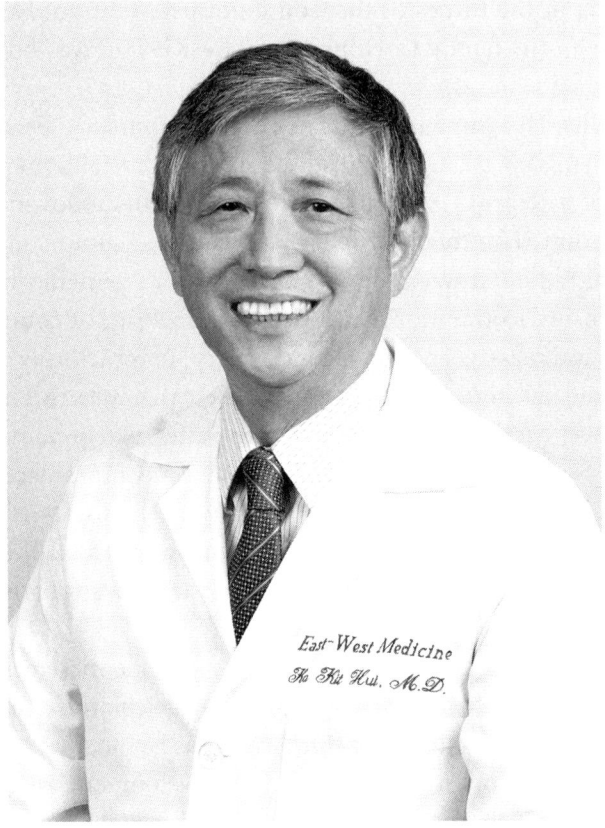

Ka-Kit Hui, the Wallis Annenberg Professor in Integrative East-West Medicine, founder and director of the
UCLA Center for East-West Medicine at the Department
of Medicine of the David Geffen School of Medicine,
and chair of the Collaborative Centers of Integrative
Medicine at UCLA. Courtesy of Ka-Kit Hui, MD, FACP,
and the UCLA Center for East-West Medicine.

and Alternative Medicine or Integrative Medicine—was becoming a
force that biomedicine could not afford to ignore.

Today, in an innocuous midlevel high-rise in Westwood, the
UCLA Center for East-West Medicine supports clinical care, education,
and research that integrate biomedical science with traditional Chinese

therapies.[5] Although it has typically served as a "clinic of last resort," receiving referrals for patients failed by Western-style biomedicine, Hui has greater ambitions. The center sponsors research collaborations that span the Pacific Ocean, bringing together scientists and practitioners, the ancient and the modern. Improved health outcomes are as paramount as issues of safety, affordability, and accessibility. Ka-Kit Hui aims to revolutionize global health care. His goal is nothing short of "building a new medicine."[6]

Hui is part of a generation of Chinese and Chinese American scientists who have constructed bridges of understanding between medical knowledge systems in the late twentieth and early twenty-first centuries. Many of them directly benefited from World War II– and Cold War–era immigration policies that favored the entry of Chinese students and scientists. Formally trained in biomedicine and at least conversant with traditional Chinese healing practices, they have dedicated their careers to proving and explaining the efficacy of Chinese medicine within biomedical paradigms. Their work has been controversial. They have faced criticism, skepticism, and outright repudiation. Biomedical scientists and traditional practitioners alike have attacked their objectivity as compromised, their methods as flawed, and their results as inconclusive. Yet today, ancient Chinese therapies occupy a small but sturdy toehold in American biomedical health care, both because of what biomedical research has been able to explain and what it has not.

De-orientalizing Chinese Medicine

Recovering from his emergency appendectomy in July 1971, James Reston expressed his gratitude and admiration for the doctors and acupuncturist who cared for him at Beijing's Anti-Imperialist Hospital. He praised their dedication to achieving a "combination of the very old and the very new"—the best of Western-style biomedicine and classical Chinese therapies—in their efforts to raise the nation's level of health care and quality of life.[7] In the decade leading up to Reston's highly publicized encounter with acupuncture, the gradual rapprochement between the United States and the People's Republic had made it possible for American scientists to learn more about new applications of ancient Chinese

therapies under Mao Zedong, a modern health care system commonly
referred to as Traditional Chinese Medicine—with capital letters. As
part of Mao's efforts to restore his regime's global reputation in the wake
of the Cultural Revolution, he invited American journalist Edgar Snow
to visit China and observe its progress, including the recent innovation
of "acupuncture anesthesia." Snow had a long relationship with Mao
and his premier Zhou Enlai. In the 1930s, the young Chinese leaders had
granted him an exclusive interview, which then became the authoritative source on Communist China when published as a book, *Red Star
over China,* in 1939. Snow remained in contact with the Communist
leadership in China, returning there in 1960 and 1965. After his 1970
visit, Snow published a series of articles in the *New Republic,* one of
which detailed his observations of the use of acupuncture anesthesia in
surgery.[8] Critics distrusted Snow, who was not a physician by training,
and they suspected that he had been duped. They held out for expert
confirmation of what Snow had seen.

In the 1960s, American biomedical doctors had tried unsuccess-
fully to secure invitations to tour the People's Republic, but the United
States' war with Vietnam opened up alternative channels of communication. Ethnic Chinese doctors were practicing traditional therapies
in Southeast Asia. In 1965, E. Grey Dimond, a cardiologist, shadowed
an acupuncturist at a rural clinic outside of Saigon and wrote up his
favorable impression of the therapy for the *New England Journal of
Medicine* (*NEJM*).[9] Around the same time, dispatches from Cambodia
reported that its premier, Lon Nol, preferred treatment from his Chinese acupuncturist to the American doctors who cared for him after a
stroke.[10]

In the fall of 1971, four American physicians—including Dimond
and his mentor, Paul Dudley White, as well as Samuel Rosen, an otolar-
yngologist, and Victor Sidel, a public health specialist and international
peace activist—received visas to travel to China. They became the
first of several American delegations of expert "witnesses" to the state
of medicine in China.[11] Richard Nixon's personal physician, Walter R.
Tkach, who joined the president on his 1972 tour of China, told journalists that he found acupuncture anesthesia superior to the anesthetics
currently in use in American hospitals.[12] In 1975, Ted J. Kaptchuk and

Dan Bensky completed training programs in acupuncture and Oriental medicine in Macao and returned to the United States to promote the study and practice of traditional Chinese therapies as reinvented during the Maoist era. While neither was an M.D. (Bensky would later get a degree in osteopathy), Kaptchuk's *The Web That Has No Weaver: Understanding Chinese Medicine* and Bensky's volumes on Chinese *materia medica* (compiled and translated with Andrew Gamble, a graduate of the New England School of Acupuncture, and Kaptchuk) first released in the 1980s, became essential English-language textbooks for American practitioners of Chinese medicine.[13]

Not all travelers to China returned with such favorable opinions of its medical system. After his 1971 tour of the major medical institutions of Beijing, Dimond published several articles about the state of Chinese medicine in both academic and popular journals. In the *Journal of the American Medical Association* (*JAMA*), Dimond was cautiously optimistic about the modern applications of traditional therapies: "We may find that there is much for *us* to learn."[14] For the readers of the popular magazine the *Saturday Review,* however, he was more dismissive, crediting acupuncture's efficacy to "the solace of a 'doctor's' attention." According to Dimond, acupuncture was no more than "an impressive psychosomatic therapy."[15] An eminent anesthesiologist and chair of the National Institutes of Health's Ad Hoc Committee on Acupuncture, John J. Bonica criticized the lack of well-controlled clinical trials of acupuncture when he visited China in 1974. He remarked, "Some of the traditional practitioners did not know what we were talking about when we inquired about clinical trials. Other acupuncturists who were younger and better educated, though cognizant of the concept . . . considered it unethical."[16] Looking back on the 1970s, sociologist Paul Root Wolpe identified a prevalent sense among eminent American physicians that acupuncture's effect was merely a placebo.[17] Nonetheless, the accumulated experiences of American physicians in the People's Republic convinced even the highly conservative American Medical Association (AMA) to concede in 1974 that acupuncture for pain relief merited additional study.[18]

Back in the United States, Chinese and Chinese American scientists rushed into their country's void of research into traditional Chinese

medicine. They leveraged their native-speaker fluency to read the studies emerging from the People's Republic and led some of the first clinical experiments conducted in American hospitals. In 1972, Dr. Wei-Chi
Liu, the director of anesthesiology at Louis A. Weiss Memorial Hospital
in Chicago, used acupuncture anesthesia in a tonsillectomy for the first
time in the United States. Liu described himself as "an anesthesiologist with some understanding of Chinese traditional medicine," which
he gleaned from reading recent books on acupuncture anesthesia published in Hong Kong. Liu's guinea pig was Gary Chinn, a young Asian
American nurse anesthetist employed by the hospital. The procedure
seems to have been a success; Chinn was sufficiently fit to wheel himself
to the recovery room after the operation.[19] Within a year, four other
hospitals had reported successes using acupuncture anesthesia in surgeries conducted by Chinese American physicians.[20] After some initial
euphoria, however, other experiments yielded negligible or negative
results, and in general surgery, acupuncture anesthesia in the United
States remained decidedly fringe.[21]

Nevertheless, Chinese and Chinese American scientists persisted
with their goal to "de-Orientalize" Chinese medicine. To secure institutional support for research and gain legitimacy among their academic
peers, they had to explain the efficacy of traditional Chinese therapies
in their community's lingua franca: conventional scientific models and
methods. Publishing a peer-reviewed journal was an important step in
this direction. In 1973, Frederick F. Kao founded the *American Journal of Chinese Medicine* (*AJCM*). Kao was a native of Beijing with an
M.D. from West China Union Medical College. An expert in respiratory physiology, he had immigrated to the United States to pursue a
Ph.D. at Northwestern University and then joined the faculty at the
State University of New York, Downstate Medical Center. Kao's journal identified the traditional Chinese therapies that had been "proven
effective" by biomedical methods and encouraged their adoption in
Western-style hospitals and medical schools.[22] In its inaugural issue,
he wrote, "'Magical' or 'miraculous' results . . . are only catch-phrases
until their worth has been proven; such 'worth' must ultimately be rig-
orously investigated and either verified, or discarded if found wanting.
It is always true that the importance of the 'magical' qualities of some

cure or principle must be secondary to its actual efficacy, rationale, and explanatory power according to the unbiased objective observer."[23] The *AJCM* would go on to publish articles, abstracts, and case reports primarily on acupuncture but also on the pharmacology of Chinese herbal medicines. Each issue presented research conducted in laboratories and clinics in the United States, China, Japan, and Europe as well as the Middle East.[24] The journal contained studies concerning the many variations of classical Chinese acupuncture, including the closely related Japanese and Korean traditional styles as well as the more recent, scientized innovations and naturopathic and homeopathic versions popularized in Europe.[25] In an early issue from 1974, Ko Kuei Chen contributed a retrospective on studies of ephedrine.[26] The *AJCM* also reported on the state of medical care in the People's Republic and regularly featured translations and histories of classical Chinese medicine. Still early in his career, the German historian and Sinologist Paul Unschuld published a two-part discourse on Chinese medical thought in 1977.[27]

Not all of the contributors to the *AJCM* had special training in traditional Chinese medicine or qualifications beyond a native-speaker fluency in Chinese. One frequent early contributor to the *AJCM* was James Y. P. Chen, an expert in clinical pharmacology and space medicine with a degree from Peking Union Medical College.[28] Born in Tianjin (Tientsin), Chen left China during World War II with his wife, Marjory Liu, and spent the next two decades teaching at prestigious medical colleges including the University of California, Tulane, and Marquette. By the 1970s, he had retired from academic medicine to focus on clinical pharmacology and space science research at Riker Laboratories and North American Aviation.[29] Throughout his career, Chen remained attentive to the changes occurring in Chinese medicine under Mao. In 1973, Chen joined Frederick Kao as part of a delegation of Chinese American physicians to China, where they had the opportunity to observe more than thirty operations conducted with acupuncture anesthesia. When the National Institutes of Health (NIH) announced plans to develop a formal research program into acupuncture, its officers enlisted Chen to lay the academic foundations.[30] In his work for the government, Chen aimed to "acquaint the American public" with "unfamiliar" remedies and practices, and to synthesize the best available scientific data on their efficacy.[31] In these ways, Chen literally and conceptually translated traditional therapies and practices for his fellow scientists and the policymakers they influenced.

Chen's work preceded the NIH's formation of an Ad Hoc Committee on Acupuncture, chaired by John Bonica. As part of its work, the committee identified twenty-six American medical schools and universities conducting research on acupuncture anesthesia and analgesia. In 1973, representative scientists from these institutions gathered for a national conference, where they presented work explaining the mechanism of classical Chinese acupuncture through biomedical models of biological information theory, energy distribution, and neurophysiology.[32] By no means did the conference "solve the mystery" of acupuncture, but it did signal the federal government's commitment to define the traditional Chinese therapy within conventional biomedical frameworks, and in so doing promote its acceptability in biomedical clinical care. In 1992, the NIH created the Office of Alternative Medicine to promote the research and regulation of irregular therapies, including those associated with Chinese medical knowledge systems. Five years later, the institutes sponsored a Consensus Meeting on Acupuncture, where a review panel of scientists identified specific conditions where biomedical research had proven acupuncture's clinical utility: postoperative and chemotherapy nausea and vomiting, and postoperative dental pain. The panel also recommended acupuncture as an adjunct or alternative treatment for select pain syndromes, headaches, asthma, addiction, and stroke rehabilitation.[33]

One can measure the success of biomedicalization by the increased inclusion of traditional Chinese medicine in major journals of academic medicine. A search of the Web of Science Core Collection, a database of peer-reviewed journals, returned nearly seven thousand articles on Chinese herbalism or acupuncture generated by American research institutes and universities since 1972. In the same period, one hundred of those articles have appeared in *JAMA* and fifty-two on the same topics in the *NEJM*, peer-reviewed, academic journals with national readerships. *JAMA* and the *NEJM* published roughly a third of those articles in the 1970s, but their coverage of these topics has not waned in subsequent decades. In 2017, ten articles on acupuncture appeared in these two journals—nine in *JAMA* and two in the *NEJM*.[34]

The burgeoning field of ethnopharmacology has combined chemical analysis of traditional Chinese remedies with sociocultural studies of their production and consumption. Although there is a long history of European bioprospecting for medicinal plants and animals in foreign lands, modern ethnopharmacology formally professionalized in the late 1960s and 1970s, bringing together pharmacologists, botanists, toxicologists, chemists, and anthropologists.[35] In 2009, Juerg Gertsch defined the essence of the interdisciplinary field as testing traditional remedies with laboratory science: "The ethnopharmacologist tries to understand the pharmacological basis of culturally important plants."[36] The end-goal of such work was often to commercialize local plants for drug development in global markets. In the late twentieth and early twenty-first centuries, researchers have concentrated on indigenous medical cultures in countries like Brazil, Mexico, South Africa, India, and—of course—China.[37] During his lifetime, Ko Kuei Chen accepted numerous honors including the AMA's Distinguished Service Award and the American Pharmaceutical Association's highest prize, the Remington Honor Medal, for his work on the traditional Chinese remedy ephedrine.[38] In 2015, a chief scientist at the China Academy of Traditional Chinese Medicine in Beijing, Tu Youyou, received the Nobel Prize in Physiology or Medicine for her discovery of Artemisnin, the active component of the traditional herb sweet wormwood (*Artemesia annua*), which has reduced the mortality rates associated with malaria. Tu used a conventional scientific method of phytochemical screening to identify and isolate Artemisnin. In bestowing the award, a Nobel committee member, Hans Forssberg, insisted, "It's very important that we are not giving a prize to traditional medicine; the award was only for the scientific work that had been inspired by it."[39] Forssberg's message was clear: biomedicalization made an ancient science worthy of international recognition.

Clinical studies of traditional Chinese medicine have complemented laboratory and fieldwork. Prominent hospitals and medical research groups like the Mayo Clinic in Minnesota; Cleveland Clinic;

University of California, San Francisco; and Mount Sinai in New York have incorporated acupuncture and herbalism into their pain management and integrative care programs.[40] American biomedical education has also cracked open the door to irregular practices, including Chinese acupuncture and herbalism. Medical students and physicians who pursue an elective or certification in integrative medicine gain familiarity with these Chinese therapies so that they know when to refer a patient to a practitioner.[41] Because of this new scholarship and training, it has become somewhat more common for major health insurance plans to cover traditional Chinese therapies. Anthem Blue Cross, Kaiser Permanente, and Aetna of California treat chiropractic medicine and acupuncture as equivalents, and Aetna has some plans that consider acupuncture "medically necessary" (and therefore reimbursable) for specific pain conditions, nausea associated with pregnancy or chemotherapy, and dental analgesia.[42] Given the middle- and upper-class demographic that tends to seek out traditional Chinese therapies, industry analysts have reasoned that attracting relatively healthy consumers to the risk pool may be the primary motivation for private health insurers, but it may also signal a longer-term strategy to reduce costs associated with chronic conditions through noninvasive and drugless treatments.[43]

Biomedical scientists seeking to explain the efficacy of traditional therapies with conventional research methods have run up against the limitations of their discipline. In the decades after World War II, American and European researchers increasingly relied on double-blind, randomized controlled studies to prove the superiority of their intervention over a placebo.[44] While other research methods like case studies and population studies retained an important place in academic medicine, by the 1960s and 1970s American and European regulatory agencies required evidence gathered by such trials to approve new drugs and other therapies for the market. Students of traditional Chinese medicine have often argued that this so-called gold standard of biomedical research is poorly suited to the therapeutic principles of their practice. In the 2000 edition of his book *The Web That Has No Weaver*, Ted Kaptchuk outlined the unique challenges that acupuncture researchers face when submitting their therapy to randomized controlled trials including the impossibility of introducing a sham control: "Most researchers worry that needling at 'non-acupuncture' [points] is not analogous to a dummy inert pill as a placebo control. The concern is that needling anywhere in the body (at both real acupuncture sites or non-acupuncture sites) may have physiological effects."[45] Recent scholarship has attempted to address the placebo problem through different study designs that can still yield measurements of efficacy. These have included single-blind, randomized controlled trials and crossover trials in which patients initially receive acupuncture for pain relief followed by a period of placebo treatment.[46] At Massachusetts General Hospital and Harvard Medical School, researchers have collaborated with scientists in China and Korea to conduct multicenter prospective cohort studies of cardiovascular disease to evaluate clinical alternatives, including Chinese and Korean medicines and yoga, for patients at risk of major cardiac arrest.[47]

Vivienne Lo's preface to the 2002 edition of Gwei-Djen Lu and Joseph Needham's *Celestial Lancets* argued that the more "intractable" problem of biomedicalization is the fundamental incompatibility between randomized controlled trials and traditional Chinese medicine. Such trials privilege therapeutics and outcomes that researchers can reduce, isolate, and replicate; traditional Chinese therapies are inherently eclectic, holistic, and particular. According to Lo, "No studies directly compare different styles of individual complementary therapies, let alone the many different forms of acupuncture that exist internationally—and even within the confines of one clinic. There are a multitude of individual styles of practice as well as individual issues of competence, all of which introduce an untenable amount of variable and undermine any trial of 'acupuncture and moxibustion' as a unitary phenomenon."[48]

Researchers have explored creative ways to reconcile seemingly irreconcilable epistemologies. In 2006, Rishma Walji and Heather Boon recommended modifying the standard approach to clinical trials by randomizing participants according to "Oriental" diagnoses rather than Western-style biomedical criteria, a step toward acknowledging the significance of taking into account the medical knowledge system from which Chinese therapies emanated.[49] Walji and Boon's proposal joined a wider movement among Complementary and Alternative Medical researchers to pursue a "mixed methods" approach, combining qualitative methodologies in the formulation of studies with quantitative methods suited to a clinical setting.[50] A search of the NIH's Research Portfolio Online Reporting Tools finds that the federal agency funded forty-seven projects between 2017 and 2019 that concern Chinese acupuncture or herbalism.[51] Such research holds out the promise that a fuller reckoning with the internal logic of traditional Chinese therapies might open up new ways of understanding the nature of human health.

Practitioners of traditional Chinese medicine have responded to biomedicalization with understandable ambivalence. Among national accrediting organizations and American schools of acupuncture and "Oriental" medicine, there is no standard curriculum; some require courses in Western-style biomedical science, others offer them as an elective or not at all.[52] Some practitioners and educators have embraced partnerships with biomedical hospitals and researchers for both the pecuniary and nonpecuniary opportunities that they generate. As medical anthropologist Hannah Flesch observed in her 2013 study of the acupuncture and "Oriental" medicine program at West Coast University, an emphasis on biomedical education and research improved students' rates of licensure and public and private insurance reimbursements. Flesch also noted that faculty and administrators felt that "science provides a common language for communication with allopathy," allowing students to become "better practitioners, proponents, and communicators of [Chinese] medicine."[53] Yet there are also practitioners who insist that their work is an alternative to biomedicine, and that forcing standardization and compatibility with biomedical epistemologies or institutions reduces the complexity of traditional therapies to the point of inefficacy. Economic and language barriers have prevented some practitioners of traditional Chinese medicine from accessing biomedical education and licensing, but others deliberately and actively reject biomedical assimilation. They have made unconventionality and exoticism the basis of their value proposition to American patient-consumers. In a 2003 article, medical anthropologist Linda Barnes named this professional dispute "The Acupuncture Wars," and it continues with no end in sight.[54]

"The Very Old and the Very New"

In the 1980s, sociologists anticipated that the biomedicalization of traditional Chinese medicine would precipitate the swift decline of Chinese acupuncture.[55] Paul Root Wolpe characterized biomedical studies of acupuncture as a "tactic pursued by the medical profession in the United States to monopolize acupuncture," and ultimately to discourage American patients from perceiving the therapy as a viable alternative to biomedical treatments. Wolpe predicted that, as a result, public interest in acupuncture would inevitably fade.[56] It did not.

Chinese acupuncture and its closely paired modalities, moxibustion and herbalism, have become mainstays in Complementary and Alternative Medicine, a modern reinterpretation of what Progressive Era Americans might have called "irregular" medicine. In some parts of the world, acupuncture continues to serve as preventative medicine for poor and rural populations unable to afford other treatments, but in the United States, it has become a hallmark of what anthropologist Mei Zhan calls "hip, middle-class, cosmopolitan lifestyles that emphasize overall well-being and mind-body health."[57] Between 2000 and 2010, an estimated 20 million Americans received acupuncture. An NIH survey in 2007 found that acupuncture was one of the fastest growing Complementary and Alternative Medical therapies in the United States.[58] A 2015 study of acupuncture users in the United States based on a 2012 NIH survey found that they tend to be older than sixty-five, women, and white, with at least a bachelor's degree or higher education.[59]

As members of a wealthy and aging society, middle-class and affluent Americans have pressured biomedical institutions to open their doors to alternative treatments. In turn, biomedical scientists have become increasingly accepting of an "integrative" approach, especially where it presents the potential to reduce costs associated with chronic conditions like heart disease, diabetes, and pain. The most popular Chinese therapies as well as cupping, scraping, and therapeutic exercise like t'ai chi and qi gong are served up in combination with Ayurvedic medicine, de-spiritualized variations of yoga, meditation, homeopathic and naturopathic remedies, chiropractic medicine, and countless other traditions that have had historically contentious relationships with Western-style scientific medicine.[60] American patient-consumers sample freely from a global buffet of health and "wellness" offerings.

After struggling through the mid-twentieth century, the Chinese herb business in the United States is thriving. The United States is the biggest importer of traditional Chinese medicine outside of Asia.[61] The 1994 Dietary Supplement Health and Education Act (DSHEA) offered a major boost to the industry. The federal legislation classified traditional Chinese remedies as "dietary" or food supplements, and as such exempted them from the approval process and regulatory scrutiny to which pharmaceuticals submit. The DSHEA did place some limits on manufacturing, marketing, and labeling of herbal products; most importantly, producers could not claim to treat or prevent diseases, but the law left ample leeway to make claims to restore, improve, or otherwise favorably affect the consumer's body.[62] By 1997, sales of herbal supplements in the United States increased 50 percent, from $8 billion to $12 billion. Medicinal plants commonly used by the Chinese like ginseng, Echinacea, and gingko biloba constituted a sizeable percentage of total revenues.[63] The Chinese herb business was becoming big business.

The expansion of the herbal supplement market has prompted not only new products on the market but also an uptick in chemical analyses of the active components of traditional herbal remedies and studies concerning toxicity and adverse drug interactions. A search of the Web of Science Core Collection for articles on Chinese herbalism between 1970 and 2018 yielded over 900 peer-reviewed citations from American research institutes and universities, nearly all of them published after the passage of the DSHEA.[64] Historically, conventional drug manufacturers ignored herbal remedies because of their limited potential for patenting, but the volume of revenues has attracted the attention of pharmaceutical companies. Traditional remedies once tucked away inside the drawers and jars of Chinatown apothecaries are now mass-produced and shipped from Chinese, Japanese, and Korean factories.[65] While manufacturers still source most of the raw ingredients in China, American farmers have found a lucrative opportunity augmenting the supply.[66] Big-box stores are just as likely to stock ancient herbal remedies as tiny, Chinese apothecaries.[67] The widening availability of Chinese herbal remedies, combined with processes of professionalization and institutionalization, has drawn Chinese medicine from the margins into the mainstream.

For American patient-consumers, the core cultural associations with Chinese medicine have proved remarkably durable over time. When "Chinese Doctor, Dr. John Howard" advertised his services in Harrisburg, Pennsylvania, in 1799, he promised to cure by "herbs and roots only," an implicit criticism of the harsh emetics and purgatives favored by his competitors. With just four words, Howard—whoever he was—foreshadowed the essential value proposition that generations of Chinese doctors would extend to their non-Chinese patients. In China, traditional therapies were wide-ranging, from drug therapy and surgery to faith healing and ancestor worship, but in the United States, they narrowed and became everything that regular medicine was not: noninvasive and "drugless." As biomedical science became increasingly technical and complex, Chinese medicine—along with other irregular medical sects—insisted on its simplicity and accessibility, its closeness to an essential nature of human health. "Nature's" laws were not just universal; they were universally comprehensible. At the same time, however, Chinese doctors traded on their unique, embodied, and racialized expertise in age-old, quasi-mystical, and altogether foreign healing arts. For more than two centuries, practitioners of Chinese medicine in the United States defined their work in a series of contradictions. Their remedies were equal parts exotic and familiar, miraculous and empirical, ancient and modern.

Today, Chinese herbal remedies remain central to debates over the meanings of nature in the realm of human health. Critics of biomedical science continue to characterize conventional pharmaceuticals as "toxic" or "unnatural." Synthesized in a laboratory, dispensed by the prescription of formally trained, licensed professionals, pharmaceuticals cannot shake their association with the discomfiting expertise and elitism of biomedical science. Chinese herbal remedies, on the other hand, are presumed to be unsynthesized or only very lightly processed and thus seem intuitively closer to their original state as plants, animals, or minerals. The historically persistent and largely unquestioned coupling of Chinese medicine and "nature" presents several troubling consequences for human and nonhuman health.

The presumed closeness to nature of Chinese remedies has not necessarily led to sustainable relationships with *materia medica.* In North America, over-foraging of wild ginseng led to its depletion and disappearance in areas of Canada and the eastern United States where it once grew. Likewise, the combination of unregulated foraging and the rapid conversion of forest to farmland across the Midwest led to a similar decline in that region. In 1865, Minnesota passed the first legislation to restrict the gathering season to May 1 to August 1, with fines up to one hundred dollars for violations. The efforts were for naught; by the end of the century, wild ginseng was vanishing.[68] Beginning in the 1870s, American and Canadian farmers experimented with growing cultivated ginseng, but Chinese buyers deemed it less potent and therefore less valuable.[69] In 1977, in an effort to protect the vestiges of wild ginseng, the Endangered Species Scientific Authority, a division of the U.S. Fish and Wildlife Service, proposed an export ban.[70] In the end, ginseng-producing states reached a compromise with the federal agency that limited diggers to harvesting mature roots five years or older during a restricted season lasting from August to December. Within the last decade, however, soaring international demand for wild ginseng has triggered a surge in illegal "poaching" across Appalachia. Extinction is a real possibility.[71]

As the market for Chinese herbal remedies has expanded since the 1980s, so has its impact on the environment. Ethnopharmacologists' search for "miracle drugs" in less-developed Asian regions has drawn attention to biodiversity and heightened public investment in conservation, but wild animals and plants still suffer from unsustainable harvesting linked to the expanding global market for traditional Chinese medicine.[72] Hunting tigers and other animals coveted for their medicinal properties has accelerated and contributed to the endangerment of the species. Poaching and smuggling have become the subject of international debate with no clear resolution. In October 2018, the Chinese government lifted a twenty-five-year ban on the use of rhinoceros horns and tiger bones in medicine. Although the new policy directive purports to restrict that use to animals raised in captivity, practically speaking, there is no way to enforce such a distinction, and legalization of rhino and tiger parts will surely spur illegal hunting among endangered, wild populations.[73] As with North American ginseng, over-foraging has imperiled other Chinese medicines traditionally grown in the wild in Asia. *Ophiocordyceps sinensis,* a combination of a caterpillar and fungus found in the high altitude mountains of Tibet, is one prime example of this problem. Recorded in both classical Chinese and Tibetan pharmacopoeia, cordyceps flourishes beneath the snowpack and has a variety of traditional medicinal uses, including treating cancers. Locals forage for cordyceps by hand, using trowels to uproot the fungus along with the soil and vegetation that surrounds it. As demand has increased, so has collection, which has damaged the vegetative cover that prevents soil erosion. A drought in 2014 exacerbated conditions and diminished the production of cordyceps by 50 percent. Global climate change has also adversely affected cordyceps by raising the snow line and shrinking the species' natural habitat. Seemingly oblivious to these changing ecological pressures, local governments have encouraged Tibetan families to increase cordyceps production as a means to integrate their communities more fully into the commercial economy.[74]

Naturalism can also pose dangers to human health. The discourse of natural medicine has created a false sense of security with regard to the consumption of herbal remedies. Since the passage of the 1994 DSHEA, the federal government has intervened in the herbal remedy market only in a few instances, most famously the 2003 ban on ephedra (the ancient Chinese remedy *ma huang*) after research connected its overconsumption to cardiac arrest and strokes. The federal ban—which followed in the wake of several independent state bans—did not affect other traditional Chinese remedies, which the Food and Drug Administration (FDA) continues to regulate as dietary supplements and conventional foods.[75] Meanwhile, across the Pacific Ocean, the Chinese government under President Xi Jinping minimized the clinical-trial requirements for traditional Chinese medicines to make it easier for companies to bring their products to market.[76] Since 2002, the American federal government has increased its funding for studies of dietary supplements that investigate issues of toxicity, cancer and tumor growth, and health claims.[77] Nonetheless, there remains a great deal of uncertainty about dosage, side effects, and drug interactions. Scientists have identified potential adverse interactions between Chinese medicinal plants and nonsteroidal anti-inflammatory drugs (for example, aspirin). Enhanced risk for bleeding, kidney damage, liver cancer, and depression have all been linked to the consumption of traditional Chinese herbal remedies.[78] In the absence of robust oversight, contamination also remains a major concern. The FDA does establish "Current Good Manufacturing Practices" for dietary supplements, but inspections have been sporadic at best.[79] As a result, a startling number of imports of Chinese herbal remedies have been found to contain bacteria, pesticides, and other adulterants hazardous to human health.[80]

The association of irregular medicine with "nature" and regular medicine with its opposite is part of a much larger problem: a climate of science skepticism that breeds misinformation at least and dire health outcomes at worst. For an example, one need only look as far as the rampant "anti-vaxxer" movement of parents who refuse to follow the vaccination schedule recommended by the Centers for Disease Control for their children. Their concerns about vaccines are not based on empirical evidence but rather a reflexive distrust of biomedical authority and its interventionism. In the case of the anti-vaxxer movement, "letting nature take its course" has allowed potentially deadly infectious diseases like measles and whooping cough to roar back to life.[81]

On the other side of the sectarian divide, biomedical scientists have been slow to adopt "alternative" therapies. Only recently (and reluctantly) have biomedical scientists considered acupuncture to address the problem of opioid over-prescription. In 2017, the American College of Physicians and the FDA approved pain management plans that include acupuncture as an alternative to prescription opioids. The announcement divided biomedical scientists.[82] An op-ed for the American Council on Science and Health scathingly criticized the FDA and Centers for Disease Control as members of a "pharmaceutical police state" whose policies inhumanely and indiscriminately restrict conventional drug treatments for pain and offer instead a useless regimen of "Advil, yoga, or acupuncture."[83] For a century, the discourse of natural medicine has divided biomedical scientists and practitioners of other healing systems, resulting in lost opportunities not only for common colloquy but, most importantly, for improved health for all.

Along with naturalism, the language of Orientalism continues to mediate American interpretations of traditional Chinese medicine. Over time, the changing relationship between China and the United States has made new demands of Orientalism. The politics of trade and empire-building in the nineteenth century insisted on Chinese racial subordination whereas Cold War–era imperatives to recruit overseas knowledge-workers and generate international goodwill invented the myth of the Asian American as model minority. Nonetheless, fundamental assumptions of Oriental alterity persisted. The Chinese, and by extension their healing practices, were alternatingly demeaned and esteemed, but their eternal otherness was never in doubt.

In today's medical marketplace, practitioners of traditional Chinese medicine continue to present their services through Orientalist frames of exoticism, mysticism, and naturalism. Step inside any Chinese American herb shop and you will find shelves of plastic pill bottles bearing pictures of bamboo, flowers, fields of grass, or birds in flight. Occasionally, a label features a male or female figure costumed in robes and caps from premodern China and framed by tree branches, a mountainous vista, or other images conveying their embeddedness in nature. The images on the outside of the bottle rarely correspond to the ingredients inside. The Plum Flower brand of Six Flavor Tea Pills contains a combination of *Rehmannia glutinosa* root, Chinese yam, and dogwood fruit while its label shows a Chinese man and woman racing a dragon boat across a bright green sea.[84] Anthropologists Emily Wu and Mei Zhan, who have shadowed Chinese acupuncturists in California at the turn of the twenty-first century, have observed in their clinics and marketing the adoption of stereotypically Oriental aesthetics that conjure images associated with nonhuman nature, otherworldliness, and miracle-working.[85]

The incentives to "de-Orientalize" are not clear. As Mei Zhan has argued, self-Orientalization is still in many ways a source of practitioners' legitimacy and power to challenge biomedical authority.[86] Practitioners of traditional Chinese medicine have translated their therapeutic practices and principles into racialized shorthand and profited from it. In the American medical marketplace, Chinese medicine has historically thrived as an alternative, not a complement, to regular medicine. Moving forward, the integration of traditional therapies with biomedical care will have to overcome a long historical campaign to define Chinese medicine as the opposite of regular medicine, a campaign in which Chinese doctors have played a significant and supportive role.

Notes

Introduction

1. "A Chinese Doctor," *Arizona Sentinel* (Yuma), October 17, 1885.

2. "Chinese Consulate at Chicago," *New York Times,* May 17, 1883; "Chinatown History," Chicago Chinatown, http://chicago-chinatown.info/chinatown-history/.

3. "Chicago Chinaman," *Elyria [Ohio] Democrat,* August 22, 1889; "A Chinese Doctor's Troubles," *Daily Alta California* (San Francisco), January 4, 1890; "Cheap Chinese Doctors," *Connersville [Ill.] Daily Examiner,* January 6, 1890.

4. "Chicago Workingmen Resolve," *Los Angeles Times,* March 21, 1882; "Anti-Chinese in Chicago," *Los Angeles Times,* April 18, 1882; "Raid on Chinese Opium-Eaters in Chicago," *Los Angeles Times,* June 6, 1883; "Chinese Consulate at Chicago," *New York Times,* May 17, 1883.

5. "A Chinese Doctor," *Arizona Sentinel,* October 17, 1885.

6. For a discussion of this terminology and periodization, see Viviane Quirke and Jean-Paul Gaudilliere, "The Era of Biomedicine: Science, Medicine, and Public Health in Britain and France after the Second World War," *Medical History* 52, no. 4 (October 2008): 441–452, and Ilana Lowy, "Historiography of Biomedicine: 'Bio,' 'Medicine,' and In Between," *Isis* 102, no. 1 (March 2011): 116–122.

7. There is an important difference between "traditional Chinese medicine" and "Traditional Chinese Medicine," with capitalized first letters. The latter refers to the regularized and simplified version of ancient therapies promoted under Mao Zedong's regime of medical modernization. I discuss Traditional Chinese Medicine in chapter 7.

8. For broad surveys of traditional Chinese medicine from its ancient and geographically varied origins to the near present, *Herbs and Roots* has relied principally on T. J. Hinrichs and Linda L. Barnes's *Chinese Medicine and Healing: An Illustrated History,* Paul U. Unschuld's *Medicine in China: A History of Ideas,* and Volker Scheid's

Currents of Tradition in Chinese Medicine, 1626–2006. Gwei-Djen Lu and Joseph Need-ham's *Celestial Lancets: A History and Rationale of Acupuncture and Moxa* offers a simi-larly comprehensive intellectual history of two closely linked traditional Chinese mo-dalities. Scheid's work on the merchant-physicians of Menghe and their influence on nineteenth-century medicine in China and Marta Hanson's analysis of scholarly debates over medical knowledge have been critical to understanding the intellectual milieu in which the early generations of Chinese immigrant doctors trained. Research by Char-lotte Furth and Yi-Li Wu on the history of obstetrics and gynecology in China sup-plied context for the services that Chinese immigrant doctors provided to women in the United States. Bridie Andrews's *The Making of Modern Chinese Medicine, 1850–1960* has traced the biomedicalization of China's health care system from its nineteenth-century origins to its Communist-era fruition. Importantly, she locates the construction of a scienticized traditional Chinese medicine in the Nationalist Era reforms to education and civil service. T. J. Hinrichs and Linda L. Barnes, *Chinese Medicine and Healing: An Illustrated History* (Cambridge, Mass.: Belknap Press of Harvard University Press, 2013); Paul U. Unschuld, *Medicine in China: A History of Ideas* (Berkeley: University of California Press, 1985); Volker Scheid, *Currents of Tradition in Chinese Medicine, 1626–2006* (Seattle: Eastland Press, 2007); Gwei-Djen Lu and Joseph Needham, *Celes-tial Lancets: A History and Rationale of Acupuncture and Moxa* (Cambridge: Cambridge University Press, 1980); Volker Scheid, "Remodeling the Arsenal of Chinese Medicine: Shared Pasts, Alternative Futures," *Annals of the American Academy of Political and So-cial Science* 583, no. 1 (2002): 136–159; Marta Hanson, "Robust Northerners and Delicate Southerners: The Nineteenth-Century Invention of a Southern Medical Tradition," *Po-sitions* 6, no. 3 (1998): 515–550; Marta Hanson, "The 'Golden Mirror' in the Imperial Court of the Qianlong Emperor, 1739–1742," *Early Science and Medicine* 8, no. 2 (2003): 111–147; Charlotte Furth, *A Flourishing Yin Gender in China's Medical History, 960–1665* (Berkeley: University of California Press, 1999); Yi-Li Wu, *Reproducing Women: Medi-cine, Metaphor, and Childbirth in Late Imperial China* (Berkeley: University of California Press, 2010); Bridie Andrews, *The Making of Modern Chinese Medicine, 1850–1960* (Van-couver: University of British Columbia Press, 2014).

9. Hinrichs and Barnes, *Chinese Medicine and Healing,* 39.

10. Ibid., 7; Unschuld, *Medicine in China,* 55–60.

11. John Kuo Wei Tchen, *New York before Chinatown: Orientalism and the Shaping of American Culture, 1776–1882* (Baltimore: Johns Hopkins University Press, 1999); Mari Yoshihara, *Embracing the East: White Women and American Orientalism* (Oxford: Oxford University Press, 2003); Karen J. Leong, *The China Mystique: Pearl S. Buck, Anna May Wong, Mayling Soong, and the Transformation of American Orien-talism* (Berkeley: University of California Press, 2005).

12. Henry Yu advances a similar argument in his study of Asian American sociolo-gists in the early twentieth century. Henry Yu, *Thinking Orientals: Migration, Contact, and Exoticism in Modern America* (Oxford: Oxford University Press, 2001), 10–11.

13. Practitioners of Chinese medicine were not all Chinese. In the United States,

immigrants from Japan, Korea, and Southeast Asia practiced herbalism, acupuncture, and other modalities that originated in China. Today, non-Asians are increasingly represented among licensed practitioners of traditional Chinese therapies, especially acupuncture. I leave the work of considering how healers of non-Chinese nativity have transformed this system of medical knowledge as it spread to the United States to other scholars. Emily S. Wu, *Traditional Chinese Medicine in the United States: In Search of Spiritual Meaning and Ultimate Health* (Lanham, Md.: Lexington Books, 2013), 21.

14. Jeffrey G. Barlow and Christine Richardson, *China Doctor of John Day* (Portland, Ore.: Binford and Mort, 1979), 66.

15. Ibid., 63.

16. Linnea Klee, "The 'Regulars' and the Chinese: Ethnicity and Public Health in 1870s San Francisco," *Urban Anthropology* 12, no. 2 (1983): 192; Will Sarvis, "Gifted Healer Ing Hay and the Chinese Medical Tradition in Eastern Oregon, 1888–1948," *Journal of the West* 44, no. 3 (2005): 65–66; Paul D. Buell, *Chinese Medicine on the Golden Mountain: An Interpretive Guide* (Seattle: Wing Luke Memorial Museum, 1984), 64–65.

17. Barlow and Richardson, *China Doctor of John Day*; Sarvis, "Gifted Healer Ing Hay and the Chinese Medical Tradition in Eastern Oregon"; Chia-lin Chen, "A Gold Dream in the Blue Mountains: A Study of the Chinese Immigrants in the John Day Area, Oregon, 1870–1910" (M.A. thesis, Portland State University, 1972); *Oregon Experience: Kam Wah Chung*, 2009, http://watch.opb.org/video/1207317935/; Haiming Liu, *The Transnational History of a Chinese Family: Immigrant Letters, Family Business, and Reverse Migration* (New Brunswick, N.J: Rutgers University Press, 2005).

18. Buell, *Chinese Medicine on the Golden Mountain*; Aminda M. Smith, "Choosing Chinese Medicine: Idaho's C. K. Ah Fong and Turn-of-the-Century Apothecaries in the American West," *Journal of the West* 48, no. 4 (2009): 96–103; Michael Devitt, "The Curious Case of Ah Fong Chuck, America's First 'Licensed' Acupuncturist," *Journal of Chinese Medicine*, no. 97 (October 2011): 5–12.

19. William M. Bowen, "The Five Eras of Chinese Medicine in California," in *The Chinese in America: A History from Gold Mountain to the Millennium*, ed. Susie Lan Cassel (Walnut Creek, Calif.: AltaMira Press, 2002), 174–192; Sue Fawn Chung, *In Pursuit of Gold: Chinese American Miners and Merchants in the American West* (Urbana: University of Illinois Press, 2011); Haiming Liu, "Chinese Herbalists in the United States," in *Chinese American Transnationalism: The Flow of People, Resources, and Ideas between China and America during the Exclusion Era*, ed. Sucheng Chan (Philadelphia: Temple University Press, 2006), 136–155; Kenneth H. Marcus and Yong Chen, "Inside and Outside Chinatown: Chinese Elites in Exclusion Era California," *Pacific Historical Review* 80, no. 3 (August 2011): 369–400; Shehong Chen, *Being Chinese, Becoming Chinese American* (Urbana: University of Illinois Press, 2002); Mary Ting Li Lui, *The Chinatown Trunk Mystery: Murder, Miscegenation, and Other Dangerous Encounters in Turn-of-the-Century New York City* (Princeton, N.J.: Princeton University Press, 2005).

20. Liu, "Chinese Herbalists in the United States," 155.

21. Mae M. Ngai, *The Lucky Ones: One Family and the Extraordinary Invention of Chinese America*, expanded ed. (2010; Princeton, N.J.: Princeton University Press, 2012).

22. Tchen, *New York before Chinatown*, xxxiii; Yoshihara, *Embracing the East*, 6–7.

23. Yu, *Thinking Orientals;* Leong, *The China Mystique;* Judy Tzu-Chun Wu, *Doctor Mom Chung of the Fair-Haired Bastards: The Life of a Wartime Celebrity* (Berkeley: University of California Press, 2005); Emma Teng, *Eurasian: Mixed Identities in the United States, China, and Hong Kong, 1842–1943* (Berkeley: University of California Press, 2013).

24. Ellen D. Wu, *The Color of Success: Asian Americans and the Origins of the Model Minority* (Princeton, N.J.: Princeton University Press, 2014); Madeline Yuan-yin Hsu, *The Good Immigrants: How the Yellow Peril Became the Model Minority* (Princeton, N.J.: Princeton University Press, 2015); Scott Kurashige, *The Shifting Grounds of Race: Black and Japanese Americans in the Making of Multiethnic Los Angeles* (Princeton, N.J.: Princeton University Press, 2008).

25. Thomas F. Gieryn, *Cultural Boundaries of Science: Credibility on the Line* (Chicago: University of Chicago Press, 1999).

26. Colleen Derkatch, *Bounding Biomedicine: Evidence and Rhetoric in the New Science of Alternative Medicine* (Chicago: University of Chicago Press, 2016).

27. Hans A. Baer, *Biomedicine and Alternative Healing Systems in America: Issues of Class, Race, Ethnicity, and Gender* (Madison: University of Wisconsin Press, 2001).

28. James C. Whorton, *Nature Cures: The History of Alternative Medicine in America* (Oxford: Oxford University Press, 2002).

29. Ibid.; Norman Gevitz, ed., *Other Healers: Unorthodox Medicine in America* (Baltimore: Johns Hopkins University Press, 1988); Susan E. Cayleff, *Nature's Path: A History of Naturopathic Healing in America* (Baltimore: Johns Hopkins University Press, 2016); Volney Steele, *Bleed, Blister, and Purge: A History of Medicine on the American Frontier* (Missoula, Mont.: Mountain Press, 2005), 105–106; Baer, *Biomedicine and Alternative Healing Systems in America.*

30. Martin Kaufman, *Homeopathy in America: The Rise and Fall of a Medical Heresy* (Ann Arbor, Mich.: UMI Books on Demand, 1995), ix.

31. Alan M. Kraut, *Silent Travelers: Germs, Genes, and the "Immigrant Menace"* (Baltimore: Johns Hopkins University Press, 1995), 5.

32. In addition to the monographs discussed in this introduction, see, for example, Klee, "The 'Regulars' and the Chinese," 181–207, and Joan B. Trauner, "The Chinese as Medical Scapegoats in San Francisco, 1870–1905," *California History* 57, no. 1 (April 1, 1978): 70–87.

33. Nayan Shah, *Contagious Divides: Epidemics and Race in San Francisco's Chinatown* (Berkeley: University of California Press, 2001), 5.

34. Guenter B. Risse, *Plague, Fear, and Politics in San Francisco's Chinatown* (Baltimore: Johns Hopkins University Press, 2012), 10–11.

35. Buell, *Chinese Medicine on the Golden Mountain;* Linda L. Barnes, "The Acupuncture Wars: The Professionalizing of American Acupuncture—A View from Massachusetts," *Medical Anthropology* 22, no. 3 (2003): 261–301; Linda L. Barnes, "The Psychologizing of Chinese Healing Practices in the United States," *Culture, Medicine and Psychiatry: An International Journal of Comparative Cross-Cultural Research* 22, no. 4 (1998): 413–443; Linda L. Barnes, "Multiple Meanings of Chinese Healing in the United States," in *Religion and Healing in America*, ed. Linda L. Barnes and Susan Starr Sered (New York: Oxford University Press, 2005), 307–332; Sarah Christine Heffner, "Exploring Health-Care Practices of Chinese Railroad Workers in North America," *Historical Archaeology* 49, no. 1 (2015): 134–147; Samir S. Patel, "America's Chinatowns," *Archaeology* 67, no. 3 (June 5, 2014): 38–43; Douglas E. Ross, *An Archaeology of Asian Transnationalism* (Gainesville: University Press of Florida, 2013); Mei Zhan, *Other-Worldly: Making Chinese Medicine through Transnational Frames* (Durham, N.C.: Duke University Press, 2009).

36. Beth Howlett, interview with author, September 8, 2011.

37. Foundational texts in the field of U.S. environmental history such as Richard White's *The Organic Machine*, Donald Worster's *Rivers of Empire* and *Dust Bowl,* and William Cronon's *Changes in the Land* and *Nature's Metropolis* have considered major human transformations of the nonhuman landscape: dams, reclamation, farming and grazing, overhunting, deforestation, and urbanization and industrialization. Richard White, *The Organic Machine* (New York: Hill and Wang, 1996); Donald Worster, *Rivers of Empire: Water, Aridity, and the Growth of the American West* (Oxford: Oxford University Press, 1992); Worster, *Dust Bowl: The Southern Plains in the 1930s* (Oxford: Oxford University Press, 1982); William Cronon, *Changes in the Land: Indians, Colonists, and the Ecology of New England* (New York: Hill and Wang, 1983); Cronon, *Nature's Metropolis: Chicago and the Great West* (New York: Norton, 1992).

38. Conevery Bolton Valencius, *The Health of the Country: How American Settlers Understood Themselves and Their Land* (New York: Basic Books, 2002); Gregg Mitman, *Breathing Space: How Allergies Shape Our Lives and Landscapes* (New Haven, Conn.: Yale University Press, 2007); Linda Nash, *Inescapable Ecologies: A History of Environment, Disease, and Knowledge* (Berkeley: University of California Press, 2006); Nancy Langston, *Toxic Bodies: Hormone Disruptors and the Legacy of DES* (New Haven, Conn.: Yale University Press, 2010).

39. Whorton, *Nature Cures.*

40. Other scholars devote attention to the spaces where American jurisdiction did not extend. To understand the global diaspora of Chinese therapeutic practices and principles in the premodern and early modern world, *Herbs and Roots* rests on the foundations of Linda L. Barnes's *Needles, Herbs, Gods, and Ghosts: China, Healing, and the West to 1848*, and Roberta E. Bivins's *Alternative Medicine? A History*, both of which survey European and—to a lesser extent—American observations and interpretations of Chinese medical practices and texts. British traders and missionaries in China served as role models for their American counterparts, and *Herbs and Roots* has depended on the robust scholarship on these subjects including Fa-ti Fan's *British Natu-*

ralists in Qing China: Science, Empire, and Cultural Encounter and G. H. Choa's *"Heal the Sick" Was Their Motto: The Protestant Medical Missionaries in China.* To understand late twentieth-century developments in the assimilation of Chinese therapies into modern national health care systems outside of China such as England, France, and Germany, *Herbs and Roots* has drawn from Kelvin Chan and Henry Lee's anthology, *The Way Forward for Chinese Medicine.* Linda L. Barnes, *Needles, Herbs, Gods, and Ghosts: China, Healing, and the West to 1848* (Cambridge, Mass.: Harvard University Press, 2005); Roberta E. Bivins, *Alternative Medicine? A History* (Oxford: Oxford University Press, 2010); Fa-ti Fan, *British Naturalists in Qing China: Science, Empire, and Cultural Encounter* (Cambridge, Mass.: Harvard University Press, 2004); G. H. Choa, *"Heal the Sick" Was Their Motto: The Protestant Medical Missionaries in China* (Shatin, N.T., Hong Kong: Chinese University Press, 1990); Kelvin Chan and Henry Lee, *The Way Forward for Chinese Medicine* (London: Taylor and Francis, 2002).

    41. "A Chinese Doctor," *Arizona Sentinel,* October 17, 1885.

ONE Herbs and Roots

    1. Advertisement, *Oracle of Dauphin and Harrisburgh [Penn.] Advertiser,* April 17, 1799.

    2. Advertisement, *Oracle of Dauphin and Harrisburgh Advertiser,* May 1, June 5, 1799; Advertisement, *Kline's Carlisle [Penn.] Weekly Gazette,* September 3, November 5, 26, 1800.

    3. C. A. Rahter, "Medical History of Dauphin County," *Pennsylvania Medical Journal* 11, no. 4 (1907): 302.

    4. Walton Look Lai and Chee-Beng Tan, *The Chinese in Latin America and the Caribbean* (Leiden: Brill, 2010), 7.

    5. In the late seventeenth and eighteenth centuries, Jesuits made it possible for some Chinese young men to travel to Europe, where they assisted with translations and language study. Barnes, *Needles, Herbs, Gods, and Ghosts,* 81–84.

    6. Lai and Tan, *The Chinese in Latin America and the Caribbean,* 14–16; Gary Y. Okihiro, *The Columbia Guide to Asian American History* (New York: Columbia University Press, 2001), 9, 12–13; Barnes, *Needles, Herbs, Gods, and Ghosts,* 227–228.

    7. Eric Jay Dolin, *When America First Met China: An Exotic History of Tea, Drugs, and Money in the Age of Sail* (New York: Liveright, 2012), 37.

    8. U.S. Census, 1800, Carlisle, Penn., reel M32, Records of the Bureau of the Census, Record Group 29, National Archives, Washington, D.C., http://search.ancestry library.com.

    9. Rahter, "Medical History of Dauphin County," 302.

    10. *Norwich [Conn.] Packet,* August 19, 1800.

    11. This chapter focuses on the European sources on Chinese medicine that Americans of the colonial period and early republic would have been most likely to encounter. For a more comprehensive and detailed survey of European reactions to

Chinese medicine from the medieval period to the mid-nineteenth century, see Barnes, *Needles, Herbs, Gods, and Ghosts,* and Bivins, *Alternative Medicine?*

12. William of Rubruck, *Account of the Mongols: The Journey of William of Rubruck to the Eastern Parts of the World, 1253–55, as Narrated by Himself, with Two Accounts of the Earlier Journey of John of Pian de Carpine,* trans. William Woodville Rockhill (London: Hakluyt Society, 1900), https://depts.washington.edu/silkroad/texts/rubruck.html.

13. Barnes, *Needles, Herbs, Gods, and Ghosts,* 9.

14. Marco Polo, *The Travels of Marco Polo,* ed. Milton Rugoff (New York: Signet Classics, 2004), 163.

15. Ibid., 161, 202.

16. Jonathan D. Spence, *To Change China: Western Advisers in China, 1620–1960* (Boston: Little, Brown, 1969), 5–6.

17. Fan, *British Naturalists in Qing China,* 95.

18. Barnes, *Needles, Herbs, Gods, and Ghosts,* 23, 40.

19. Ibid., 75.

20. Ibid., 87–107.

21. Lu and Needham, *Celestial Lancets,* 270.

22. Reproduced without annotation, the plates were probably mystifying to Cleyer's audience. Ibid., 277.

23. James Morss Churchill, *A Treatise on Acupuncturation* (London: Simpkin and Marshall, 1821), 10–11; Jules Cloquet, *Treatise on Acupuncture* (Paris: Chez Béchet Jeune, 1826), 278–279, copy in Historical Medical Library of the College of Physicians of Philadelphia; Lu and Needham, *Celestial Lancets,* 292–293.

24. Fan, *British Naturalists in Qing China,* 13.

25. Ibid., 19.

26. Barnes, *Needles, Herbs, Gods, and Ghosts,* 109.

27. Dolin, *When America First Met China,* 37–41.

28. Fan, *British Naturalists in Qing China,* 78–79.

29. Sia Jia Jane and Dong Shaoxin, "Humanistic Approach of the Early Protestant Medical Missionaries in Nineteenth-Century China," *Zygon* 51, no. 1 (March 2016): 103.

30. Choa, *"Heal the Sick" Was Their Motto,* 7–8; Si and Dong, "Humanistic Approach of the Early Protestant Medical Missionaries in Nineteenth-Century China," 104.

31. Fan, *British Naturalists in Qing China,* 22.

32. Barnes, *Needles, Herbs, Gods, and Ghosts,* 295–296.

33. Fan, *British Naturalists in Qing China,* 79–80.

34. Barnes, *Needles, Herbs, Gods, and Ghosts,* 41.

35. Dave Wang, "Confucius in the American Founding: The Founders' Efforts to Use Confucian Moral Philosophy in Their Endeavor to Create New Virtue for the New Nation," *Virginia Review of Asian Studies* 16 (2014): 11.

36. Dolin, *When America First Met China*, 62–64.

37. Paul Starr, *The Social Transformation of American Medicine* (New York: Basic Books, 1982), 38; Barnes, *Needles, Herbs, Gods, and Ghosts*, 310–312; John Harley Warner, *Against the Spirit of System: The French Impulse in Nineteenth-Century American Medicine* (Princeton, N.J.: Princeton University Press, 2014), 3.

38. Lu and Needham, *Celestial Lancets*, 299.

39. Bivins, *Alternative Medicine?* 7–9.

40. Hinrichs and Barnes, *Chinese Medicine and Healing*, 21.

41. Michael Sappol, *A Traffic of Dead Bodies: Anatomy and Embodied Social Identity in Nineteenth-Century America* (Princeton, N.J.: Princeton University Press, 2004), 53; Warner, *Against the Spirit of System*, 3–5.

42. Starr, *The Social Transformation of American Medicine*, 39–47; Rosemary Stevens, *American Medicine and the Public Interest* (New Haven, Conn.: Yale University Press, 1971), 16–26.

43. In cities, more affluent patients might have had access to trained physicians, but elsewhere, women took primary responsibility for maintaining a stock of medicine and caring for the sick in their households. They exchanged recipes for remedies with family and friends or studied almanacs and other domestic medical manuals. Starr, *The Social Transformation of American Medicine*, 32.

44. William G. Rothstein, "The Botanical Movements and Orthodox Medicine," in Gevitz, ed., *Other Healers*, 32.

45. Starr, *The Social Transformation of American Medicine*, 48–49.

46. Sharla M. Fett, *Working Cures: Healing, Health, and Power on Southern Slave Plantations* (Chapel Hill: University of North Carolina Press, 2002), 111–141; Wonda L. Fontenot, *Secret Doctors: Ethnomedicine of African Americans* (Westport, Conn.: Bergin and Garvey, 1994), 31–32.

47. Starr, *The Social Transformation of American Medicine*, 51–52; Whorton, *Nature Cures*, 32; Susan Strasser, "A Historical Herbal: Household Medicine and Herbal Medicine in a Developing Consumer Society," in *Decoding Modern Consumer Societies*, ed. Hartmut Berghoff and Uwe Spiekermann (New York: Palgrave Macmillan, 2012), 214.

48. Joseph M. Gabriel, *Medical Monopoly: Intellectual Property Rights and the Origins of the Modern Pharmaceutical Industry* (Chicago: University of Chicago Press, 2014), 9.

49. Rothstein, "The Botanical Movements and Orthodox Medicine," 32–33.

50. Bivins, *Alternative Medicine?* 31–32; Strasser, "A Historical Herbal," 213–214.

51. David A. Taylor, *Ginseng, the Divine Root* (Chapel Hill, N.C.: Algonquin Books of Chapel Hill, 2006), 41.

52. Anthony Florian Madinger Willich, *The Domestic Encyclopedia; or, A Dictionary of Facts and Useful Knowledge* (Philadelphia: William Young Birch and Abraham Small, 1803–1804), 383; M. K. Hard, *Woman's Medical Guide: Being a Complete Review of the Peculiarities of the Female Constitution and the Derangements to Which*

It Is Subject, with a Description of Simple Yet Certain Means for Their Cure (Mount Vernon, Ohio: W. H. Cochran, 1848), 280.

53. M. Mattson, *The American Vegetable Practice, of a New and Improved Guide to Health, Designed for the Use of Families* (Boston: Daniel L. Hale, 1841), 258–262.

54. Gideon Harvey, *The Family Physician, and the House Apothecary* (London: T. Rooks, 1676), 50–53.

55. William H. Harding, "On the Chinese Snake-Stone and Its Operation as an Antidote to Poison," *Medical Repository* 4 (1807): 248; James Harvey Young, *The Toadstool Millionaires: A Social History of Patent Medicines in America before Federal Regulation* (Princeton, N.J.: Princeton University Press, 1972), 17.

56. *Federal Republican and Commercial Gazette* (Baltimore, Md.), August 17, 1810; *The Star* (Raleigh, N.C.), October 4, 1810; *Alexandria [Va.] Daily Gazette, Commercial, and Political,* November 22, 1810; *Public Advertiser* (New York), November 23, 1810; *Salem [Mass.] Gazette,* December 7, 1810; *Hampshire Federalist* (Springfield, Mass.), December 13, 1810; Kai Schultz, "Demand for Himalayan Viagra Fungus Heats Up, Maybe Too Much," *New York Times,* June 26, 2016, http://www.nytimes.com/2016/06/27/world/asia/himalayan-viagra-climate-change.html?smid=fb-nytimes&smtyp=cur&_r=0.

57. Dolin, *When America First Met China,* 49–50.

58. Ibid., 102; Thomas Beddoes, *Hygëia; or, Essays, Moral and Medical, on the Causes Affecting the Personal State of Our Middling and Affluent Classes* (Bristol, England: J. Mills, 1802), 1:32; Samuel Auguste David Tissot, *An Essay on Diseases Incident to Literary and Sedentary Persons* (London: James Williams, 1769), 148–152.

59. Sir John Sinclair, *The Code of Health and Longevity; or, A Concise View, of the Principles Calculated for the Preservation of Health, and the Attainment of Long Life* (Edinburgh: Arch. Constable, 1807), 290.

60. Jonas Hanaway, *Advice from Farmer Trueman, to His Daughter Mary* (Boston: Munroe and Francis, 1810), 133.

61. A. F. M. Willich, *Lectures on Diet and Regimen: Being a Systematic Inquiry into the Most Rational Means of Preserving Health and Prolonging Life* (Boston: Manning and Loring, 1800), 2:125–126.

62. Young, *The Toadstool Millionaires,* 63.

63. Ibid., 173; *The General Family Directory: Showing the Remedies Which Every Family Should Keep in Their Houses, and the Manner of Using Them* (New York: Comstock, 1842), 25.

64. John C. Gunn, *Gunn's New Family Physician; or, Home Book of Health* (Cincinnati: Moore, Wilstach, and Baldwin, 1864), 165; James Bryan, *The Druggist's Price Book, Containing a List of All the Articles Generally Kept for Sale by Druggists* (Rochester, N.Y.: James Bryan, 1850), 41; *Bragg's Arctic Liniment Almanac for the Year 1860* (Boston: Bragg and Burrowes, 1859), 9; Joseph Burnett, *Burnett's Floral Handbook: Ladies Calendar for 1866* (Boston: Joseph Burnett, 1865).

65. See, for example, William Barton, "Observations on the Probabilities of the Duration of Human Life, and the Progress of Population, in the United States of

America; in a Letter from William Barton, Esq. to David Rittenhouse, L.L.D. President, A.P.S.," *Transactions of the American Philosophical Society* 3 (1793): 46–47; Willich, *Lectures on Diet and Regimen,* 72–73; "Longevity of Women in China," *The Democrat* (Boston), July 12, 1806, 2; and Jay Sokolovsky, *The Cultural Context of Aging: Worldwide Perspectives* (Westport, Conn.: Bergin and Garvey, 1990), 509.

66. *The General Family Directory,* 15.

67. Stephen Freeman, *The Good Samaritan and Domestic Physician* (Albany, N.Y.: E. Andrews, 1780), 2.

68. Kristin Johannsen, *Ginseng Dreams: The Secret World of America's Most Valuable Plant* (Lexington: University Press of Kentucky, 2006), 17.

69. Taylor, *Ginseng, the Divine Root,* 98; Johannsen, *Ginseng Dreams,* 17–18.

70. Jonathan Edwards, *The Works of Jonathan Edwards, A.M.* (London: William Ball, 1834), cxcv.

71. *New-York Gazette,* September 18, 1752.

72. Taylor, *Ginseng, the Divine Root,* 118–119.

73. Ibid., 131.

74. Dolin, *When America First Met China,* 19; Taylor, *Ginseng, the Divine Root,* 132.

75. Dolin, *When America First Met China,* 15–16.

76. Johannsen, *Ginseng Dreams,* 22.

77. *Loudon's New-York Packet,* June 8, 1786; "The Following Observations upon the Article of Ginseng We Find in the Pennant's Outlines of the Globe," *Farmers' Museum, or Literary Gazette* (Walpole, N.H.), June 1, 1802.

78. Advertisement, *Vermont Gazette or Freemen's Depository* (Bennington), July 10, 1783; Advertisement, *Vermont Journal and the Universal Advertiser* (Windsor), January 4, 1785; Advertisement, *Thomas's Massachusetts Spy; or, Worcester Gazette,* April 1, 1784; Advertisement, *New York Packet and the American Advertiser,* August 12, 1784.

79. Johannsen, *Ginseng Dreams,* 20–21.

80. "A Short Account of Crown-Point and Niagara," *Boston Evening-Post,* December 24, 1759; *New-York Gazette,* December 3, 1759.

81. *Freemen's Journal; or, The North-American Intelligencer* (Philadelphia), December 5, 1787.

82. See, for example, "Extract from the Third Volume of Medical Transactions Published by the College of Physicians in London," *Essex Journal and New Hampshire Packet* (Newburyport, Mass.), June 27, 1787; Joseph James, *A System of Exchange with Almost All Parts of the World* (New York: John Furman, 1800), 136–137; and "The Following Observations upon the Article of Ginseng We Find in Pennant's Outlines of the Globe," *Farmer's Museum; or, Literary Gazette* (Walpole, N.H.), June 1, 1802.

83. "Philadelphia, July 27," *New-York Weekly Journal,* August 21, 1738; *New-York Gazette,* September 18, 1752; Jean-Baptiste du Halde, *A General History of China,* 2nd ed. (1735; London: J. Watts, 1739), 263.

84. William Cullen, *A Treatise of the* Materia Medica (Philadelphia: J. Crukshank and R. Campbell, 1789), 109.

85. Robert Hooper, *A Compendious Medical Dictionary* (Boston: Manning and Loring, 1801), 122.

86. Jacob Bigelow, *American Medical Botany, Being a Collection of the Native Medicinal Plants of the United States* (Boston: Cummings and Hilliard, 1817–1820), 2:94.

87. John Bell, "Journey of John Bell, Esq. from St. Petersburg to Peking," in William Fordyce Mavor, *An Historical Account of the Most Celebrated Voyages, Travels, and Discoveries from the Time of Columbus to the Present Period* (Philadelphia: Samuel F. Bradford, 1802), 253.

88. John Wilson, *Medical Notes on China* (London: Churchill, 1846), 256.

89. "London, March 4," *Maryland Journal* (Baltimore), April 29, 1785; "Extract from a Letter from a Swedish Supra-Cargo at Canton to His Friend in London, February 25, 1785," *American Recorder and the Charlestown Advertiser* (Boston), February 10, 1786.

90. Barnes, *Needles, Herbs, Gods, and Ghosts*, 215.

91. Dolin, *When America First Met China*, 41–43.

92. Ibid., 123, 155.

93. Elizabeth Sinn, *Pacific Crossing: California Gold, Chinese Migration, and the Making of Hong Kong* (Hong Kong: Hong Kong University Press, 2013), 383.

94. Choa, *"Heal the Sick" Was Their Motto*, 4–5.

95. Michael C. Lazich, "Seeking Souls through the Eyes of the Blind: The Birth of the Medical Missionary Society in Nineteenth-Century China," in *Healing Bodies, Saving Souls: Medical Missions in Asia and Africa*, ed. David Hardiman (Amsterdam: Rodopi, 2006), 62.

96. Charles (Karl) Gutzlaff, "Journal of a Residence in Siam, and of a Voyage along the Coast of China to Mantchou Tartary," *Chinese Repository* 1 (May 1832–April 1833): 181.

97. Lazich, "Seeking Souls through the Eyes of the Blind," 62–63; Si and Dong, "Humanistic Approach of the Early Protestant Medical Missionaries in Nineteenth-Century China," 105.

98. Dolin, *When America First Met China*, 251–252.

99. Lazich, "Seeking Souls through the Eyes of the Blind," 65–66.

100. Choa, *"Heal the Sick" Was Their Motto*, 56.

101. Quoted in "The Advantages of Medical Missions to China," *Chinese and General Missionary Gleaner* 1–2 (1851–1852): 42, http://hdl.handle.net/2027/coo.31924007186392.

102. See, for example, "Brief Remarks on the Qualifications of Medical Practitioners to Labor among the Chinese," *Chinese Repository* 4 (1835–1836): 575–576, http://hdl.handle.net/2027/njp.32101048166969, and "E Tsung Kin Keeun Yu Tsaon; or, The Golden Mirror of Eminent Medical Authors, Compiled by Imperial Authority," *Chinese Repository* 9 (1840): 487, http://hdl.handle.net/2027/mdp.39015025535942.

103. Spence, *To Change China*, 36.

104. Edward Vose Gulick, *Peter Parker and the Opening of China* (Cambridge, Mass.: Harvard University Press, 1973), 19; George Barker Stevens and William Fisher Markwick, *The Life, Letters, and Journals of the Rev. and Hon. Peter Parker* (Boston: Congregational Sunday-School and Publishing Society, 1896), 94–95.

105. Spence, *To Change China*, 46.

106. Choa, *"Heal the Sick" Was Their Motto*, 23.

107. Stevens and Markwick, *The Life, Letters, and Journals of the Rev. and Hon. Peter Parker*, 128.

108. Choa, *"Heal the Sick" Was Their Motto*, 17; Stevens and Markwick, *The Life, Letters, and Journals of the Rev. and Hon. Peter Parker*, 134–135.

109. Andrews, *The Making of Modern Chinese Medicine*, 111.

110. *Medical Missionary Society in China, Address with Minutes of Proceedings* (Canton: Office of the Chinese Repository, 1838), 17–18, copy in Historical Medical Library of the College of Physicians of Philadelphia.

111. Ibid., 18–19.

112. Thomas Richardson Colledge, "Suggestions with Regard to Employing Medical Practitioners as Missionaries to China," *Chinese Repository* 4 (1835–1836): 387, http://hdl.handle.net/2027/njp.32101048166969.

113. Spence, *To Change China*, 36.

114. Gulick, *Peter Parker and the Opening of China*, 33.

115. Quoted in Stevens and Markwick, *The Life, Letters, and Journals of the Rev. and Hon. Peter Parker*, 128.

116. Colledge, "Suggestions with Regard to Employing Medical Practitioners as Missionaries to China," 387.

117. E. C. Bridgman, Eliza J. Gillett Bridgman, and Asa D. Smith, *The Pioneer of American Missions in China: The Life and Labors of Elijah Coleman Bridgman* (New York: Anson D. F. Randolph, 1864), 97.

118. Wilson, *Medical Notes on China*, 180–181.

119. Ibid. 233.

120. Ibid., 234.

121. See, for example, "Description of a Chinese Anatomical Plate, Illustrative of the Human Body, with Explanations of the Terms," *Chinese Repository* 6–10 (1937–1942): 200, http://hdl.handle.net/2027/mdp.39015025535942.

122. Robert Morrison, *Dictionary of the Chinese Language*, part 3 (London: Black, Parbury, and Allen, 1822), 273.

123. Ibid., 318.

124. Ibid., 344.

125. William Lockhart, *The Medical Missionary in China: A Narrative of Twenty Years' Experience* (London: Hurst and Blackett, 1861), 58–59.

126. Ibid., 112.

127. Ibid., 114–115.

128. Quoted in ibid., 154.

129. Quoted in ibid., 155.

130. Si and Dong, "Humanistic Approach of the Early Protestant Medical Missionaries in Nineteenth-Century China," 106–107.

131. *Medical Missionary Society in China, Address with Minutes of Proceedings*, 16–17.

132. John Parascandola, "Chaulmoogra Oil and the Treatment of Leprosy," *Pharmacy in History* 45, no. 2 (2003): 47–57; Si and Dong, "Humanistic Approach of the Early Protestant Medical Missionaries in Nineteenth-Century China," 107.

133. Lockhart, *The Medical Missionary in China*, 113–114.

134. C. Toogood Downing, *The Fan-Qui in China, in 1836–7* (London: H. Colburn, 1838), 167.

135. Ibid., 143.

136. Barnes, *Needles, Herbs, Gods, and Ghosts*, 296.

137. Lazich, "Seeking Souls through the Eyes of the Blind," 81; Spence, *To Change China*, 52.

TWO Transplanted

1. "Dr. Li's Ghost Is Now at Rest," *Morning Call* (San Francisco), May 8, 1897.

2. "Li Po Tai Is Dead," *Morning Call*, March 21, 1893; Bowen, "The Five Eras of Chinese Medicine in California," 185.

3. Advertisement, *Daily Alta California*, March 1865; Bowen, "The Five Eras of Chinese Medicine in California," 185.

4. "How a Mongolian Works upon the Caucasian Credulity," *The Courier* (Waterloo, Iowa), December 26, 1883; "A Fortunate Chinese," *Sacramento Daily Union*, March 15, 1865; *Goshen [Ill.] Times*, September 9, 1869.

5. "Li Po Tai's Testament," *San Francisco Call*, March 31, 1893; "Dr. Li's Ghost Is Now at Rest," *San Francisco Call*, May 8, 1897.

6. "Lined with Gems: The Dead Chinese Doctor's Last Bed," *Morning Call*, March 23, 1893; "Li Po Tai's Funeral," *San Francisco Chronicle*, March 23, 1893; "Death of a Chinese Doctor," *Los Angeles Times*, March 21, 1893.

7. Nancy Tomes, *Remaking the American Patient: How Madison Avenue and Modern Medicine Turned Patients into Consumers* (Chapel Hill: University of North Carolina Press, 2016), 82–84.

8. Barbara Berglund, *Making San Francisco American: Cultural Frontiers in the Urban West, 1846–1906* (Lawrence: University Press of Kansas, 2007), 97.

9. For a fuller discussion of the Chinatown travel literature in the late nineteenth century, see ibid., 100–136.

10. Barbara Berglund writes about Chinese participation in the tourism industry in San Francisco in her article "Chinatown's Tourist Terrain," *American Studies* 46, no. 2 (Summer 2005): 10–12.

11. In southern California, Chinese doctors, along with other irregular medical practitioners, built up the health tourism industry, a major driver of regional economic

growth in the late nineteenth century. Advertisement, *Los Angeles Herald*, March 4, 1900; John E. Baur, *The Health Seekers of Southern California, 1870–1900* (San Marino, Calif.: Huntington Library, 1959), 153.

12. "Oakland Business Man Here since 1915," *Oakland [Calif.] Tribune*, February 15, 1939.

13. Gustavus L. Simmons, "Remarks on Chinese Pharmacy," *New York Daily Times*, July 22, 1854. French and British travelers often referred to China as the "Celestial Empire" or "Celestial Kingdom," a literary translation of a Chinese word for "China" (天朝, heavenly kingdom or kingdom ruled in accord with Heaven).

14. "Dr. Li Po Tai Borrowing," *Daily Alta California*, July 3, 1871; "John as Doctor," *Wellsville [N.Y.] Free Press*, August 31, 1870.

15. J. W. Ames, "A Day in Chinatown," *Lippincott's Magazine*, October 1875, 500.

16. Ibid., 501.

17. J. Thomas Scharf, "Chinaman's Medicines," *Salt Lake Herald* (Salt Lake City), January 9, 1893.

18. "Hit or Miss: Healing Art among the Chinese," *Los Angeles Times*, July 5, 1908.

19. See, for example, "A Victim of Misplaced Confidence," *Sacramento Daily Union*, August 9, 1864, and "In the Circuit Court," *Evening Capital Journal* (Sacramento, Calif.), February 16, 1894.

20. "A Chinese Aesculapius," *New York Herald*, May 18, 1880.

21. "Doctors with Pigtails," *The World* (New York), August 9, 1891.

22. Madeline Yuan-yin Hsu, *Dreaming of Gold, Dreaming of Home* (Stanford, Calif.: Stanford University Press, 2000), 27–31; Erika Lee, *At America's Gates: Chinese Immigration during the Exclusion Era, 1882–1943* (Chapel Hill: University of North Carolina Press, 2003), 25.

23. Hsu, *Dreaming of Gold, Dreaming of Home*, 32–33.

24. Peter Huston, *Tongs, Gangs, and Triads: Chinese Crime Groups in North America* (San Jose: Author's Choice Press, 2001), 73–78.

25. Steele, *Bleed, Blister, and Purge*, 88–89.

26. Bruce Hallmark, "Chinese Health Hazards and Traditional Chinese Medicine in the Frontier Northwest," *Pacific Northwest Forum* 6, no. 1 (1993): 62.

27. See, for example, Jean Pfaelzer, *Driven Out: The Forgotten War against Chinese Americans* (New York: Random House, 2007), and Scott Zesch, *The Chinatown War: Chinese Los Angeles and the Massacre of 1871* (New York: Oxford University Press, 2012).

28. "Memorial of Chinese Laborers, Resident at Rock Springs, Wyoming Territory, to the Chinese Consul at New York" (1885), reprinted in Cheng-Tsu Wu, ed., *Chink!* (New York: World Publishing, 1972), 152–164; Alexander Saxton, *The Indispensable Enemy: Labor and the Anti-Chinese Movement in California* (Berkeley: University of California Press, 1995), 72; Beth Lew-Williams, *The Chinese Must Go: Violence,*

Exclusion and the Making of the Alien in America (Cambridge, Mass.: Harvard University Press, 2018), 17-52.

29. Bowen, "The Five Eras of Chinese Medicine in California," 176.

30. "Wharves and Waves," *San Francisco Chronicle,* July 21, 1882.

31. In her history of Chinese miners in Nevada and Oregon, Sue Fawn Chung names one book—the *Golden Mirror of Medicine*—that cost just $2.25. This "self-help" book may have been a volume or distillation of the eighteenth-century medical compendium *The Imperially Commissioned Golden Mirror of the Orthodox Lineage of Medicine,* whose mnemonics and illustrations aimed to make diagnosis and treatment accessible to physicians with varying levels of education. Chung, *In Pursuit of Gold,* 110; Hanson, "The 'Golden Mirror' in the Imperial Court of the Qianlong Emperor," 111-112.

32. Bowen, "The Five Eras of Chinese Medicine in California," 176.

33. Chung, *In Pursuit of Gold,* 110; Heffner, "Exploring Health-Care Practices of Chinese Railroad Workers in North America," 142.

34. Chung, *In Pursuit of Gold,* 160; Patel, "America's Chinatowns," 42.

35. William Harland Boyd and Mary Sue Ming, *The Chinese of Kern County, 1857-1960* (Bakersfield, Calif.: Kern County Historical Society, 2002), 171-172.

36. Chung, *In Pursuit of Gold,* 160; Patel, "America's Chinatowns," 42; Bowen, "The Five Eras of Chinese Medicine in California," 176; Ross, *An Archaeology of Asian Transnationalism,* 162, 175.

37. According to the company website, the brand Cuticura had been used to sell "medicated" soap and ointment since 1865. http://www.cuticura.com/main_frame.htm.

38. Louise Leung Larson, *Sweet Bamboo: A Memoir of a Chinese American Family* (Berkeley: University of California Press, 2001), 58, 159.

39. In a notable exception, according to historian Joan Trauner, "In the 1880s, a few church missions in Chinatown began offering the services of white female physicians for pediatric and obstetrical care." Trauner, "The Chinese as Medical Scapegoats in San Francisco," 82.

40. Liu, "Chinese Herbalists in the United States," 141-142; Trauner, "The Chinese as Medical Scapegoats in San Francisco," 72-73.

41. "Chinese Hospital," *Sacramento Daily Union,* January 20, 1872.

42. Trauner, "The Chinese as Medical Scapegoats in San Francisco," 81-83.

43. Public health campaigns against San Francisco's Chinatown have been the subject of significant scholarly work. See, for example, Shah, *Contagious Divides;* Risse, *Plague, Fear, and Politics in San Francisco's Chinatown;* Trauner, "The Chinese as Medical Scapegoats in San Francisco," 70-87; Susan Craddock, *City of Plagues: Disease, Poverty, and Deviance in San Francisco* (Minneapolis: University of Minnesota Press, 2000); Kraut, *Silent Travelers;* and Juily Iyn Vo Phun, "Contours of Care: The Influenza Pandemic, Public Health and Asian American Communities in Southern California, 1918-1941" (Ph.D. diss., University of California, Irvine, 2016).

44. Shah, *Contagious Divides*, 20; Klee, "The 'Regulars' and the Chinese," 207.

45. Risse, *Plague, Fear, and Politics in San Francisco's Chinatown,* 74–76.

46. Trauner, "The Chinese as Medical Scapegoats in San Francisco," 81.

47. Steele, *Bleed, Blister, and Purge,* 104.

48. "Chinese Hospital," *San Francisco Chronicle,* June 2, 1888.

49. "Organization of an Oriental Hospital Association," *San Francisco Chronicle,* February 19, 1899.

50. Risse, *Plague, Fear, and Politics in San Francisco's Chinatown,* 92–93.

51. "For Ill Chinamen," *Los Angeles Herald,* July 9, 1892.

52. Ibid.; Kraut, *Silent Travelers,* 198; Risse, *Plague, Fear, and Politics in San Francisco's Chinatown,* 53–56.

53. "Oregon Chinese Will Build Home for Sick," *Indianapolis Star,* April 9, 1910.

54. Harriet Quimby, "The Chinese Hospital," *San Francisco Chronicle,* August 24, 1902.

55. Risse, *Plague, Fear, and Politics in San Francisco's Chinatown,* 161.

56. Colin Quock, *Chinese Hospital Medical Staff Archives, 1978–1981* (San Francisco: Chinese Hospital, 1978), 2–3.

57. "A Chinese Hospital Association," *New York Times,* December 29, 1890; "For Ill Chinamen," *Los Angeles Herald,* July 9, 1891; "A Chinese Puzzle," *Christian Union,* January 30, 1892, 214; Louis J. Beck, *New York's Chinatown: An Historical Presentation of Its People and Places* (New York: Bohemia Publishing, 1898), 268.

58. "A Chinese Hospital," *Brooklyn Daily Eagle,* September 22, 1907.

59. Liping Bu, *Public Health and the Modernization of China, 1865–2015* (Abingdon, U.K.: Routledge, 2017), 36.

60. K. Chimin Wong, *History of Chinese Medicine, Being a Chronicle of Medical Happenings in China from Ancient Times to the Present Period* (Tientsin, China: Tientsin Press, 1933), 394; "New Woman of China, Dr. Mary 'Stone' Is on Tour," *San Francisco Call,* March 6, 1907; "A New Woman," *Hawaiian Gazette* (Honolulu), September 7, 1897; Donald MacGillivray, *A Century of Missions in China, 1807–1907: Being the Centenary Conference Historical Volume* (Shanghai: American Presbyterian Mission Press, 1907) 466; Connie Anne Shemo, *The Chinese Medical Ministries of Kang Cheng and Shi Meiyu, 1872–1937: On a Cross-Cultural Frontier of Gender, Race, and Nation* (Bethlehem, Penn.: Lehigh University Press, 2011).

61. Lui, *The Chinatown Trunk Mystery,* 133.

62. "Commencement Exercises of the College of Medicine," *Southern California Practitioner* 11 (1896): 231.

63. Advertisements, *Anaconda Standard* (Butte, Mont.), June 11, 1905; October 8, 1910; February 20, 1922.

64. "Chinamen Want to Practice Medicine," *Great Falls [Mont.] Tribune,* October 2, 1901.

65. "A Chinese Physician," *Philadelphia Record,* September 20, 1891.

66. "Many Chinamen Approve," *New York Times*, April 12, 1893; "St. Bartholomew's Work," *New York Times*, December 13, 1895; "City and Vicinity," *New York Times*, March 21, 1896.

67. "Directory of Deceased American Physicians, 1804–1929," ancestry.com; "U.S. Consular Reports of Marriages, 1910–1949," ancestry.com.

68. Dr. Herbert Yee, interview with Nancy Wey, June 4, 1978, Nancy Wey Papers, carton 2, folder 16, Asian American Studies Archive, Ethnic Studies Library, University of California, Berkeley; Larson, *Sweet Bamboo*, 109.

69. "Chew Kee Store," Fiddletown Preservation Society, Fiddletown, Calif., http://www.fiddletown.info/buildings; Liu, *The Transnational History of a Chinese Family*, 47.

70. U.S. Census, 1860, population schedule, reel M653.

71. This count of Chinese occupations is combined with that of the Japanese, but a closer look at census manuscript data for the Japanese shows that the fifty-five individuals identified were primarily farm laborers, domestic servants, and college students. Thus, it seems likely that all 193 physicians and surgeons counted by census takers were Chinese.

72. Liu Boji Zhu, *Meiguo Hua Qiao Shi* (Taibei: Li Ming Wen Hua Shi Ye Gong Si, 1976), 314.

73. *A Compendium to the Ninth Census* (Washington, D.C.: Government Printing Office, 1872), 617.

74. *Ninth Census—Volume I, The Statistics of the Population of the United States* (Washington, D.C.: Government Printing Office, 1872), xvii, 707; *Statistics of the Population of the United States at the Tenth Census* (Washington, D.C.: Government Printing Office, 1883), xxxvii, 738.

75. U.S. Census, 1860, Forrestville, Jackson County, Oregon, reel M653_1055.

76. It was common for Chinese physicians to be employed on "coolie" ships to reduce voyage mortality rates. After 1855, an act of Parliament required British ships with more than twenty Chinese passengers to provide medicine to Chinese workers leaving Hong Kong on voyages longer than seven days. Later amendments to the law stipulated that a "medical officer" had to be aboard, a responsibility that often fell to a Chinese doctor either because Chinese passengers preferred to consult with native-Chinese speakers or because Chinese doctors were less expensive than their European colleagues. See "Regulations Respecting Chinese Passenger Ships, Schedule (A)," *The Chronicle and Directory for China, Japan, and the Philippines* (Hong Kong: Daily Press Office, 1875), 233–235, and "Chinese Passengers Act and Hong Kong Ordinances," *Colonization Circular,* nos. 30–32 (1873): 97–98. See also John McDonald and Ralph Shlomowitz, "Mortality on Chinese and Indian Voyages to the West Indies and South America, 1847–1874," *Social and Economic Studies* 41 (1992): 203–240, and Sinn, *Pacific Crossing*, 78–79.

77. "The Chinese Physician Question," *Pacific Commercial Advertiser* (Honolulu, Hawaii), September 8, 1859.

78. "Chinese Physician," *Pacific Commercial Advertiser,* September 24, 1859.

79. *The Polynesian* (Honolulu, Hawaii), September 15, 1860.

80. Lily Lim-Chong and Harry V. Ball, "Opium and the Law," *Chinese America: History and Perspectives* (2010): 64.

81. *Hawaiian Gazette,* March 29, 1887.

82. Lai and Tan, *The Chinese in Latin America and the Caribbean,* 14–16.

83. "All Canadian Census Collection, 1851–1916," Ancestry.com, http://search .ancestrylibrary.com/search/group/canadiancensus#databases.

84. U.S. Census, 1880, ancestry.com; Chung, *In Pursuit of Gold,* 109.

85. Chung, *In Pursuit of Gold,* 82–83.

86. U.S. Census, 1880.

87. Chen, "A Gold Dream in the Blue Mountains," 33, 51, 69.

88. Barlow and Richardson, *China Doctor of John Day,* 9–12.

89. Ibid., 35.

90. Chung, *In Pursuit of Gold,* 60.

91. U.S. Census, 1880.

92. Sarvis, "Gifted Healer Ing Hay and the Chinese Medical Tradition in Eastern Oregon," 62.

93. Barlow and Richardson, *China Doctor of John Day,* 6.

94. Ibid., 14.

95. Barlow and Richardson, *China Doctor of John Day,* 54–55.

96. Ibid., 17–21.

97. Ibid., 18–19, 57.

98. U.S. Census, 1880.

99. U.S. Census, 1900, Boise, Idaho, reel 231.

100. Smith, "Choosing Chinese Medicine," 98.

101. Buell, *Chinese Medicine on the Golden Mountain,* 52; Idaho State Historical Society Reference Series: C. K. Ah Fong—1845–1927, January 1996, http://www.history .idaho.gov/sites/default/files/uploads/reference-series/1130.pdf.

102. Smith, "Choosing Chinese Medicine," 98.

103. Buell, *Chinese Medicine on the Golden Mountain,* 73–74; Smith, "Choosing Chinese Medicine," 98.

104. Idaho State Historical Society Reference Series: C. K. Ah Fong—1845–1927.

105. U.S. Census, 1880, Ogden, Utah, reel 1339.

106. "Gun Wah in Trouble," *Pittsburgh Dispatch,* December 24, 1889; Advertisement, *Weekly Wisconsin* (Milwaukee), March 15, 1890.

107. "Ogden Jottings," *Daily Tribune* (Salt Lake City), January 7, 1885.

108. *Salt Lake Herald,* March 3, 1890; "Brigham City Department," *The Standard* (Ogden, Utah), December 9, 1891; *Daily Tribune,* November 9, 1893; *Salt Lake Telegram* (Salt Lake City), December 24, 1902.

109. "A Fortunate Chinese," *The Union,* March 15, 1865.

110. Tomes, *Remaking the American Patient,* 52–55; Gabriel, *Medical Monopoly,* 61–63.

111. Andrews, *The Making of Modern Chinese Medicine,* 9–10.

112. Ibid., 197.

113. Hinrichs and Barnes, *Chinese Medicine and Healing,* 234.

114. In a biography of Los Angeles herbalist Tom Leung, his daughter claimed that "Papa knew about acupuncture, but he didn't know how to practice it." Larson, *Sweet Bamboo,* 74.

115. Devitt, "The Curious Case of Ah Fong Chuck," 7.

116. Thomas W. Wing, Carolyn Wing Greenlee, and Duncan Chin, *Son of South Mountain and Dust* (Kelseyville, Calif.: Earthen Vessel Productions, 2001), 75–76.

117. Paul D. Buell, "Chinese Medicine on the 'Gold Mountain': Tradition, Adaptation, and Change," in *Disease and Medical Care in the Mountain West: Essays on Region, History, and Practice,* ed. Martha Lee Hildreth and Bruce T. Moran (Reno: University of Nevada Press, 1998), 107.

118. U.S. Census, 1870, San Francisco, California, reel 221.

119. Garding Lui, *Inside Los Angeles Chinatown* (Los Angeles: Garding Lui, 1948), 203; Boyd and Ming, *The Chinese of Kern County,* 171.

120. Bowen, "The Five Eras of Chinese Medicine in California," 178; Tomes, *Remaking the American Patient,* 52–53.

121. Ted J. Kaptchuk, *The Web That Has No Weaver: Understanding Chinese Medicine,* rev. ed. (1983; Chicago: Contemporary Books, 2000), 110; William Tisdale, "Chinese Physicians in California," *Lippincott's Magazine,* March 1899, 415; Heffner, "Exploring Health-Care Practices of Chinese Railroad Workers in North America," 141–142.

122. Beth Howlett, interview with author, September 8, 2011.

123. Liu, "Chinese Herbalists in the United States," 138.

124. Lin Ken to Ing Hay, Baker City, Oregon, May 24,1907, translated and reprinted in Chia-lin Chen, "The Kam Wah Chung Company Papers," 1974, Oregon Historical Society, Portland; Lee Miller to Ing Hay and Lung On, Izee, Oregon, June 15, 1903; W. E. Freeman to Lung On, Drewsey, Ore., May 9, 1905, Kam Wah Chung Papers, reels 1–2, Oregon Historical Society.

125. "Lee Has a Chinese Farm," *New York Times,* October 31, 1898.

126. Johannsen, *Ginseng Dreams,* 8; Taylor, *Ginseng, the Divine Root,* 144–145.

127. "Local Ginseng Culture Promises Rich Returns," *Oxnard Courier,* May 27, 1904; "Queer Chinese Medicines," *Los Angeles Times,* August 11, 1907.

128. *Sacramento Daily Union,* March 27, 1880; "Chinese Medicos," *Los Angeles Times,* September 27, 1900.

129. Fred Masier to Lung On, November 28, 1902, Kam Wah Chung Papers.

130. Heffner, "Exploring Health-Care Practices of Chinese Railroad Workers in North America," 142, 144.

131. "The Pacific Coast Trade in Chinese Medicines and How a Celestial Pharmacist Makes Drugs out of Horned Toads," *San Francisco Chronicle Magazine,* March 29, 1903, 2.

132. Heffner, "Exploring Health-Care Practices of Chinese Railroad Workers in North America," 141.

133. Li Wing Fawn and B. C. Platt, "A Step in Advance," *Los Angeles Times,* May 26, 1896.

134. "Do the Chinese Manage It Better Than Caucasian Physicians?" *Daily Alta California,* January 9, 1869.

135. Smith, "Choosing Chinese Medicine," 96.

136. "An Interesting Medical Case," *Daily Alta California,* February 9, 1878. Dr. Loo was later arrested for practicing medicine without a license. "A Chinese Doctor's License," *San Francisco Chronicle,* July 17, 1879.

137. "Cheap Chinese Doctors," *Connersville Daily Examiner,* January 6, 1890.

138. Risse, *Plague, Fear, and Politics in San Francisco's Chinatown,* 49–50.

139. After Fan-Chung Yee's death in 1904, his paper son, You Fong (Jimmy) Chow, stayed on as caretaker, fulfilling a promise he made to "guard the shop," but the Chinese population was dwindling, lured away by jobs in other places or compelled to leave the country by Chinese exclusion. In 1900, the U.S. Census manuscripts reveal that just over 150 Chinese people continued to live in all of Amador County. By 1920, their community numbered fewer than forty. Jimmy Chow became the sole Chinese resident of Fiddletown. He worked odd jobs around town and left the store intact, with Yee's bottles and personal effects gathering dust. Upon Chow's death in 1965, Amador County took over the property, leaving its contents undisturbed. When the Fiddletown Preservation Society and Yee's great-grandson, a Sacramento dentist named Herbert Yee, raised the funds to restore the historic shop in 1987, preservationists found Yee's belongings largely untouched since his death eighty-three years earlier. Charles Hillinger, "Fiddletown Finds a Cure for Its Crumbling Old Herb Shop," *Los Angeles Times,* February 19, 1987, http://articles.latimes.com/1987–02–19/news/mn-4474_1_herb-shop.

140. Chew Kee Store Catalog of Items, Nancy Wey Papers, carton 2, folder 14.

141. Students of Oregon's history are well acquainted with the story of Ing Hay, purveyor of Kam Wah Chung, a Chinese apothecary in a remote eastern town on the John Day River. When Ing died in a nursing home in Portland, Oregon, in 1952, his heir and nephew, Bob Wah, used the property as storage for his own herb shop, conveniently located across the street, but he left his uncle's personal papers and other belongings in place. The city of John Day eventually negotiated to lease and then to purchase the building with the agreement that it would be maintained as a museum. The state lovingly restored Ing's apothecary, registered it as a National Historic Landmark, and opened it to the public. The correspondence, business records, and personal objects that Ing Hay left behind have inspired several biographies of the herbalist and of his business partner Lung On, as well as an Emmy-nominated episode of Oregon Public Broadcasting's *Oregon Experience.* Barlow and Richardson, *China Doctor of John Day,* 29–33; Chen, "A Gold Dream in the Blue Mountains," 89–90.

142. Chen, "A Gold Dream in the Blue Mountains," 88.

143. Ibid., 89.

144. Barlow and Richardson, *China Doctor of John Day,* 28–29.

145. Lung On to Liang Kwang-jin, March 2, 1905; Liang to Lung, May 14, 1906; Liang to Lung, May 15, 1906, translated and reprinted in Chen, "The Kam Wah Chung Company Papers."

146. Barlow and Richardson, *China Doctor of John Day*, 21.

147. Ing Tow to Ing Hay, November 25, 1913, translated and reprinted in Chen, "The Kam Wah Chung Company Papers."

148. Larson, *Sweet Bamboo*, 69.

149. Ibid., 52–53.

150. Ibid., 157.

151. "Action for Debt—Chinese Wages," *Daily Alta California*, February 12, 1869.

152. *Oregon Sentinel* (Jacksonville), December 19, 1885; "Went Broke on Mines," *Morning Oregonian* (Portland), July 25, 1886.

153. "Dr. Woo [*sic*] Sing, the Head of the Chinese Underground Railroad System," *Los Angeles Herald*, April 22, 1890; "Who Smuggles Chinese?" *Los Angeles Herald*, April 22, 1890.

154. Tom was a more common family name among the San Diego Chinese community so it is likely that the man identified as San Diego doctor "Wo Sing" was really Tom Li Chung. "United States Courts," *Los Angeles Herald*, February 21, 1891; Gilbert Hom, interview with author, March 29, 2016.

155. Lui, *The Chinatown Trunk Mystery*, 124–125.

156. "Many Chinamen Approve," *New York Times*, April 12, 1893; "St. Bartholomew's Work," *New York Times*, December 13, 1895.

157. "City and Vicinity," *New York Times*, March 21, 1896.

158. "Dr. Jin Moy Arrested," *New York Times*, May 3, 1911.

159. The 1870 federal census lists Li Po Tai as residing with fourteen dependents, including nine druggists, three "domestics," and possibly two wives. U.S. Census, 1870, San Francisco, reel M593.

160. "Chinese Doctors Given a Flaying," *Oakland Tribune*, December 24, 1909; "Two Chinamen Claim Partnership," *Boston Globe*, June 20, 1918; "Chinese Claim Part of Dead Doctor's Estate," *Boston Globe*, June 21, 1918; Larson, *Sweet Bamboo*, 69.

161. Larson, *Sweet Bamboo*, 19; *Chinese Herbal Science; Its Principles and Methods, Comprising Its Treatment of Various Prevalent Diseases, Useful Information on Matters of Diet and Testimonials; a Guide to Health* (Los Angeles: T. Leung Herb Company, 1928), 7.

162. Liu, *The Transnational History of a Chinese Family*, 54; Larson, *Sweet Bamboo*, 99.

163. Larson, *Sweet Bamboo*, 70, 167.

164. See Lynn Bragg, *More than Petticoats: Remarkable Washington Women* (Guilford, Conn.: Globe Pequot, 2011), chap. 4.

165. Larson, *Sweet Bamboo*, 19.

166. Wing, Greenlee, and Chin, *Son of South Mountain and Dust*, 1–3.

167. Liu, *The Transnational History of a Chinese Family,* 29–30.

168. Ibid., 34.

169. Lao Chi-Kwang to Ing Hay, June 6, 1905, Kam Wah Chung Papers.

170. Ng See Poy to Ing Hay, October 30, 1903; Lin Zu-hsiang to Ing Hay, n.d., Kam Wah Chung Papers.

171. Advertisement, *Los Angeles Times,* February 29, 1892; *Los Angeles City Directory* (Los Angeles: W. H. L. Corran, 1891–1893), Historic City and Business Directories Collection, Los Angeles Public Library, http://rescarta.lapl.org/ResCarta-Web/jsp/RcWebBrowse.jsp;jsessionid=2DE0F3C75D4C72FB109FAED5274F92BF.

172. Analysis of advertisements in the *Los Angeles Times* and city directories from Historic City and Business Directories Collection, 1901–1942.

173. Wing Lee, Record Group 85: Records of the Immigration and Naturalization Service, entry 137, box 27, casefile 54007/22, National Archives; Chung, *In Pursuit of Gold,* 62.

174. Chang Gee Wo, *Things Chinese,* 5th ed. (Portland: Oregon Historical Society, 1924), 26–28.

175. Gilbert Hom, interview with author, March 29, 2016.

176. "World's Columbian Exposition Illustrated," *Campbell's Illustrated Weekly,* vol. 3, no. 1 (1893): 131.

177. U.S. Census, 1920, Portland, Oregon, reel T625_1502.

178. "Chinese Herb Specialist to Start Offices," *Idaho Evening Times* (Twin Falls), January 15, 1938; Biography, Chan Doo Sung Papers, H.Mss 1016, Special Collections, Honnold Mudd Library, Claremont University Consortium, Claremont, Calif.

179. Lee had the unusual distinction of being a third-generation Chinese American. Her mother, Wong Yut, was the American-born daughter of a Chinese wagon driver and a much younger Chinese woman who had worked in a gambling house, likely as a prostitute. U.S. Census, 1880, San Francisco, Calif., reel M593.

180. "Chinese Herb Specialist to Start Offices," *Idaho Evening Times,* January 15, 1938.

181. Anna Don, e-mail correspondence with author, June 19, 2018.

182. Anna Don, interview with author, October 12, 2013; Advertisement, *Idaho Evening Times,* January 17, 1938.

183. Anna Don, interview with author, October 12, 2013.

THREE Translated

1. U.S. Census, 1900, Berkeley, California, reel 83; Walter and Emma Fong Collection (SC0994), Department of Special Collections and University Archives, Stanford University Libraries, Stanford, Calif.

2. Calvin Fong, interviews with author, November 30, 2017, December 5, 2017.

3. Fong Wan Herb Company, *Herb Lore,* 5th ed. (1924; Oakland, Calif.: Fong Wan, 1936), 138.

4. Calvin Fong, interviews with author, November 30, December 5, 2017; Walter Fong and Emma Howse, marriage certificate, 1897; Yoshi S. Kuno and Emma Fong, marriage certificate, 1907, "Colorado, County Marriages and State Indexes, 1862–2006," ancestry.com; Fong Wan, Berkeley High School report cards, 1908, 1909, Calvin Fong personal collection.

5. Advertisements, *Santa Rosa [Calif.] Republican,* 1912–1915, Calvin Fong personal collection.

6. Calvin Fong, interview with author, November 30, 2017.

7. "China Doctor," *Wide West* (San Francisco, Calif.), March 8, 1857.

8. Liu, *The Transnational History of a Chinese Family,* 50.

9. Advertisements, *Sacramento Daily Union,* February 24, 1860; September 3, 1860.

10. "Chinese Medication," *Marysville [Calif.] Daily Appeal,* December 11, 1860.

11. Advertisement, *Marysville Daily Appeal,* July 4, 1865.

12. The first federal regulation of medical advertising—the 1906 Pure Food and Drug Act—only concerned the accurate labeling of the ingredients of proprietary medicines. Until the major revision of the law in 1938, the Food and Drug Administration and the Federal Trade Commission were largely powerless to regulate direct-to-consumer advertising of drugs. Young, *The Toadstool Millionaires,* 249–250.

13. Gabriel, *Medical Monopoly,* 79–80.

14. Young, *The Toadstool Millionaires,* 100–101.

15. T. J. Jackson Lears, *Fables of Abundance: A Cultural History of Advertising in America* (New York: Basic Books, 1994), 142.

16. Ann Anderson, *Snake Oil, Hustlers and Hambones: The American Medicine Show* (Jefferson, N.C.: McFarland, 2000), 39–41.

17. Lears, *Fables of Abundance,* 142–143.

18. Charles E. Rosenberg, *Every Man His Own Doctor: Popular Medicine in Early America: An Exhibition Drawn from the Collections of Charles E. Rosenberg, William H. Helfand, and the Library Company of Philadelphia* (Philadelphia: Library Company of Philadelphia, 1998), 22–47; Young, *The Toadstool Millionaires,* 165–189.

19. Advertisement, *Omaha [Neb.] Daily Bee,* August 31, 1890.

20. Advertisement, *Los Angeles Times,* January 1, 1899.

21. Advertisement, *San Francisco Chronicle,* April 9, 1905.

22. Advertisement, *Bisbee [Ariz.] Daily Review,* April 12, 1914.

23. Advertisement, *Los Angeles Times,* June 4, 1882.

24. Advertisement, *Sunday Oregonian* (Portland, Ore.), December 27, 1903; Advertisement, *Idaho Evening Times,* January 17, 1938.

25. Advertisement, *Los Angeles Times,* May 3, 1896.

26. Advertisement, *Los Angeles Times,* December 17, 1907.

27. In the 1920s and 1930s, advertisements for Chinese medicine began to appear in Japanese-language newspapers in San Francisco. Haiming Liu, "The Resilience of Ethnic Culture: Chinese Herbalists in the American Medical Profession," *Journal of Asian American Studies* 1, no. 2 (1998): 181.

28. Translation: All the sick cured here. Advertisement, *Los Angeles Times*, December 11, 1881.

29. Tom She Ben (Bin) Trade Card, Los Angeles County Medical Association Collection, Huntington Library, San Marino, Calif.; Advertisement, *Los Angeles Times*, April 14, 1891. This card transliterates the doctor's name as "Tom She Ben," but he was more commonly known as "Tom She Bin."

30. Phun, "Contours of Care"; George J. Sánchez, *Becoming Mexican American: Ethnicity, Culture, and Identity in Chicano Los Angeles, 1900–1945* (New York: Oxford University Press, 1995), 176.

31. Lui, *Inside Los Angeles Chinatown*, 204.

32. Advertisement, *Daily Dramatic Chronicle* (San Francisco), March 31, 1865.

33. Advertisement, *Daily Dramatic Chronicle*, September 2, 1865.

34. Advertisement, *Daily Alta California*, March 3, 1865.

35. "Employing an Interpreter," *Daily Alta California*, March 2, 1865.

36. Advertisement, *Los Angeles Times*, June 4, 1882.

37. Advertisement, *Los Angeles Times*, February 11, 1887.

38. Analysis of advertisements from the *San Francisco Chronicle*, 1894, and San Francisco Public Library City Directories Online, https://sfpl.org/?pg=2000540401.

39. Analysis of advertisements from the *San Francisco Chronicle* and the *San Francisco Call*, 1910–1912, and San Francisco Public Library City Directories Online.

40. Analysis of advertisements from the *San Francisco Chronicle*, 1912, and San Francisco Public Library City Directories Online.

41. Analysis of advertisements from the *Los Angeles Times* and Los Angeles City Directories, 1875–1945, Historic City and Business Directories Collection.

42. Lui, *Inside Los Angeles Chinatown*, 202.

43. Larson, *Sweet Bamboo*, 21–22.

44. Advertisement, *Los Angeles Times*, January 1, 1903.

45. Wing, Greenlee, and Chin, *Son of South Mountain and Dust*, 77.

46. Beverly Chan, interview with Arthur W. Chung, October 23, 25, 1979, Southern California Chinese American Oral History Project, Chinese Historical Society of Los Angeles; Liu, "Chinese Herbalists in the United States," 144–145.

47. Liu, "Chinese Herbalists in the United States," 144–145.

48. Beverly Chan, interview with Arthur W. Chung, October 23, 25, 1979, Southern California Chinese American Oral History Project.

49. "Gun Wa's Great Fake," *Anaconda Standard*, June 23, 1890.

50. "Doctor Gun Wa," *Daily Alta California*, June 23, 1890; "Was Medical Fraud," *Daily Leader* (Davenport, Iowa), August 2, 1894.

51. "Gun Wah in Trouble," *Pittsburgh Dispatch*, December 24, 1889.

52. Advertisement, *Weekly Wisconsin*, March 15, 1890.

53. Advertisement, *Daily Californian* (Berkeley), February 22, 1907.

54. Reproduced in Smith, "Choosing Chinese Medicine," 101.

55. "A Great Event in History," *Los Angeles Herald*, February 9, 1896.

56. "The Courts," *Los Angeles Herald*, February 14, 1894; "Record of B. C. Platt," *Los Angeles Herald*, October 19, 1896.

57. "Oriental Medicine in America," *Los Angeles Times*, October 27, 1895.

58. "Chinese Physicians," *Los Angeles Times*, August 15, 1895.

59. Ibid.; "Chinese Physicians Again," *Los Angeles Times*, September 1, 1895; "Oriental Medicine in America," *Los Angeles Times*, October 27, 1895; "Exponents of Prejudice," *Los Angeles Times*, January 19, 1896.

60. "Given Unusual Treatment," *San Francisco Chronicle*, January 8, 1896.

61. "The Public Service," *Los Angeles Times*, November 21, 1896; "At the Court House," *Los Angeles Times*, November 21, 1896.

62. C. B. Pinkham, California Board of Medical Examiners, "News Items," *California and Western Medicine* 26, no. 3 (March 1927): 387.

63. "A Doctor's Manager," *Los Angeles Times*, March 20, 1897; "Where's That Warrant?" *Los Angeles Times*, March 26, 1897.

64. Larson, *Sweet Bamboo*, 21.

65. Dr. Wong Company, articles of incorporation, July 18, 1901, book 133, p. 2, Office of the Secretary of State, Los Angeles County.

66. "Courthouse Notes," *Los Angeles Times*, June 26, 1904; "Toy Kee Herb Company," *Los Angeles Herald*, September 14, 1906.

67. "Courthouse Notes," *Los Angeles Times*, June 26, 1904.

68. Advertisement, *Los Angeles Times*, November 19, 1890; Advertisement, *Los Angeles Times*, November 21, 1890.

69. Advertisement, *Los Angeles Herald*, May 1, 1902; Advertisement, *Los Angeles Times*, December 17, 1907.

70. Anna Don, interview with author, October 12, 2013.

71. Advertisement, *Daily Dramatic Chronicle*, March 31, 1865; Advertisement, *Daily Dramatic Chronicle*, September 2, 1865.

72. "John as Doctor," *Wellsville Free Press*, August 31, 1870.

73. There are many examples: "From Hip to Hip," *San Francisco Call*, February 7, 1892; "Death of Dr. Yee," *San Francisco Call*, February 8, 1892; "San Francisco Highbinders," *Los Angeles Herald*, February 10, 1892; "Fong's Murder," *San Francisco Call*, June 26, 1894; "A Chinese Murder Revived," *San Francisco Chronicle*, June 25, 1894; "A Chinese Doctor Dead," *San Francisco Call*, October 10, 1895; "Chinese Doctor Shot," *San Francisco Chronicle*, January 16, 1902; "Lured Victim to His Death," *San Francisco Chronicle*, June 26, 1903; "Is Accused of Murder of Fellow Countryman," *San Francisco Call*, August 21, 1903; "Lured into a Den and Shot," *San Francisco Chronicle*, January 27, 1904; "Chink 'Doctor' Is Caught in Dope Dragnet," *Billings [Mont.] Gazette*, March 23, 1924.

74. "Chinese Poisons," *New York Times*, May 20, 1883.

75. "Chinese Shot by Highbinder," *Daily Call* (San Francisco), January 27, 1904.

76. "Highbinders at War," *San Francisco Chronicle*, February 3, 1893.

77. "Shot in the Back," *Los Angeles Herald*, April 12, 1898.

78. "Hit by Assassin," *Morning Oregonian*, September 7, 1904; "Saw Fatal Blow," *Morning Oregonian*, September 9, 1904; "He Saw the Crime," *Morning Oregonian*, October 7, 1904.

79. "Found Dead," *Daily Alta California*, January 31, 1855; "Murder and Robbery," *Los Angeles Star*, February 8, 1855; "Matters in Carson," *Sacramento Daily Union*, July 22, 1864; "A Victim of Misplaced Confidence," *Sacramento Daily Union*, August 9, 1864; "Drugged and Robbed," *San Francisco Call*, January 7, 1893; "A Chinatown Mystery," *San Francisco Call*, December 10, 1893; "Josshouse Funds Stolen," *Los Angeles Times*, January 7, 1893; "Believed to Have Been Poisoned," *San Francisco Chronicle*, October 10, 1895; *Arizona Weekly Journal-Miner* (Prescott), October 16, 1895; "Clue Sought in Chinese Murder," *Idaho Times* (Twin Falls), December 12, 1933.

80. "Chinese Doctor Shot and Killed," *San Francisco Chronicle*, December 25, 1901; "Chinese Doctor Murdered," *Los Angeles Times*, December 25, 1901.

81. "Is Strangled with His Own Queue," *San Francisco Chronicle*, July 10, 1905; "Chinese Physician: Strangled to Death," *Los Angeles Herald*, July 10, 1905; "Loved Too Many," *Oakland Tribune*, July 10, 1905.

82. "Opium Is Seized in Visalia Raid," *Oakland Tribune*, May 7, 1911; "Dope Raiders Seize Woman, Chinese Doctor, and Actor," *Los Angeles Times*, December 13, 1936; "Third Narcotic Suspect Taken," *Los Angeles Times*, January 27, 1937.

83. W. E. Freeman to Lung On, May 9, 1905, Kam Wah Chung Papers; Chow Kee Store Catalog of Items, Nancy Wey Papers, carton 2, folder 14.

84. For a discussion of the possible causes of increased rates of opiate addiction, see David T. Courtwright, *Dark Paradise: A History of Opiate Addiction in America* (Cambridge, Mass.: Harvard University Press, 2001), 43–60.

85. Diana L. Ahmad, *The Opium Debate and Chinese Exclusion Laws in the Nineteenth-Century American West* (Reno: University of Nevada Press, 2007), 51.

86. "Heathen Pretenders," *Anaconda Standard*, August 30, 1890.

87. "Not Brown-Sequard's but Said to Be as Good, if Not Better," *Boston Globe*, August 16, 1889.

88. *Hawaiian Gazette*, March 29, 1887.

89. "An Act to Amend an Act Entitled An Act Relating to the Practice of Medicine by Chinese," *Hawaiian Gazette*, December 13, 1887.

90. "Before His Honor Today," *Salt Lake Democrat* (Salt Lake City), July 21, 1885; "A Batch of Chinese," *Los Angeles Herald*, April 25, 1890; "Opium Joint Raided," *Daily Journal* (Salem, Ore.), August 20, 1902; "Did He Kill Girl?" *Morning Oregonian*, June 29, 1904; "Chinese Eager to See Juries Work," *Los Angeles Herald*, June 5, 1907; "Catch Alleged Opium Venders," *Hawaiian Gazette*, July 15, 1910; "Opium Is Seized in Visalia Raid," *Oakland Tribune*, May 7, 1911; "Chinks Convicted," *Arizona Republican* (Phoenix), March 7, 1912; "Find Smoke, Opium Odor," *Los Angeles Times*, April 24, 1912; "Opium Doctor Fined," *San Francisco Call*, January 21, 1913; "Chinese Taken in Raid," *Morning Oregonian*, January 26, 1915; "Chinese Doctor Jailed," *Morning Oregonian* (Portland), July 9, 1922; "Chinese Doctor Is Again Accused on Drug Charge," *Salt Lake Tribune* (Salt Lake City), February 15, 1923; "'Chink Doctor' Is Caught in Dope

Dragnet," *Billings Gazette,* March 23, 1924; "Dope Raiders Seize Woman, Chinese Doctor, and Actor," *Los Angeles Times,* December 13, 1936; "Third Narcotic Suspect Taken," *Los Angeles Times,* January 27, 1937.

91. *Daily Alta California,* September 20, 1885.

92. "Before His Honor Today," *Salt Lake Democrat,* July 21, 1885.

93. "A Chinese Quack," *San Francisco Chronicle,* July 24, 1870.

94. "Dr. Li Po Tai Borrowing," *Daily Alta California,* July 3, 1871, Him Mark Lai Papers, box 23, folder 18.

95. "Celestial Quacks," *San Francisco Chronicle,* December 5, 1880. Nineteenth-century Americans often referred to Chinese immigrants as "celestials." The term referenced the literary translation of the Chinese word for "China," but it quickly took on pejorative associations. Anti-Chinese reformers perceived the Chinese as "heathens" and employed the term "celestial" ironically.

96. *Li Po Tai, 1817–1893: Translated from a History of the Sam Yup Benevolent Association in the United States, 1850–1979* (San Francisco: Sam Yup Association, 1974), 180; Him Mark Lai Papers, box 22, folder 11; "Curious Chinese Medicines," *Racine [Wisc.] Daily Journal,* November 23, 1906.

97. "Celestial Quacks," *San Francisco Chronicle,* December 5, 1880.

98. *Anaconda Standard,* July 14, 1890.

99. "Ways That Are Dark," *Anaconda Standard,* October 30, 1891.

100. "Dr. Lamb in Butte," *Anaconda Standard,* September 20, 1909.

101. *Los Angeles Times,* November 17, 1890.

102. "In a Frock Coat and High Hat," *Los Angeles Times,* March 10, 1908.

103. "Herb 'Doctors' Taken," *Los Angeles Times,* December 10, 1913.

104. "Doctor Chan Talks Fight," *Los Angeles Times,* July 31, 1907.

105. "Herb Quacks in Law Net," *Los Angeles Times,* June 4, 1907.

106. Ibid.

107. "Chinese Doctors Answer in Court," *Los Angeles Herald,* June 5, 1907.

108. "Potter Death Still a Mystery," *Los Angeles Times,* August 31, 1912.

109. "Peach Poison Killed Potter," *New York Times,* September 1, 1912.

110. Stewart Culin, "Chinese Drug Stores in America," *American Journal of Pharmacy* 59 (December 1887): 593–598; Stewart Culin, "The Practice of Medicine by the Chinese in America," *Medical and Surgical Reporter,* March 19, 1887, 1–3.

111. "Old and New Medicine," *Los Angeles Times,* June 18, 1916.

112. "I Doctored by a Celestial," *New York Sun,* September 26, 1886.

113. Tisdale, "Chinese Physicians in California," 412.

114. Ibid., 414.

115. Ibid.

116. Ibid., 416.

117. Mrs. Fred Deardorff to Ing Hay, n.d., Kam Wah Chung Papers.

118. Liu, "Chinese Herbalists in the United States," 151.

119. Mrs. M. J. Baker to Ing Hay, November 3, 1911, Kam Wah Chung Papers. See also James F. Draplan to Ing Hay, October 8, n.d., Kam Wah Chung Papers.

120. "Two Others Fined," *Anaconda Standard,* August 6, 1897.

121. Advertisement, *Los Angeles Times,* April 7, 1910; Advertisement, *Bakersfield Californian,* July 5, 1911; Advertisement, *Los Angeles Times,* February 6, 1927.

122. See, for example, Advertisement (Wong Tack Fun), *Daily Independent* (Helena, Mont.), August 11, 1881; Advertisement (Jim Yen), *Los Angeles Times,* January 8, 1893; Advertisement (H. C. Wong), *Anaconda Standard,* August 23, 1901; Advertisement (Chang Gee Wo), *Billings Gazette,* September 25, 1910; and business card from Dr. Chin Man Sui's Chinese herbal medicine clinic, ca. 1911, MS 2/1287, Idaho State Historical Society, Boise, reproduced in Smith, "Choosing Chinese Medicine," 101.

123. Buell, "Chinese Medicine on the 'Gold Mountain,'" 104.

124. Sarah Stage, *Female Complaints: Lydia Pinkham and the Business of Women's Medicine* (New York: Norton, 1979), 82–83.

125. Andrea Tone, *Devices and Desires: A History of Contraceptives in America* (New York: Hill and Wang, 2001), 94–95.

126. Historians have often assumed that non-Chinese patients enjoyed the anonymity and geographic separation from their community that a Chinese physician provided. That may have been true for offices located in Chinatowns like those of Boise doctors C. K. Ah Fong and Chin Man Sui—both of whom claimed a specialty in "private diseases"—but probably did not hold true for the many Chinese physicians who set up shop in predominantly European American neighborhoods. Smith, "Choosing Chinese Medicine," 101–102; Buell, *Chinese Medicine on the Golden Mountain,* 65; Steele, *Bleed, Blister, and Purge,* 92.

127. Gynecology as a distinct field of study within Chinese medicine first developed in the Song Dynasty (960–1279). For more on the history of gynecology in China, see Furth, *A Flourishing Yin.*

128. Stage, *Female Complaints,* 87; Linda Gordon, *Woman's Body, Woman's Right: A Social History of Birth Control in America* (New York: Grossman, 1976), 23–24.

129. Stage, *Female Complaints,* 85.

130. The earliest example of a claim to specialize in gynecological disorders that I have found is Jock Toon's advertisement in the *Livermore Herald,* where he claimed "women and children a specialty." Advertisement, *Livermore [Calif.] Herald,* May 13, 1880. In the 1880s and 1890s, several Los Angeles doctors also explicitly advertised their services to women. For example, see Advertisement (Soo Nong), *Los Angeles Times,* February 11, 1885; Advertisement (Dr. Sing), *Los Angeles Times,* July 31, 1887; Advertisement (Dr. Qwong), *Los Angeles Times,* November 19, 1890; Advertisement (Le Po Ti), *Los Angeles Times,* December 17, 1890.

131. Foo and Wing Herb Company, *The Science of Oriental Medicine: A Concise Discussion of Its Principles and Methods, Biographical Sketches of Its Leading Practitioners, and Its Treatment of Various Prevalent Diseases, Useful Information on Matters of Diet, Exercise, and Hygiene* (Los Angeles: G. Rice and Sons, 1897), 113.

132. Chang, *Things Chinese,* 49.

133. The "Cult of True Womanhood" is a nineteenth-century phrase first revived in historical scholarship by Barbara Welter, "The Cult of True Womanhood, 1820–1860," *American Quarterly* 18, no. 2 (Summer 1966): 152. For a discussion of how the Cult of True Womanhood intersected with and influenced the lives of women in the late nineteenth- and early twentieth-century American West, see Elizabeth Jameson, "Women as Workers, Women as Civilizers: True Womanhood in the American West," in *The Women's West,* ed. Susan Armitage and Elizabeth Jameson (Norman: University of Oklahoma Press, 1984), 145–164. The doctors' emphasis on motherhood was undeniably out of touch with the "New Woman" of the 1920s. In the wake of the Nineteenth Amendment, a new icon of white femininity burst onto the scene. Sexually liberated, empowered by the right to vote, and often depicted in a "flapper" costume, the New Woman seemed omnipresent in popular media. Did Chinese doctors' emphasis on true womanhood attract or repel the New Woman? In the absence of first-person accounts, it is difficult to say. We do know that the New Woman of the 1920s did not wholly replace Victorian true womanhood, with its emphasis on sexual purity and pious domesticity. Many middle-class white women in the 1920s continued to base their claims to authority and rights to self-determination on principles of maternalism. Ellen Carol DuBois and Lynn Dumenil, *Through Women's Eyes: An American History with Documents* (Boston: Bedford/St. Martins, 2005), 483.

134. Reprinted in Chia-lin Chen, "The Golden Flower of Prosperity," October 1, 1971, Kam Wah Chung Papers.

135. Ing Hay cared for some prominent local families including the Deardorffs, the Keerins, the Van Bibbers, and one-time mayor of Burns, Oregon, J. C. Welcome, among others. Scrapbook 21, p. 59; Scrapbook 48, p. 126, Oregon Historical Society; J. Southworth, *A History of Grant County* (Dallas: Taylor, 1983), 55, 87–88; Kam Wah Chung Papers, reels 1–2; U.S. Census, 1910, John Day, Oregon, reel T624.

136. Perhaps the earliest example of a woman's name appearing in a patient testimonial is from 1869, when Mrs. C. H. Webb and her husband jointly vouched for San Francisco doctor Ho Chum. Advertisement, *San Francisco Chronicle,* August 25, 1869.

137. Advertisement, *Los Angeles Times,* March 28, 1909.

138. Gordon, *Woman's Body, Woman's Right,* 164.

139. Klee, "The 'Regulars' and the Chinese," 181–207.

140. Keith T. Downing, "Uterine Prolapse: From Antiquity to Today," *Obstetrics and Gynecology International* 2012, no. 4 (2012): 1–9; Marlene B. Goldman and Maureen Hatch, *Women and Health* (San Diego: Academic Press, 2000), 253.

141. Stage, *Female Complaints,* 77–78.

142. Ibid., 79–82; Regina Markell Morantz-Sanchez, *Conduct Unbecoming a Woman: Medicine on Trial in Turn-of-the-Century Brooklyn* (New York: Oxford University Press, 2000), 106–107.

143. Foo and Wing Herb Company, *The Science of Oriental Medicine* (Los Angeles: Times-Mirror, 1902), 167.

144. Chang, *Things Chinese,* 49–50.

145. *Gouy Shong* [Shang] *v. Chew Shee et al.*, Massachusetts Supreme Judicial Court, Suffolk County, January 7, 1926.

146. Larson, *Sweet Bamboo*, 58, 69, 111–112.

147. "Seid Gain Married," *Oregonian*, January 26, 1900; "Fiddle Versus Organ," *Oregonian*, April 6, 1903; "Entertainment at Mission in Honor of Bishop Moore," *Oregon Daily Journal* (Portland), July 28, 1906; *Oregon Daily Journal*, August 26, 1906; Marie Rose Wong, *Sweet Cakes, Long Journey: The Chinatowns of Portland, Oregon* (Seattle: University of Washington Press, 2004), 185.

148. Advertisement, *Morning Oregonian*, June 5, 1902.

149. Advertisement, *Oregon Daily Journal*, March 18, 1907.

150. Wing, Greenlee, and Chin, *Son of South Mountain and Dust*, 76.

151. Advertisement, *Goshen Times*, August 16, 1894.

152. Advertisement (Le Po Ti), *Los Angeles Times*, December 17, 1890. The earliest example I have found of pulsology illustrated is an 1890 advertisement for Dr. Kwong of Los Angeles; see Advertisement (Dr. Kwong), *Los Angeles Times*, October 8, 1890, and Advertisement (Lee Chin), *Los Angeles Times*, May 11, 1913.

153. See, for example, Advertisement (Foo and Wing), *Los Angeles Herald*, May 1, 1902; Advertisement (Le Po Tei), *Sunday Oregonian*, October 13, 1901; and Advertisement (Tom Leung), *Los Angeles Times*, August 5, 1928.

154. Version with male patient: Advertisement (no. 21), *Los Angeles Times*, March 2, 1904. Versions with female patients: Advertisement, *Los Angeles Herald*, May 1, 1902, and Advertisement, *Los Angeles Times*, November 17, 1912.

155. Stage, *Female Complaints*, 88; Judith Walzer Leavitt, *Brought to Bed: Childbearing in America, 1750 to 1950* (New York: Oxford University Press, 1986), 38–39.

156. Leavitt, *Brought to Bed*, 174–175.

157. There is a rich historiography of American midwifery including monographs that detail the vital role played by African American, indigenous, and Japanese American women. For example, see Fett, *Working Cures;* Susan Lynn Smith, *Japanese American Midwives: Culture, Community, and Health Politics, 1880–1950* (Urbana: University of Illinois Press, 2005); and Helen Varney and Joyce Beebe Thompson, *A History of Midwifery in the United States: The Midwife Said Fear Not* (New York: Springer, 2016).

158. Steele, *Bleed, Blister, and Purge*, 105–106.

159. Boyd and Ming, *The Chinese of Kern County*, 172.

160. "A Doctor Accused," *Daily Journal*, October 9, 1899; "That Albany Baby," *Daily Journal*, October 10, 1899.

161. Furth, *A Flourishing Yin*, 60–61, 66–67.

162. Wu, *Reproducing Women*, 58–59.

163. Ibid., 65–67, 167.

164. Gordon, *Woman's Body, Woman's Right*, 22.

165. Janet Farrell Brodie, *Contraception and Abortion in Nineteenth-Century America* (Ithaca, N.Y.: Cornell University Press, 1994), 254, 266–272; Leslie J. Reagan,

When Abortion Was a Crime: Women, Medicine, and Law in the United States, 1867–1973 (Berkeley: University of California Press, 1997), 10–14.

166. Gordon, *Woman's Body, Woman's Right,* 272.

167. Chen, "A Gold Dream in the Blue Mountains," 123.

168. "Another Complaint Issued against Lun," *Salt Lake Tribune,* October 26, 1913.

169. Dr. Herbert Yee, interview with Nancy Wey, June 4, 1978, Nancy Wey Papers, carton 2, folder 16.

170. U.S. Census, 1900, Sacramento, California, reel T623; "Asks for Representation," *Sacramento Daily Union,* February 29, 1894.

171. "Dr. Wah Hing," *Reno [Nev.] Evening Gazette,* September 14, 1886; Advertisement, *Daily Nevada State Journal* (Reno), July 7, 1891.

172. Advertisement, *Sacramento Daily Record-Union,* December 12, 1891.

173. U.S. Census, 1900, Sacramento, California, reel T623; "Chinese Boy Treads the Primrose Path," *Oakland Tribune,* August 9, 1910; Lawrence Tom, Brian Tom, and the Chinese American Museum of Northern California, *Sacramento's Chinatown* (Charleston, S.C.: Arcadia, 2010), 26.

174. Dr. Herbert Yee, interview with Nancy Wey, June 4, 1978, Nancy Wey Papers, carton 2, folder 16.

175. This process—from the initial consultation to the in-office procedure and postoperative medication—seems to have been typical of abortion practices at the turn of the twentieth century. The payment of $25 requested also falls within the normal range ($10 to $175) and well below the average of $48. Reagan, *When Abortion Was a Crime,* 71–72.

176. *Report of Cases Determined in the District Courts of Appeal of the State of California,* vol. 15 (San Francisco: Bancroft-Whitney, 1911), 206–207.

177. *The People, Respondent v. T. Wah Hing, Appellant,* Criminal no. 132, Court of Appeal of California, Third Appellate District, January 24, 1911, California State Archives, Sacramento, Calif.

178. "Chinese Physician Claims an Alibi," *San Francisco Call,* November 6, 1909; "Further Evidence to Prove Alleged Alibi," *San Francisco Call,* November 10, 1909; "Juggled," *San Francisco Call,* November 11, 1909; "Safe in Prison Walls," *Los Angeles Times,* December 12, 1909.

179. "Fail to Convict Chinese Doctor," *San Francisco Chronicle,* November 14, 1909.

180. "Safe in Prison Walls," *Los Angeles Times,* December 12, 1909.

181. "Admits to Seeking to Send Witness Away," *San Francisco Call,* December 10, 1909; "Burglary Charged in Wah Hing Trial," *San Francisco Call,* December 11, 1909.

182. "Witness Charges Bribe Was Offered," *San Francisco Call,* December 9, 1909.

183. "Chinese Doctor Gets Three Years in Prison," *San Francisco Call,* December 15, 1909.

184. "Grand Jury Refuses to Indict Dr. Hing," *Sacramento [Calif.] Union,* July 3, 1917; "Chinese Doctor Sued for $50,000 for Alleged Illegal Operation," *Sacramento Union,* December 13, 1922.

185. U.S. Census, 1860, reel M653_60; Mary Tongere Westfall, memorial no. 33106186, www.findagrave.com.

186. Susan Lee Johnson, *Roaring Camp: The Social World of the California Gold Rush* (New York: Norton, 2000), 125–126.

187. Andrew T. Urban, "The Advantages of Empire: Chinese Servants and Conflicts over Settler Domesticity in the 'White Pacific,' 1870–1900," in *Making the Empire Work: Labor and United States Imperialism,* ed. Daniel E. Bender and Jana K. Lipman (New York: NYU Press, 2015), 185.

188. Wong, *Sweet Cakes, Long Journey,* 211–212.

189. "Small Pox in San Francisco," *Sacramento Daily Union,* May 24, 1876.

190. W. B. Gratzer, *Terrors of the Table: The Curious History of Nutrition* (Oxford: Oxford University Press, 2005), 36.

191. Anne Mendelson, *Stand Facing the Stove: The Story of the Women Who Gave America the Joy of Cooking* (New York: Scribner, 2003), 260–261; Harvey Levenstein, *Paradox of Plenty: A Social History of Eating in Modern America* (Oxford: Oxford University Press, 1994), 13–15.

192. Gratzer, *Terrors of the Table,* 188–210.

193. Foo and Wing Herb Company, *The Science of Oriental Medicine* (1902 ed.), 20–72.

194. Ibid., 154.

195. For example, Yee and York advertisement, *Evening Statesman* (Walla Walla, Wash.), October 11, 1908.

196. Hinrichs and Barnes, *Chinese Medicine and Healing,* 14.

197. Fong Wan Herb Company, *Herb Lore,* 181–188.

198. Ibid., 189; Advertisement, *Oakland Tribune,* February 15, 1939.

199. Advertisement, *Oakland Tribune,* February 15, 1939.

200. Fong Wan Herb Company, *Herb Lore,* 19.

FOUR   Chinese Quacks

1. Samuel Hall would later achieve notoriety for committing criminal malpractice and murder. "Delayed Justice," *San Francisco Call,* November 30, 1893.

2. "The Doctor," *San Francisco Chronicle,* October 17, 1878; "Around the City," *Daily Alta California,* October 17, 1878.

3. The *Chronicle* identified them as Ah Wing, Ting Chee Lou, Chang Lou Farn, Jook Toon, Tsuen Luen, and Wong Tsok Toon. "Chinese Doctors Arrested," *San Francisco Chronicle,* August 22, 1879; *Daily Alta California,* February 10, 1880.

4. Starr, *The Social Transformation of American Medicine,* 106.

5. William Rothstein offers an extensive discussion of this movement in his book *American Physicians in the Nineteenth Century,* including a comparative look at how individual states organized their various licensing agencies. He writes, "Non-regular physi-

cians participated in some way in the licensing processing of at least 33 of the 45 states with licensing laws in 1900." William Rothstein, *American Physicians in the Nineteenth Century: From Sects to Science* (Baltimore: Johns Hopkins University Press, 1992), 305–310.

6. James G. Burrow, *Organized Medicine in the Progressive Era: The Move toward Monopoly* (Baltimore: Johns Hopkins University Press, 1977), 12; Whorton, *Nature Cures*, 135.

7. Professional medicine in Europe was at that time far more developed and hierarchical with elite diplomates acting as the profession's gatekeepers. Starr, *The Social Transformation of American Medicine*, 38; Roy Porter, *The Greatest Benefit to Mankind: A Medical History of Humanity* (New York: Norton, 1998), 352–355.

8. Starr, *The Social Transformation of American Medicine*, 44–46.

9. Ibid., 58.

10. Samuel Thomson, *New Guide to Health* (Brockville, Ontario: W. Willes, 1831), 9.

11. Ibid., 42.

12. John Harley Warner, *The Therapeutic Perspective: Medical Practice, Knowledge, and Identity in America, 1820–1885* (Cambridge, Mass.: Harvard University Press, 1986), 7.

13. There is ample scholarship on anti-monopolist movements in the Gilded Age and Progressive Era including Daniel T. Rodgers, "In Search of Progressivism," *Reviews in American History* 10, no. 4 (1982): 123–124. Recent monographs on anti-monopolism in the Gilded Age include Richard R. John, *Network Nation: Inventing American Telecommunications* (Cambridge, Mass.: Belknap Press of Harvard University Press, 2010), 8; Charles Postel, *The Populist Vision* (Oxford: Oxford University Press, 2007), 4; Richard White, *Railroaded: The Transcontinentals and the Making of Modern America* (New York: Norton, 2011), xxxiv, 493; and Tamara Venit Shelton, *A Squatter's Republic: Land and the Politics of Monopoly in California* (San Marino, Calif.: Huntington Library Press, 2013).

14. Whorton, *Nature Cures*, 69.

15. Ibid., 155.

16. Starr, *The Social Transformation of American Medicine*, 56; Warner, *The Therapeutic Perspective*, 7.

17. Porter, *The Greatest Benefit to Mankind*, 308–312.

18. Ibid., 320–322.

19. Ibid., 344.

20. Ibid., 388.

21. William G. Rothstein, *American Medical Schools and the Practice of Medicine: A History* (New York: Oxford University Press, 1987), 71.

22. Nancy Tomes, *The Gospel of Germs: Men, Women, and the Microbe in American Life* (Cambridge, Mass.: Harvard University Press, 1998), 45–46.

23. Ibid., 28; Porter, *The Greatest Benefit to Mankind*, 428–448.

24. Tomes, *The Gospel of Germs*, 33; Rothstein, *American Medical Schools and the Practice of Medicine*, 74.

25. Porter, *The Greatest Benefit to Mankind*, 344.

26. Rothstein, *American Medical Schools and the Practice of Medicine*, 71.

27. Starr, *The Social Transformation of American Medicine*, 115–116; Rothstein, *American Medical Schools and the Practice of Medicine*, 89–93, 153.

28. Starr, *The Social Transformation of American Medicine*, 117–118; Rothstein, *American Medical Schools and the Practice of Medicine*, 144.

29. Rothstein, *American Medical Schools and the Practice of Medicine*, 144–146.

30. Burrow, *Organized Medicine in the Progressive Era*, 42–43; Starr, *The Social Transformation of American Medicine*, 104–106.

31. Quoted in Rothstein, *American Medical Schools and the Practice of Medicine*, 148–149.

32. Norman Gevitz, "Three Perspectives on Unorthodox Medicine," in Gevitz, ed., *Other Healers*, 9–10.

33. Pharmacists and other drug peddlers who did not diagnose patients were exempt from the new law. "Correspondence," *New England Medical Gazette*, June 1876, 278–281.

34. Linda A. McCready and Billie Harris, "From Quackery to Quality Assurance: The First Twelve Decades of the Medical Board of California," Medical Board of California, 1995, 3–8, http://www.mbc.ca.gov/publications/quackery.pdf.

35. "The Heathen Chinese as a Doctor," *Wisconsin State Journal* (Madison), December 31, 1870.

36. "First Shot at Medico Quacks," *Los Angeles Times*, August 2, 1911.

37. *Journal of the Senate and the House of the Legislative Assembly of the State of Oregon*, sess. 25 (Salem, Ore.: [The State], 1909), 89; "Bill Aimed at Chinese Doctors Beaten in Senate," *San Francisco Chronicle*, March 24, 1911.

38. James Harvey Young, *The Medical Messiahs: A Social History of Quackery in Twentieth-Century America* (Princeton, N.J.: Princeton University Press, 1992), 83.

39. "They Will Approve It," *Anaconda Standard*, May 19, 1891.

40. *Los Angeles Times*, November 13, 1887.

41. "Crusade against Quacks," *Morning Oregonian*, October 4, 1907.

42. *Western Liberal* (Lordsburg, N.M.), August 4, 1893.

43. "Chinese Doctors Answer in Court," *Los Angeles Herald*, June 5, 1907; "Chinese Eager to See Juries Work," *Los Angeles Herald*, June 7, 1907.

44. "Druggist Deplores Oriental Methods," *San Francisco Call*, August 20, 1909.

45. Kraut, *Silent Travelers*, 5.

46. "Druggists Put under Arrest," *Los Angeles Times*, June 13, 1914.

47. "Arrest of a Chinese Doctor," *San Francisco Chronicle*, December 14, 1883.

48. Annual Reports of the Board of Medical Examiners, *Appendix to the Journals of the Senate and Assembly* (Sacramento, Calif.: State Printing, 1914–1942).

49. In this case, the newspaper article presents the case as though it were the same person arrested under two separate complaints, but it is impossible to verify. See "Arrest Quack Again," *Los Angeles Times*, June 6, 1919.

50. J. A. Crawshaw, "Prosecution of Illegal Practitioners," *California State Journal of Medicine* 8 (May 1910): 155.

51. "Chinese Doctor Fined," *Los Angeles Times*, December 5, 1909.

52. Crawshaw, "Prosecution of Illegal Practitioners."

53. "Assessments Are Not Lien," *Los Angeles Times*, February 2, 1910.

54. Ibid.

55. "China Frees Dr. L. T. Sue of Hanford," *Los Angeles Times*, July 10, 1923.

56. *Daily Alta California*, June 12, 1884; "Dr. Kwai Ding Kwai," *New York Times*, September 10, 1887; "Dr. Bow Chang Tong," *Anaconda Standard*, September 25, 1895; "Want a Chinese Hospital," *New York Tribune*, November 22, 1902.

57. *Daily Alta California*, November 10, 1880.

58. "An Official in Trouble," *Sacramento Daily Union*, December 3, 1891.

59. *The Medical Standard* 15 (January–June 1894): 95; "Kansas," *Journal of the American Medical Association* 38 (May 17, 1902): 1311; "The Talk of the Day," *New York Tribune*, August 27, 1902.

60. "A Chinese Physician," *Connersville Daily Examiner*, June 6, 1892; *Crown Point [Ind.] Register*, May 4, 1894; "Dr. Don Sang Dead," *New York Times*, March 11, 1903.

61. "Chinese Doctor," *Fort Wayne [Ind.] Daily Gazette*, July 18, 1897.

62. "Don Sang Wants a License," *Kansas City Journal*, August 31, 1897; "Temporarily," *Fort Wayne Daily Gazette*, August 31, 1897.

63. Losing his appeal was just the beginning of the doctor's woes. Swindled by his business manager, Sang lost the savings he had amassed over his fifty years in the United States. His wife, a Chinese woman half his age, ran off to Mexico with their cook. The lovers were subsequently tracked down by Chinese gangsters—presumably at Dr. Sang's behest—and the young man was murdered in Yucatán. Sang did not live to see his vengeance enacted; he had died four months earlier. "Doctor Don Sang Victim of a Plot," *Oroville [Calif.] Weekly Mercury*, February 21, 1902; "Killed by Highbinders," *The World*, July 6, 1903; U.S. Census, 1900, Chicago, Ill., reel T623; Dr. Don Sang, memorial no. 145613850, www.findagrave.com.

64. There are a few other examples of Chinese physicians requesting to be grandfathered into new licensing legislation because of their record of practicing medicine in the United States. See, for example, *C. Gee Wo v. State of Nebraska*, February 15, 1893, no. 5485, in *Reports of Cases in the Supreme Court of Nebraska*, vol. 36, *January Term* (Lincoln, Neb.: State Journal, 1893), 241–247, and "A Chinese Doctor," *Arizona Republican*, February 6, 1900. Ah Fong's Boise colleague Char Man Sui also applied for a license based on his years of service in Idaho before the passage of the 1899 law. "Is Chinaman Legal Practitioner?" *Evening Statesman*, October 14, 1905.

65. Devitt, "The Curious Case of Ah Fong Chuck," 5.

66. "Dr. Kwai Ding Kwai," *New York Times*, September 10, 1887.

67. *C. Gee Wo v. State of Nebraska*.

68. See, for example, *The People, Respondent v. Boo Doo Hong, Appellant*, Crim. no. 420, Supreme Court of California, Department 2, December 8, 1898; *The People,*

Respondent v. Ah Fong, Appellant, Crim. no. 525, Court of Appeal of California, First Appellate District, November 10, 1914; *The People, Respondent v. Tom J. Chong, Appellant,* Crim. no. 549, Court of Appeal of California, First Appellate District, July 21, 1915; and *The People, Respondent* v. *T. Wah Hing, Appellant,* Crim. no. 503, Court of Appeal of California, Third Appellate District, May 3, 1920.

69. "Medical Act Is Attacked," *Los Angeles Times,* October 20, 1915.

70. "Chinese Herb Doctors Denied Habeas Corpus," *San Francisco Chronicle,* September 12, 1916.

71. "Chinese Charge He Bribed Them," *Los Angeles Herald,* December 2, 1908.

72. "Says Sanitary Inspector Was Punished Unjustly," *Los Angeles Herald,* December 6, 1908.

73. "Chinese Doctor Faces Bribe Charge," *Oakland Tribune,* May 27, 1919; "Chinese Cleared of Bribery Charge," *Oakland Tribune,* September 12, 1919.

74. *Gouy Shong v. Chew Shee et al.*

75. Gilbert Hom, interview with author, April 19, 2016.

76. "No Chinese Provision in Law," *Journal of the American Medical Association* 48 (May 1902): 1311.

77. Larson, *Sweet Bamboo,* 73.

78. "In re: Pang Suey, merchant returning, March 1, 1905," Pang Suey Jew, National Archives and Records Administration, Record Group 85, Case File no. 2008/168, Riverside, Calif.

79. Advertisement, *Boston Globe,* March 26, 1904; Gilbert Hom, interview with author, April 18, 2016; "Chinatown's Only Doctor," *Boston Globe,* May 16, 1904.

80. "Two Chinamen Claim Partnership," *Boston Globe,* June 20, 1918; U.S. Census, 1910, Boston, Massachusetts, reel T624.

81. "Boston Women Rush to Consult," *New York Tribune,* September 29, 1912; "Dr. Holds Hand," *New York Sun,* October 3, 1912.

82. "Eastern Medicine in Calcium of the West," *Boston Globe,* March 9, 1916.

83. "Want to Allow Chinese Herb Doctor to Register," *Boston Globe,* February 24, 1916.

84. "Pang Suey Bill Killed," *New England Journal of Medicine* 174 (January–June 1916): 659; "To Relieve Pang Suey," *Boston Globe,* March 31, 1916.

85. "Women Hissed a Near-Fight," *Boston Globe,* March 6, 1917; "Pang Suey Bill Debaters Near Fistic Clash," *Boston Journal,* March 7, 1917.

86. "Eng Hen Enters Plea of Not Guilty," *Boston Globe,* November 23, 1917.

87. "Testify to Cures Pang Suey Made," *Boston Globe,* March 8, 1920.

88. Kyle D. Palmer, "Air Charges of Bribery," *Los Angeles Times,* February 26, 1925; "Hearing Today on Bribe Rumor," *Los Angeles Times,* March 2, 1925; "Herb-Bill Bribe Scheme Denied," *Los Angeles Times,* March 4, 1925.

89. Chen, *Being Chinese, Becoming Chinese American,* 162.

90. Larson, *Sweet Bamboo,* 71.

91. Ibid., 71–72.

92. "Oroville Doctor Becomes S.F. Porter," *Better Health,* February 1921, 10.

93. *California State Journal of Medicine* 18, no. 9 (September 1920): 345.

94. *California State Journal of Medicine* 18, no. 10 (October 1920): 374.

95. Wing, Greenlee, and Chin, *Son of South Mountain and Dust*, 76.

96. Larson, *Sweet Bamboo*, 71.

97. Wing, Greenlee, and Chin, *Son of South Mountain and Dust*, 77.

98. Fong Wan Herb Company, *Herb Lore*, 156.

99. Advertisement, *San Francisco Chronicle*, May 6, 1934, http://www.sfmuseum .org/hist8/fongwan.html.

100. Dick Hemp, "Fong Wan, Chinese Herbalist," *San Francisco Chronicle*, June 19, 20, 1949, http://www.sfmuseum.org/hist8/fongwan1.html; Advertisement, *Oakland Tribune*, February 12, 1940.

101. Lee, *At America's Gates*, 138–141.

102. Kraut, *Silent Travelers*, 91–95.

103. See, for example, "Says He's No Doctor," *Spokane [Wash.] Press*, January 5, 1907; "Chinese Doctor Walks into Prosecutor's Trap," *Los Angeles Herald*, January 15, 1909; "Chinese Doctor Fined," *Los Angeles Times*, December 5, 1909; "Technicality Frees Chinese Physician," *Oakland Tribune*, November 16, 1910; "Unlicensed 'Doctors' Are Hauled into Court," *San Francisco Call*, August 30, 1912; "Chink Doctors Up in Court," *Los Angeles Times*, February 4, 1911; "Charge Practicing without a License," *Salt Lake Tribune*, May 15, 1912; and "Chinese Doctor Arrested for Violating Stated Law," *Bakersfield Californian*, October 18, 1913.

104. "Acquitted," *Sacramento Daily Union*, October 27, 1879.

105. *The People, Respondent v. Lee Wah, Appellant*, no. 20217, Supreme Court of California, Department 1, September 24, 1886; "Consulting a Chinese Doctor," *San Francisco Chronicle*, September 25, 1886.

106. Advertisement, *Salt Lake Tribune*, May 4, 1913.

107. *State v. Yee Foo Lun*, no. 2702, Supreme Court of Utah, March 19, 1915; "Another Complaint Issued against Lun," *Salt Lake Tribune*, October 26, 1913.

108. *The People, Respondent v. Poo On, Appellant*, Crim. no. 794, Court of Appeal of California, Third Appellate District, September 24, 1924; "Herb Doctor Restricted," *Altoona [Penn.] Mirror*, April 22, 1938.

109. *State v. Yee Foo Lun*.

110. "Charge Practicing without a License," *Salt Lake Tribune*, May 15, 1913.

111. *State v. Yee Foo Lun*.

FIVE   Oriental Healers

1. C. B. Pinkham, "The Chinese Herbalist and the Medical Practice Act," *California and Western Medicine* 23, no. 6 (June 1927): 737–738.

2. "Testify to Cures Pang Suey Made," *Boston Globe*, March 8, 1920.

3. See for example, Gevitz, ed., *Other Healers*; Natalie S. Robins, *Copeland's Cure: Homeopathy and the War between Conventional and Alternative Medicine* (New York: Knopf, 2009); Rothstein, *American Physicians in the Nineteenth Century*;

Rothstein, *American Medical Schools and the Practice of Medicine;* Steele, *Bleed, Blister, and Purge;* Whorton, *Nature Cures;* and Young, *The Toadstool Millionaires.*

4. "Go to the Chinaman," *Anaconda Standard,* March 15, 1891.

5. "Queer Chinese Medicines," *Los Angeles Times,* August 11, 1907.

6. "Chinese Medicos," *Los Angeles Times,* September 27, 1900.

7. Leo Marx, *The Machine in the Garden: Technology and the Pastoral Ideal in America* (New York: Oxford University Press, 1964), 343.

8. T. J. Jackson Lears, *No Place of Grace: Antimodernism and the Transformation of American Culture, 1880–1920* (Chicago: University of Chicago Press, 1994), xv.

9. Henry George, *The Fiftieth Anniversary Edition of Progress and Poverty* (1879; New York: Robert Schaleknbach Foundation, 1929), 7.

10. Ibid., 446.

11. Charles E. Rosenberg has an extensive discussion of hospitals and medical income in *The Care of Strangers* in which he details the difficult position of nonprofit hospitals, attempting to maintain their mission of public service in a medical marketplace. Charles E. Rosenberg, *The Care of Strangers: The Rise of America's Hospital System* (Baltimore: Johns Hopkins University Press, 1987), 252–261.

12. Starr, *The Social Transformation of American Medicine,* 32.

13. Whorton, *Nature Cures,* 32.

14. Cayleff, *Nature's Path,* 2–3.

15. Stuart Anderson, *Making Medicines: A Brief History of Pharmacy and Pharmaceuticals* (London: Pharmacy Press, 2005), 180–182.

16. As John Harley Warner argues in *The Therapeutic Perspective,* "The dearth of research in the history of therapeutics is a reflection of the methodological difficulties inherent in determining what nineteenth-century physicians actually did at the bedside." Warner, *The Therapeutic Perspective,* 2.

17. United States Pharmacopoeia Convention, *The Pharmacopoeia of the United States of America: Ninth Decennial Revision* (Philadelphia: P. Blakiston's Son, 1916); Shizhen Li and Xiwen Luo, *Compendium of Materia Medica: Bencao Gangmu* (Beijing: Foreign Languages Press, 2003).

18. Julius Kohl, "The Physician of the Past, the Present, and the Future—A Definition of His Social Position," *Journal of the American Medical Association* 24 (1895): 969.

19. J. C. Wilson, "A Century of Medicine in America," *Journal of the American Medical Association* 32 (January–June 1899): 1279.

20. "Chinese Doctors," *Los Angeles Times,* September 30, 1894.

21. "How Physicians Aid Charlatans," *Journal of the American Medical Association* 43 (1904): 208.

22. William B. Dewees, "Eulogy on Jenner," *Journal of the American Medical Association* 27 (1896): 1130.

23. Wilhelm Hotz, "Cleanliness: The First Principle of Hygiene," *Journal of the American Medical Association* 28 (January–June 1897): 251.

24. H. J. Herrick, "Have We in Nature a Basis for a Science and Art in Medicine?" *Journal of the American Medical Association* 34 (January–June 1900): 411.

25. J. A. Work, "Discussion of Infant Feeding," *Journal of the American Medical Association* 51 (July–December 1908): 1223.

26. Historian John Harley Warner has shown that therapeutic practices and principles changed gradually in this period. Warner, *The Therapeutic Perspective*, 6.

27. James F. Hibbed, "A Plea for Greater Simplicity in Practical Medicine," *Journal of the American Medical Association* 2 (January–June 1884): 50.

28. E. P. Hurd, "The Mental Hygiene of Physicians," *Journal of the American Medical Association* 13 (July–December 1889): 349.

29. Edwin J. Gardiner, "The Non-Surgical Treatment of Strabismus Convergens," *Journal of the American Medical Association* 14 (January–June 1890): 44.

30. Laurence Turnbull, "On the Value of Antiseptic Treatment and Protection for the Membrana-Tympani in Perforations the Result of Otorrhoea," *Journal of the American Medical Association* 13 (July–December 1889): 841.

31. Warner, *The Therapeutic Perspective*, 18–19.

32. W. H. Myer, "Notes on Tracheotomy, with Cases," *Journal of the American Medical Association* 1 (January–June 1883): 423.

33. J. O. Malsberry, "Advice to the Prospective Mother," *Journal of the American Medical Association* 28 (January–June 1897): 932.

34. "Therapeutics: Diet in Typhoid Fever," *Journal of the American Medical Association* 55 (1910): 1382.

35. August Andrew Erz, *The Medical Question: The Truth about Official Medicine and Why We Must Have Medical Freedom* (Butler, N.J.: B. Lust, 1914), cited in Whorton, *Nature Cures*, 9.

36. E. H. Bowman, "Medical Ethics," *Journal of the American Medical Association* 2 (January–June 1884): 543–544.

37. Choa, *"Heal the Sick" Was Their Motto*, 90–91.

38. Andrews, *The Making of Modern Chinese Medicine*, 55–56; F. Porter Smith, *Contributions towards the Materia Medica and Natural History of China; for the Use of Medical Missionaries and Native Medical Students* (Shanghai: American Presbyterian Mission Press, 1871); F. Porter Smith and G. A. Stuart, *Chinese Materia Medica; Vegetable Kingdom* (Shanghai: American Presbyterian Mission Press, 1911).

39. "Obituary: John Dudgeon, M.D.," *British Medical Journal* 1, no. 2098 (1901): 679.

40. J. Dudgeon, "Chinese Arts of Healing," *Chinese Recorder and Missionary Journal* 2 (May 1869–April 1870): 333.

41. J. Dudgeon, "Chinese Arts of Healing," *Chinese Recorder and Missionary Journal* 2 (May 1869–April 1870): 267

42. Ibid., 267–268

43. J. Dudgeon, "Chinese Arts of Healing," *Chinese Recorder and Missionary Journal* 2 (November 1869–October 1870): 163–164.

44. Harold Balme, *China and Modern Medicine: A Study in Medical Missionary Development* (London: United Council for Missionary Education, 1921), 15–16.

45. Ibid., 83.

46. Wong, *History of Chinese Medicine,* 142.

47. Ibid., 191–192.

48. Barnes, *Needles, Herbs, Gods, and Ghosts,* 220.

49. "Chinese Medicine," *Journal of the American Medical Association* 28 (January–June 1897): 992; "Unaltered and Barbarous Medical Practice in the Orient," *Journal of the American Medical Association* 30 (January–June 1898): 935.

50. "Prof. Fluckiger," "Chinese Peppermint Oil," *American Journal of Pharmacy* 43 (December 1871): 551; John M. Maisch, "On an Asserted Specific for Ague," *American Journal of Pharmacy* 44 (July 1872): 295; F. Porter Smith, "The Oils of Chinese Pharmacy and Commerce," *American Journal of Pharmacy* 46 (September 1874): 431; Charles E. Munsell, "Analysis of Sam-Shu, a Chinese Liquor," *American Journal of Pharmacy* 58 (February 1886): 94; "Pharmaceutical Associations," *American Journal of Pharmacy* 62 (September 1890): 474.

51. Wong, *History of Chinese Medicine,* 205.

52. Ibid., 333–334; "A Chinese Doctress," *San Francisco Call,* September 16, 1896.

53. Wong, *History of Chinese Medicine,* 394; "Chinese Woman Physician, Dr. Yamei Kin, to Lecture," *Los Angeles Herald,* February 23, 1902; "Dr. Yamei Kin, China's Foremost Woman Physician, Now in the U.S.," *Arizona Daily Star* (Tucson), February 26, 1911; "Chinese Women Doctors," *New York Times,* July 21, 1915; Minute Books, Los Angeles County Medical Association, March 6, 1903, Los Angeles County Medical Association Collection.

54. Los Angeles County Medical Association, minutes, March 6, 1903, vol. 4, Los Angeles County Medical Association Collection.

55. "Cures Wrought by Chinese," *Buffalo [N.Y.] Bulletin,* November 11, 1912.

56. "Chinese Doctors," *Los Angeles Times,* September 30, 1894.

57. A. W. Loomis, "Medical Art in the Chinese Quarter," *Overland Monthly,* June 1869, 497.

58. Ibid., 498.

59. Ibid., 499.

60. Ibid., 502.

61. Lui, *The Chinatown Trunk Mystery,* 133.

62. J. C. Thoms, "Chinese Medicines," *Pittsburgh Dispatch,* June 23, 1889.

63. Ibid.

64. "Chinese Doctors," *Los Angeles Times,* September 30, 1894.

65. "Dr. Holds Hand," *New York Sun,* October 3, 1912.

66. Michael Devitt has called the period between 1860 and 1970 the "Dark Age of Acupuncture in the United States" because so few physicians—Chinese or American—practiced it. Devitt, "The Curious Case of Ah Fong Chuck," 5.

67. Andrews, *The Making of Modern Chinese Medicine,* 200–205.

68. *Daily Alta California,* May 15, 1887.

69. "The Needle Cure," *Daily Call,* February 3, 1893.

70. "It Makes Huie Kin Smile," *New York Sun,* December 6, 1897.

71. "Image Which Tells Chinese Needle Doctor Where to Punch Holes So Devils Can Escape," *Evening Herald* (Klamath Falls, Ore.), April 15, 1919.

72. "Celestial Quacks," *San Francisco Chronicle*, December 5, 1880.

73. "Casting Out Devils," *Sunday Oregonian*, February 25, 1900.

74. "Healing Art among the Chinese," *Los Angeles Times*, July 5, 1908.

75. According to James Harvey Young, in 1859, the proprietary medicine industry had revenues of $3.5 million. By 1904, it claimed over twenty times that amount. Young, *The Medical Messiahs*, 25.

76. Porter, *The Greatest Benefit to Mankind*, 395–396.

77. "Doctors with Pigtails," *The World*, August 9, 1891.

78. W. Hamilton Jefferys and James L. Maxwell, *The Diseases of China, Including Formosa and Korea* (Philadelphia: P. Blakiston's, 1910), 16.

79. Advertisement, *Daily Californian*, February 22, 1902.

80. Platt had already severed ties to the company by the time the book was published. A newspaper article made reference to Platt's contribution to the work in progress; see "A Step in Advance," *Los Angeles Times*, May 26, 1896.

81. Foo and Wing Herb Company, *The Science of Oriental Medicine* (1902 ed.), 8–9.

82. Unschuld, *Medicine in China*, 78.

83. "Discrepancy Is Trifle Too Big," *Evening Statesman*, April 14, 1910.

84. Advertisement, *Bisbee Daily Review*, April 12, 1914.

85. Advertisement, *Los Angeles Times*, January 1, 1903.

86. Advertisement, *San Francisco Chronicle*, July 21, 1912.

87. Fong Wan Herb Company, *Herb Lore*, 30.

88. Advertisement, *Oracle of Dauphin and Harrisburgh Advertiser*, April 17, 1799.

89. Advertisement, *Oakland [Calif.] Evening Tribune*, June 21, 1877.

90. Starr, *The Social Transformation of American Medicine*, 106.

91. Advertisement, *Omaha Daily Bee*, August 31, 1890; Advertisement, *Goshen Times*, August 16, 1894.

92. Chang, *Things Chinese*, 30.

93. Quoted in Smith, "Choosing Chinese Medicine," 98.

94. See, for example, Advertisement (Dr. Kwong), *Los Angeles Times*, October 8, 1890; Advertisement (Dr. Woh), *Los Angeles Times*, November 21, 1890; Advertisement (Le Po Ti), *Los Angeles Times*, December 17, 1890; Advertisement (Lee Wing), *Hutchinson [Kans.] Daily News*, September 14, 1892; Advertisement (Lou Luke), *Arizona Republican*, October 8, 1892; and Advertisement (Yee and York), *Evening Statesman*, October 11, 1909.

95. Foo and Wing Herb Company, *The Science of Oriental Medicine* (1902 ed.), 15.

96. Warner, *The Therapeutic Perspective*, 5–6; Rosenberg, *The Care of Strangers*, 148–149.

97. *Chinese Herbal Science*, 9.

98. Ibid., 1.

99. Advertisement, *Bisbee Daily Review,* April 12, 1914.

100. Advertisement, *Oakland Tribune,* November 12, 1922.

101. S. P. Lee and Sons, *Health Herbs: Nature's Great Gift to All,* n.d. [1920s?], Los Angeles County Medical Association Collection.

102. Advertisements (T. B. Chew and Best Herb Company–Lee Brothers), *Los Angeles Times,* September 17, 1939; Advertisement (Dr. Ipp), *Los Angeles Times,* September 26, 1948.

103. Fong Wan Herb Company, *Herb Lore,* 20.

104. Advertisement, *Goshen Times,* August 16, 1894; Chang, *Things Chinese,* 23, 28–30, 38–40.

105. Garding Lui, "Herbs for the Ills of China," *Los Angeles Times,* February 9, 1936.

106. Garding Lui, *Secrets of Chinese Physicians* (Los Angeles: B. N. Robertson, 1943), 10.

107. Char Miller, "A Sylvan Prospect," in *American Wilderness: A New History,* ed. Michael Lewis (Oxford: Oxford University Press, 2007), 131–147.

108. Advertisement, *Los Angeles Herald,* April 16, 1897.

109. Advertisement, *Evening Statesman,* October 11, 1909.

110. Fawn and Platt, "A Step in Advance."

111. Advertisement, *Los Angeles Times,* January 12, 1902.

112. Chang, *Things Chinese,* 28.

113. *Chinese Herbal Science,* 61.

114. Ibid., 8.

115. Foo and Wing Herb Company, *The Science of Oriental Medicine* (1902 ed.), 70.

116. Chang, *Things Chinese,* 47–48.

117. Matthew Roth, *Magic Bean: The Rise of Soy in America* (Lawrence: University Press of Kansas, 2018), 55–60.

118. "Woman Off to China as Government Agent to Study Soy Bean," *New York Times,* June 10, 1917.

119. See, for example, Gifford Pinchot, *The Fight for Conservation* (New York: Doubleday, Page, 1910).

120. "Woman Off to China as Government Agent to Study Soy Bean," *New York Times,* June 10, 1917.

121. *Oy Wo Tong Co., et al. v. United States,* United States Customs Court, Third Division, August 16, 1940.

122. Ibid.

123. *Him Sing Chong & Co. et al. v. United States,* in *Treasury Decisions under Customs and Other Laws,* vol. 38, *January–December 1920* (Washington, D.C.: Government Printing Office, 1921), 671–672.

124. *Oy Wo Tong Co., et al. v. United States.*

125. Ibid.

126. Chew Kee Store Catalog of Items, Nancy Wey Papers, carton 2, folder 14; Barlow and Richardson, *China Doctor of John Day*, 13; Chen, "A Gold Dream in the Blue Mountains," 79–80; Sarvis, "Gifted Healer Ing Hay and the Chinese Medical Tradition in Eastern Oregon," 63.

127. *Oy Wo Tong Co., et al. v. United States.*

128. Ibid.

129. Nash, *Inescapable Ecologies*, 11–12.

130. Nathan Sivin, *Traditional Medicine in Contemporary China* (Ann Arbor: Center for Chinese Studies, University of Michigan, 1987), 14.

131. Hinrichs and Barnes, *Chinese Medicine and Healing*, 155–156; Porter, *The Greatest Benefit to Mankind*, 154–155.

132. Hanson, "Robust Northerners and Delicate Southerners," 520.

133. Ibid., 538.

134. Volker Scheid, "Restructuring the Field of Chinese Medicine: A Study of the Menghe and Ding Scholarly Currents, 1600–2000, Part 2," *East Asian Science, Technology, and Medicine* 23 (2005): 100.

135. Ibid., 102.

136. Yumei Sun, "San Francisco's *Chung Sai Yat Po* and the Transformation of Chinese Consciousness, 1900–1920," in *Print Culture in a Diverse America*, ed. James Philip Danky and Wayne A. Wiegand (Urbana: University of Illinois Press, 1998), 86.

137. The date range reflects the editions of the periodical digitized by the Ethnic Studies Library at the University of California, Berkeley, available online, or on microfilm at the Asian Pacific Resource Center in Rosemead, California. Future research might extend the sample (*Chung Sai Yat Po* was published up until 1951) and consider advertisements in rival publications such as *Sai Gai Yat Po* (世界日報), which was in print from 1909 to 1969.

138. *Chung Sai Yat Po*, January 23, 1901; January 9, 1904, http://oac.cdlib.org/items/ark:/13030/ktog5016h6.

139. *Chung Sai Yat Po*, August 16, 1900; May 31, 1901, http://oac.cdlib.org/items/ark:/13030/ktog5016h6.

140. *Chung Sai Yat Po*, May 31, 1901, http://oac.cdlib.org/items/ark:/13030/ktog5016h6.

141. *Chung Sai Yat Po*, May 31, 1901; April 30, August 16, 1902; July 17, 1903; January 9, June 22, 1904, http://oac.cdlib.org/items/ark:/13030/ktog5016h6.

142. Advertisement, *Los Angeles Times*, June 1, 1889; Advertisement, *Los Angeles Herald*, October 18, 1893; Advertisement, *San Francisco Chronicle*, February 25, 1894; Advertisement, *Sacramento Record-Union*, July 14, 1898.

143. *Chung Sai Yat Po*, April 30, 1902; January 9, 1904, http://oac.cdlib.org/items/ark:/13030/ktog5016h6.

144. Advertisement, *Los Angeles Times*, June 11, 1906.

145. Advertisement, *Sacramento [Calif.] Record-Union*, July 14, 1898.

146. Advertisement, *Los Angeles Times*, December 17, 1907.

six Decline

1. Courtney Gallant, "Chinese Medicine in Boise," online exhibit, 2012, http://boisechinatown.blogspot.com/p/blog-page_9839.html.

2. U.S. Bureau of the Census, *1970 Census of Population* (Washington, D.C.: U.S. Bureau of the Census, 1973), 14–41, https://hdl.handle.net/2027/uva .x030347745?urlappend=%3Bseq=45; U.S. Bureau of the Census, *Race of the Population for Standard Metropolitan Statistical Areas, Urbanized Areas, and Places of 50,000 or More: 1970* (Washington, D.C.: U.S. Bureau of the Census, 1973), 1–324, https://hdl .handle.net/2027/mdp.39015051824715?urlappend=%3Bseq=5.

3. U.S. Bureau of the Census, *1970 Census of Population*, 14–39.

4. L. J. Davis, "Tearing Down Boise," *Harper's Magazine*, November 1974, 34.

5. John T. Reuter, "Razed and Confused: Boise's Turbulent History of Urban Renewal," *Boise [Idaho] Weekly*, August 4, 2010.

6. Devitt, "The Curious Case of Ah Fong Chuck," 61; Buell, *Chinese Medicine on the Golden Mountain*, 76.

7. Liu makes this claim in "Chinese Herbalists in the United States," 155, and Liu, "The Resilience of Ethnic Culture," 187.

8. In a 1982 essay, John C. Burnham described the first half of the twentieth century as a "Golden Age" of American medicine, an era characterized by the high level of esteem and trust enjoyed among biomedical doctors. Other historians of medicine have applied this term to a period in which the science of chemotherapy—particularly the discovery and mass production of antibiotics in the 1930s and 1940s—moved forward at an astounding pace and spurred important innovations in drug therapy, surgical interventions, and other health practices. John C. Burnham, "American Medicine's Golden Age: What Happened to It?" in *Sickness and Health in America: Readings in the History of Medicine and Public Health*, 2nd ed., ed. Judith Walzer Leavitt and Ronald L. Numbers (1978; Madison: University of Wisconsin Press, 1985), 284; Allan M. Barndt and Martha Gardner, "The Golden Age of Medicine?" in *Companion to Medicine in the Twentieth Century*, ed. Roger Cooter and John Pickstone (London: Routledge, 2003), 29–30.

9. Lui, *Inside Los Angeles Chinatown*, 199–200, 202.

10. Advertisement, *Los Angeles Times*, April 18, 1948.

11. Advertisement, *Los Angeles Times*, April 18, 1943.

12. Some examples of companies running advertisements in English-language newspapers from this period include Master Herb Company (Los Angeles), Chew & Chew (Los Angeles), Dr. Chan (Long Beach, Calif.), G. S. Wong (Huntington Park, Calif.), Lee Brothers Best Herb Company (Los Angeles and San Bernardino, Calif.), Ipp Hong Lin (Los Angeles), Dr. Wing's Herbs (Los Angeles), Nature's Herb Company (San Francisco), and Wong's Herbalik (Bend, Ore.; San Francisco; and Twin Falls, Idaho). Advertisement, *Los Angeles Times*, September 17, 1939; November 11, 1946; December 2, 1946; September 26, 1948; July 10, 1949; Advertisement, *Twin Falls [Idaho] News*, July 25, 1940.

13. Devitt, "The Curious Case of Ah Fong Chuck," 10.

14. Larson, *Sweet Bamboo*, 167.

15. "California, Death Index, 1940–1997," ancestry.com.

16. Liu, *The Transnational History of a Chinese Family.*

17. Barlow and Richardson, *China Doctor of John Day,* 90.

18. Wing, Greenlee, and Chin, *Son of South Mountain and Dust,* 136.

19. Pomona, City Directory, 1959, p. 132, in "U.S. City Directories, 1822–1995," ancestry.com.

20. Larson, *Sweet Bamboo*, 167.

21. Ibid., 174.

22. Anna Don, interview with author, October 12, 2013.

23. Liu, "The Resilience of Ethnic Culture," 187.

24. Devitt, "The Curious Case of Ah Fong Chuck," 61; Buell, *Chinese Medicine on the Golden Mountain,* 76.

25. *Los Angeles City Directory* (Los Angeles: Los Angeles Directory Company, 1942), 2769; *Los Angeles City Directory* (Los Angeles: Western Directory, 1948), 26–29.

26. Lui, *Inside Los Angeles Chinatown,* 204.

27. "San Francisco City Directories Online," https://sfpl.org/?pg=2000540401.

28. Lui, *Inside Los Angeles Chinatown,* 204.

29. Beverly Chan, interview with Arthur W. Chung, October 23, 25, 1979, Southern California Chinese American Oral History Project.

30. "About New York: Snakes and Wildcats Now Available in the City for Chinese Elders," *New York Times,* June 22, 1953.

31. Lui, *Inside Los Angeles Chinatown,* 204.

32. Barlow and Richardson, *China Doctor of John Day,* 94.

33. By then Wah's wife had passed away and his children were grown up, so he decided to move himself and his uncle to Portland. Sarvis, "Gifted Healer Ing Hay and the Chinese Medical Tradition in Eastern Oregon," 69; Barlow and Richardson, *China Doctor of John Day,* 93.

34. Photo of raid, ca. 1950s, Fang Family San Francisco Examiner Photograph Archive Negative Files, ca. 1930–2000, box 1267, BANC PIC 2006.029—NEG, codes: 135479–135494, Bancroft Library, University of California, Berkeley.

35. "10 Hunted by U.S. in Herb Smuggling," *New York Times,* August 4, 1959.

36. Lui, *Inside Los Angeles Chinatown,* 204.

37. Advertisement, *Los Angeles Times,* December 2, 1946.

38. See, for example, Barnes, "Multiple Meanings of Chinese Healing in the United States"; Buell, *Chinese Medicine on the Golden Mountain;* Barnes, "The Psychologizing of Chinese Healing Practices in the United States"; and Heffner, "Exploring Health-Care Practices of Chinese Railroad Workers in North America."

39. Advertisement, *Los Angeles Times,* April 18, 1943.

40. T. B. Chew, interview with Suellen Cheng, January 5, November 8, 1979, Southern California Chinese American Oral History Project.

41. Ibid.

42. U.S. Census, 1940, Los Angeles, California, reel T627.

43. "Herbalist Indicted for Tax Evasion," *Los Angeles Times,* February 18, 1944.

44. Advertisement, *Los Angeles Times,* July 10, 1949.

45. Ed Fishbein, "Chinese Herb Medicine: U.S. Doctors Wary," *Los Angeles Times,* November 9, 1972.

46. John E. Lesch, *The First Miracle Drugs: How the Sulfa Drugs Transformed Medicine* (Oxford: Oxford University Press, 2007), 5.

47. Chapters 2 and 4 of Swann's *Academic Scientists and the Pharmaceutical Industry* provide a succinct overview of collaborative pharmacological research among university scientists and corporations from the 1920s to 1940s. Chapter 4 of Harry M. Marks's *The Progress of Experiment* speaks to the major role that federal agencies, including the U.S. military, played in supporting and advancing biomedical research in the mid-twentieth century. John Lesch's *The First Miracle Drugs* traces the rise of sulfa drug research in Germany and the United States, and locates the origins of this "therapeutic revolution" in the buildup of chemical industries in the late nineteenth century and the exigencies of global war during the first half of the twentieth century. John Patrick Swann, *Academic Scientists and the Pharmaceutical Industry: Cooperative Research in Twentieth-Century America* (Baltimore: Johns Hopkins University Press, 1988); Harry M. Marks, *The Progress of Experiment: Science and Therapeutic Reform in the United States, 1900–1990* (Cambridge: Cambridge University Press, 1997); Lesch, *The First Miracle Drugs.*

48. David S. Jones and Nicholas L. Tilney both discuss the connections among mobilization for war, mid-twentieth-century drug discoveries, and the advances in cardiology and cardio-thoracic surgery. For a global perspective on transplant surgery and its relationship to military medicine, see David Hamilton, Clyde F. Barker, and Thomas E. Starzl's *A History of Organ Transplantation*. David S. Jones, *Broken Hearts: The Tangled History of Cardiac Care* (Baltimore: Johns Hopkins University Press, 2013); Nicholas L. Tilney, *Invasion of the Body: Revolutions in Surgery* (Cambridge, Mass.: Harvard University Press, 2011); David Hamilton, Clyde F. Barker, and Thomas E. Starzl, *A History of Organ Transplantation: Ancient Legends to Modern Practice* (Pittsburgh: University of Pittsburgh Press, 2012).

49. Andrews, *The Making of Modern Chinese Medicine,* 83; Scheid, *Currents of Tradition in Chinese Medicine,* 205–206.

50. Scheid, *Currents of Tradition in Chinese Medicine,* 199–200.

51. See Andrews, *The Making of Modern Chinese Medicine,* chap. 5.

52. Ibid., 154–155.

53. Volker Scheid offers a biographical portrait of the different strains of medical reforms during the Republican period. See Scheid, *Currents of Tradition in Chinese Medicine,* 208–219.

54. Ibid., 207–208.

55. Risse, *Plague, Fear, and Politics in San Francisco's Chinatown,* 56.

56. Boyd and Ming, *The Chinese of Kern County,* 172.

57. *Chung Sai Yat Po,* August 16, 1900; January 23, 1901, http://oac.cdlib.org/items/ ark:/13030/kt0g5016h6.

58. *Chung Sai Yat Po,* January 9, 1904, http://oac.cdlib.org/items/ark:/13030/ kt0g5016h6.

59. *Chung Sai Yat Po,* December 9, 1901, http://oac.cdlib.org/items/ark:/13030/ kt0g5016h6.

60. Sun, "San Francisco's *Chung Sai Yat Po,*" 86.

61. Alvin Yiu-Cheong So, "Ethnic Doctors in Los Angeles Chinatown," *Journal of Ethnic Studies* 11, no. 4 (Winter 1984): 80.

62. Ibid., 76–77.

63. Chun-Wai Chan and Jade K. Chang, "The Role of Chinese Medicine in New York City's Chinatown," *American Journal of Chinese Medicine* 4, no. 1 (1976): 129.

64. Franklin D. Roosevelt, "Statement on Signing the Bill to Repeal the Chinese Exclusion Laws," December 17, 1943, in Gerhard Peters and John T. Woolley, The American Presidency Project, http://www.presidency.ucsb.edu/ws/?pid=16354.

65. "Americans All," *Ladies' Home Journal,* December 1943, 104–105.

66. Ibid.

67. Hsu, *The Good Immigrants,* 109–111; Erika Lee, *The Making of Asian America: A History* (New York: Simon and Schuster, 2015), 269–270.

68. Hsu, *The Good Immigrants,* 107–112.

69. Lui, *Inside Los Angeles Chinatown,* 204–205.

70. Hsu, *The Good Immigrants,* 126.

71. Eram Alam, "Cold War Crises: Foreign Medical Graduates Respond to US Doctor Shortages, 1965–1975," *Social History of Medicine* (March 8, 2018): 1–20.

72. Hsu, *The Good Immigrants,* 200.

73. As Ellen D. Wu notes, income parity between comparably educated whites and Asians remained elusive. Wu, *The Color of Success,* 147.

74. Lee, *The Making of Asian America,* 374.

75. The matriculation rates of Chinese Americans in this period are not available for the University of California, San Francisco. At Stanford School of Medicine, it seems that most Chinese Americans who enrolled did graduate. Out of a sample of sixty-four between 1928 and 1978, only seven did not graduate. At least one of the seven transferred to the University of California, San Francisco—the late Edmund Jung, related to me by marriage. Jung's father was an herbalist in Visalia, California.

76. Wing, Greenlee, and Chin, *Son of South Mountain and Dust,* 134.

77. Calvin Fong, interview with author, November 30, 2017.

78. Beverly Chan, interview with Arthur W. Chung, October 23, 25, 1979, Southern California Chinese American Oral History Project.

79. Bernice Sam, interview with Paul Tom, April 28, May 21, 1980, Southern California Chinese American Oral History Project.

80. Wu, *Doctor Mom Chung of the Fair-Haired Bastards,* 82.

81. Ibid., 97–99.

82. Quock, *Chinese Hospital Medical Staff Archives,* 25.

83. Ibid., 63.

84. Chinese American Medical Society, constitution and bylaws, November 7, 2015, http://chineseamericanmedicalsociety.cloverpad.org/resources/Documents/CAMS%20ByLaws%20Amendments%202015%20Approved%2011–7-2015.pdf.

85. *CAMS at 40: 1963–2000: A History of the Chinese American Medical Society,* ed. John K. Li (New York: Chinese American Medical Society, 2003), 6, http://chineseamericanmedicalsociety.cloverpad.org/Resources/Documents/CAMS%20at%2040.pdf.

86. See, for example, Rockville Health Services Administration, Bureau of Community Health Services, *Home Health in Chinatown* (Washington, D.C.: Superintendent of Documents, Government Printing Office, 1973); P. R. Murphy, "Tuberculosis Control in San Francisco's Chinatown," *American Journal of Nursing* 70, no. 5 (1970): 1044–1046; and Stuart H. Cattell and Community Service Society of New York, Department of Public Affairs, *Health, Welfare, and Social Organization in Chinatown, New York City: A Report Prepared for the Chinatown Public Health Nursing Demonstration of the Department of Public Affairs, Community Service Society of New York* (New York: Community Service Society of New York, 1962).

87. Elaine Shiang and Frederick P. Li, "The Yin-Yang (Cold-Hot) Theory of Disease," *Journal of the American Medical Association* 217, no. 8 (August 23, 1971): 1108.

SEVEN Rediscovery

1. Yale University sociologist Paul Root Wolpe was the first academic to consider the "sudden, large-scale importation of acupuncture into the United States" with his 1984 article in *Social Problems.* Since then, medical anthropologists like Hans A. Baer, Linda L. Barnes, and Mei Zhan have chronicled the related processes of "acculturation" and professionalization of acupuncture in the United States. Historian James C. Whorton devotes a chapter of his book *Nature Cures* to acupuncture in the context of a "holistic health explosion" that took place in the 1970s. Each of these texts identifies Reston's appendectomy as a major contingent event in America's "rediscovery" of acupuncture and Chinese medicine more broadly. None of these scholars embeds their analysis of this moment in a continuous history of Chinese medicine in the United States. They therefore fail to notice the labor that Chinese doctors did to make rediscovery possible. Paul Root Wolpe, "The Maintenance of Professional Authority: Acupuncture and the American Physician," *Social Problems* 32, no. 5 (1985): 409–424; Baer, *Biomedicine and Alternative Healing Systems in America,* 94; Barnes, "The Acupuncture Wars," 261–301; Barnes, "The Psychologizing of Chinese Healing Practices in the United States," 413–443; Zhan, *Other-Worldly;* Whorton, *Nature Cures,* 257.

2. Robert Dallek, *Nixon and Kissinger: Partners in Power* (New York: HarperCollins, 2007), 296.

3. "Reston 3d Times Writer Given a Visa by Peking," *New York Times,* May 22, 1971.

4. James Reston, "Now, About My Operation in Peking," *New York Times,* July 26, 1971, http://www.nytimes.com/1971/07/26/archives/now-about-my-operation -in-peking-now-let-me-tell-you-about-my.html?_r=0.

5. Andrews, *The Making of Modern Chinese Medicine,* 200–205.

6. Hinrichs and Barnes, *Chinese Medicine and Healing,* 246–247.

7. Ibid., 250–252.

8. Reston, "Now, About My Operation in Peking."

9. Hinrichs and Barnes, *Chinese Medicine and Healing,* 234.

10. "A Matter of Fact," *New York Times,* March 16, 1947.

11. For example, Henry R. Lieberman, "Peiping Promotes Old Herb Therapy," *New York Times,* November 14, 1954.

12. "Herbs, Leaves, and Eel's Blood Fill Medicine Gap in Red China," *New York Times,* March 20, 1966.

13. P. K. Padmanabhan, "Red China Fails to Curb Herb Doctors," *Los Angeles Times,* June 10, 1959.

14. "Herbs, Leaves, and Eel's Blood Fill Medicine Gap in Red China," *New York Times,* March 20, 1966.

15. Lieberman, "Peiping Promotes Old Herb Therapy."

16. Peggy Durdin, "Medicine in China: A Revealing Story," *New York Times,* February 28, 1960.

17. Medical anthropologists and historians of medicine in China have debated to what extent Maoist reforms to medical education and research invented a new form of Traditional Chinese Medicine that coexisted with ancient therapies and modern biomedicine. Scheid, "Remodeling the Arsenal of Chinese Medicine," 136–159; E. I. Karchmer, "Chinese Medicine in Action: On the Postcoloniality of Medical Practice in China," *Medical Anthropology* 29, no. 3 (2010): 226–252; Kim Taylor, *Chinese Medicine in Early Communist China, 1945–63: A Medicine of Revolution* (London: Routledge Curzon, 2005).

18. Lieberman, "Peiping Promotes Old Herb Therapy"; E. Gray Dimond, "Medical Education and Care in People's Republic of China," *Journal of the American Medical Association* 218, no. 10 (December 1971): 1552–1557; E. Gray Dimond, "Acupuncture Anesthesia, Western Medicine, and Chinese Traditional Medicine," *Journal of the American Medical Association* 218, no. 10 (December 1971): 1558–1563; "Acupuncture Free, Common in China," *Los Angeles Times,* June 4, 1971; "Chinese Treat Mental Ills with Acupuncture," *Los Angeles Times,* December 16, 1971.

19. *Chinese Medical Journal,* http://www.cmj.org/aboutus.asp; Lu and Needham, *Celestial Lancets,* 347–381.

20. Hinrichs and Barnes, *Chinese Medicine and Healing,* 304–307; E. Grey Dimond, *More Than Herbs and Acupuncture* (New York: Norton, 1975), 116.

21. For an extensive discussion of the premodern transmission of Chinese acupuncture and moxibustion to Japan, see Lu and Needham, *Celestial Lancets.*

22. See, for example, "The Growth of Medical Science," *Sacramento Daily Union,* October 1, 1881; "Acupuncture for Cholera," *Sausalito [Calif.] News,* March 19,

1885; "Cholera in Japan," *Daily Alta California,* November 23, 1890; and "Acupuncture," *New York Times,* June 12, 1887.

23. Lu and Needham, *Celestial Lancets,* 301–302.

24. Ibid., 199.

25. T. Nakayama and G. Soulié de Morant, *Acupuncture et médecine chinoise: Vérfiées au Japon* (Paris: Éditions Hippocrate, 1934).

26. C. Flandin, P. Ferreyrolles, and H. Khoubesserian, "Traitement de la maladie de dupuytren et des rétractions tendineuses par l'acupuncture," *Bulletins et mémoires de La Société Médicale des Hopitaux de Paris* 66, nos. 19–20 (1950): 963; C. Flandin, P. Ferreyrolles, and H. Khoubesserian, "Une observation d'acupuncture paraissant vérifier la thèse chinoise de la circulation d'énergie suivant des méridiens," *Bulletins et mémoires de La Société Médicale des Hopitaux de Paris* 66, nos. 19–20 (1950): 965–967; C. Flandin, P. Ferreyrolles, and H. Khoubesserian, "Traitement des chéloïdes par l'acupunture," *Bulletins et mémoires de La Société Médicale des Hopitaux de Paris* 66, nos. 19–20 (1950): 964; C. Flandin et al., *Traitement des algies par l'acupuncture chinoise, par MM. Ch. Flandin, Ferreyrolles et A. Macé de Lépinay* (Clermont-Fd, France: Impr. de G. Mont-Louis, 1933); Paul Ferreyrolles and Charles Flandin, *Dr Paul Ferreyrolles. L'Acupuncture chinoise: Thérapeutique énergétique* (Lille, France: Éditions S.L.E.L., 1951); Paul Ferreyrolles and Charles Flandin, *L'Acupuncture chinoise: Thérapeutique énergétique* (Lille, France: Éditions S.L.E.L, 1951).

27. Ilza Veith, "A Note on Acupuncture," *Proceedings of the Institute of Medicine of Chicago* 18, no. 16 (October 1951): 365–356.

28. Franz Hubotter, "La médecine chinoise au cours des siècles: Pierre Huard, Ming Wong," *Isis* 52, no. 4 (1961): 601–602; Pierre Huard, Zensetson Ohya, and Ming Wong, "La Médecine japonaise des origines à nos jours," *Medical History* 20, no. 1 (1976): 89–90. For a full list of Huard's publications on East Asian medicine, see http://www.gera.fr/modules.php?name=Downloads&d_op=viewdownload&cid=4907.

29. R. De La Fuye and R. Faure, "Observations et communications: Deux ans d'acupuncture au Val-De-Grâce (statistiques)," *Bulletin Mensuel* 51, no. 4 (1957): 152–153.

30. Ilza Veith, "Acupuncture Therapy—Past and Present, Verity or Delusion," *Journal of the American Medical Association* 180 (June 17, 1962): 136; "Medicine: Quick, the Needle!" *Time Magazine,* July 2, 1952, http://content.time.com/time/subscriber/article/0,33009,857242,00.html.

31. Howard A. Rusk, "Old Chinese Medicine," *New York Times,* July 23, 1967.

32. See, for example, G. Bachmann, "Acupuncture: Indication and Technique," *Hippokrates* 22, no. 13 (1951): 360–363; G. Bachmann, "Acupuncture and Its Effect on M. Curry's Reaction Depositions," *Hippokrates* 23, no. 23 (December 15, 1952): 664–665; J. H. Bennett, "Acupuncture and Moxibustion," *Journal of the College of General Practitioners* 13, no. 2 (March 1967): 251–253; M. Finlay, "Acupuncture," *Manchester Medical Gazette* 49, no. 4 (July 1970): 11–13; W. Rott, "Acupuncture in Clinical Therapy," *Acta Neurovegetativa* 1, no. 5 (1950): 518–529; R. Wachsmuth, "The Acupuncture," *Medizinische Klinik* 48, no. 31 (July 31, 1953): 1123–1124; and H.

Schmidt, "Fundamentals in Acupuncture," *Hippokrates* 22, no. 17 (September 15, 1951): 475–478.

33. Thomas Ots, "50 Jahre Deustche Zeitschrift für Akupunktur—Das Forum der Auseinandersetzung," *Deustche Zeitschrift für Akupunktur* 45, no. 4 (December 2002): 274–279.

34. R. Bivins, "The Needle and the Lancet: Acupuncture in Britain, 1683–2000," *Acupuncture in Medicine: Journal of the British Medical Acupuncture Society* 19, no. 1 (2001): 12.

35. K. K. Chen and Carl F. Schmidt, "The Action of Ephedrine, the Active Principle of the Chinese Drug *Ma Huang*," *Journal of Pharmacology and Experimental Therapeutics* 24, no. 5 (December 1924): 339–357; K. K. Chen et al., *Pharmacology of Oriental Plants* (Oxford: Pergamom Press, 1965).

36. James H. Madison, *Eli Lilly, a Life, 1885–1977* (Indianapolis: Indiana Historical Society, 1989), 66–67.

37. Michael Goldstein, "The Emerging Socioeconomic and Political Support for Alternative Medicine in the United States," *Annals of the American Academy of Political and Social Science* 583, no. 1 (September 2002): 52; Chan and Lee, *The Way Forward for Chinese Medicine,* 355.

38. Albert Fields, "Physiotherapy in Ancient Chinese Medicine," *American Journal of Surgery* 79, no. 4 (April 1950): 613–616; Albert Fields, "Medical Officer in China," *Military Surgeon* 103, no. 299 (October 1948): 299–304; China Society of Sothern California Collection, University of Southern California, http://digitallibrary.usc.edu/cdm/search/searchterm/China%20Society%20of%20Southern%20California%20Collection/field/relatig/mode/exact/page/1.

39. Albert Fields, "Yin and Yang in Ancient Chinese Medicine," *Western Journal of Surgery, Obstetrics, and Gynecology* 59, no. 1 (1951): viii.

40. Albert Fields, "The Pulse in Ancient Chinese Medicine," *California Medicine* 66, no. 5 (May 1947): 305.

41. William W. Cadbury, "Medicine as Practised by the Chinese," *Medical Record* 90 (August 26, 1916): 364–367.

42. Jerome D. Waye, "From the Little Toe to the Root of the Tongue: A Short Account of Chinese Medicine," *Boston Medical Quarterly* 2, no. 2 (June 1958): 52.

43. Veith, "Acupuncture Therapy," 139.

44. John Saar, "A Visit to the Friendly Neighborhood Sorcerer," *Life,* August 13, 1971, 34–35.

45. C. Robert Jennings, "The Needle Epidemic," *Los Angeles Times,* October 1, 1972.

46. "Acupuncture: Myth or Miracle," *Newsweek,* August 14, 1972, 48–52.

47. "All About Acupuncture," *Newsweek,* August 14, 1972, 49.

48. "Nation's First Acupuncture Clinic Slated," *Los Angeles Times,* July 6, 1972; "First Acupuncture Clinic Shut," *Los Angeles Times,* July 20, 1972.

49. "Quick, Nagayama, the Needle," *Sports Illustrated,* June 5, 1972, https://www.si.com/vault/1972/06/05/612876/quick-nagayama-the-needle; "Acupuncture: Myth or Miracle," 49; Wolpe, "The Maintenance of Professional Authority," 412.

50. Wolpe, "The Maintenance of Professional Authority," 410–411; Barbara J. Culliton, "Acupuncture: Fertile Ground for Faddists and Serious NIH Research," *Science* 177, no. 4049 (1972): 592.

51. Lillian Africano, "Acupuncture: Child of the Media," *The Nation*, May 31, 1975, 657.

52. "NBC Obtains Acupuncture Surgery Film," *Los Angeles Times*, July 4, 1972; "A Nation of Human Pincushions," *The Bold Ones: The New Doctors*, aired October 3, 1972, http://www.imdb.com/title/tt0528597/; Cecil Smith, "Glancing Back at TV Happenings," *Los Angeles Times*, January 1, 1973.

53. *Golden Needles*, 1974, http://www.imdb.com/title/tt0071568/.

54. Advertisement, *New York Amsterdam News*, April 25, 1981.

55. Tomes, *Remaking the American Patient*, 159.

56. Ibid., 182.

57. Ibid., 221; Rock Brynner and Trent D. Stephens, *Dark Remedy: The Impact of Thalidomide and Its Revival as a Vital Medicine* (New York: Basic Books, 2001), 103–104.

58. Starr, *The Social Transformation of American Medicine*, 336.

59. James C. Whorton partially attributes the rise of a 1970s holistic medicine movement as a response to "exasperating" levels of specialization among biomedical doctors. Whorton, *Nature Cures*, 248–249, 253.

60. Some examples of companies offering such a range of services at this time include T. B. Chew (Los Angeles, Calif.), Dr. G. S. Wong (Huntington Park, Calif.), and Dr. Chan (Los Angeles, Calif.). Advertisements, *Los Angeles Times*, April 25, 1943; February 17, 1947; December 5, 1948.

61. Stefanie Syman, *The Subtle Body: The Story of Yoga in America* (New York: Farrar, Straus and Giroux, 2010), 235; June S. Lowenberg, *Caring and Responsibility: The Crossroads between Holistic Practice and Traditional Medicine* (Philadelphia: University of Pennsylvania Press, 1989), 66–78; Baer, *Biomedicine and Alternative Healing Systems in America*, 98–99; Anne Harrington, *The Cure Within: A History of Mind-Body Medicine* (New York: Norton, 2009), 213–222; Jane Naomi Iwamura, *Virtual Orientalism: Asian Religions in American Popular Culture* (New York: Oxford University Press, 2011), chaps. 2–3.

62. Joy James, *Imprisoned Intellectuals: America's Political Prisoners Write on Life, Liberation, and Rebellion* (Lanham, Md.: Rowman and Littlefield, 2003), 193.

63. Christopher Sellers provides an excellent discussion of the links among naturalism, surburbanization, and the emergence of modern environmentalism in mid-twentieth-century California. Christopher Sellers, *Crabgrass Crucible: Suburban Nature and the Rise of Environmentalism in Twentieth-Century America.* (Chapel Hill: University of North Carolina Press, 2012), 80–82.

64. Li and Luo, *Compendium of Materia Medica*.

65. Whorton, *Nature Cures*, 425–426; Lowenberg, *Caring and Responsibility*, 18.

66. Steven Rosenblatt and Keith Kirts, *The Birth of Acupuncture in America: The White Crane's Gift* (Bloomington, Ind.: Balboa Press, 2016), 17; Harrington, *The Cure Within*, 222–224.

67. Africano, "Acupuncture: Child of the Media," 659.

68. "All About Acupuncture," 49.

69. Jennings, "The Needle Epidemic."

70. Whorton, *Nature Cures*, 463.

71. Jennings, "The Needle Epidemic."

72. "SF Man Held on Violation of Acupuncture Law," *Los Angeles Times*, December 17, 1972.

73. Emily S. Wu, "History of Traditional Chinese Medicine in California," in *Chinese America: History and Perspectives*, ed. Chinese Historical Society of America (San Francisco: Chinese Historical Society of America, 2012), 11–12.

74. Miriam Lee, *Insights of a Senior Acupuncturist: One Combination of Points Can Treat Many Diseases* (Boulder, Col.: Blue Poppy Press, 1992), ix.

75. "Prominent Palo Alto Acupuncturist Dies," *The Argus* (Fremont, Calif.), July 1, 2009.

76. Lee, *Insights of a Senior Acupuncturist*, x.

77. Narda Z. Trout, "Woman Doctor Faces Charges over Practice of Acupuncture," *Los Angeles Times*, July 27, 1973.

78. Lee, *Insights of a Senior Acupuncturist*, x.

79. Susan Johnson, "In Memorium: Doctor Miriam Lee (1926–2009)," *Acupuncture Today*, September 2009, http://www.acupuncturetoday.com/mpacms/at/article.php?id=32021.

80. Fishbein, "Chinese Herb Medicine."

81. "All About Acupuncture," 49.

82. Jennings, "The Needle Epidemic"; Dorothy Townsend, "Chinese Acupuncture Shown: Volunteers Get the Needle—Onlookers See the Point," *Los Angeles Times*, January 28, 1972; Culliton, "Acupuncture," 592.

83. Barnes, "The Acupuncture Wars," 265; Laurel Kao Skurko, "Legalizing Acupuncture in California—The Story of a Suffragette," Healthy.net, http://www.healthy.net/Health/Essay/Legalizing_Acupuncture_in_California/50/2; "About J. R. Worsley and Worsley Five-Element Acupuncture," Cambridge Health Associates, http://www.cambridgehealthassociates.com/bill-and-jim/worsley.

84. Jean Harrison Osgrod, "Regulating the Practice of Acupuncture: Recent Developments in California," *University of California, Davis Law Review* 7 (1973): 398; *1970 United States Census—Subject Reports: Japanese, Chinese, and Filipinos in the United States* (Washington, D.C.: Government Printing Office, July 1973), 60, https://www2.census.gov/library/publications/decennial/1970/pc-2-1g/42043783v2p1d1gch5.pdf.

85. Osgrod, "Regulating the Practice of Acupuncture," 398.

86. "Acupuncturist Faces N.Y. Licensing Charges," *Los Angeles Times*, November 29, 1972; "First U.S. Acupuncture Clinic Shut," *Los Angeles Times*, July 20, 1972.

87. Osgrod, "Regulating the Practice of Acupuncture," 396–398.

88. Lee, *Insights of a Senior Acupuncturist,* xi.

89. Ginger McRae, "A Critical Overview of U.S. Acupuncture Regulation," *Journal of Health Politics, Policy, and Law* 7, no. 1 (Spring 1982): 179.

90. Ibid., 173.

91. "Clinic Established for Acupuncture," *Los Angeles Times,* December 7, 1972.

92. Myrna Oliver, "Doctor, 2 Patients Go to Court: Suit Seeks Lifting of Limits on Acupuncture," *Los Angeles Times,* November 29, 1973.

93. Steve Emmons, "Acupuncture Clinic Will Open," *Los Angeles Times,* September 27, 1973.

94. "Riverside Gets Acupuncture Clinic," *Los Angeles Times,* May 1, 1973; Emmons, "Acupuncture Clinic Will Open."

95. Morton W. Barke, interview with author, June 15, 2017.

96. Myrna Oliver, "Suit Challenges Law Limiting Availability of Acupuncture," *Los Angeles Times,* November 29, 1973.

97. Myrna Oliver, "Pact Ends Acupuncture Suit," *Los Angeles Times,* November 30, 1973.

98. Morton W. Barke, interview with author, June 15, 2017.

99. Sue Fawn Chung, *The Chinese in Nevada* (Charleston, S.C.: Arcadia, 2011), 96–98. In 1970, the U.S. Census recorded 966 people of Chinese descent living in Nevada, which ranked the state thirty-first in size of Chinese population. *1970 United States Census—Subject Reports: Japanese, Chinese, and Filipinos in the United States,* 60.

100. Anton P. Sohn and Robert M. Daugherty, *150 Years of Nevada Medicine (and More): Nevada's Men and Women Healers* (Reno, Nev.: Greasewood Press, 2014), 27–28.

101. Richard G. Pugh, *Serving Medicine: The Nevada State Medical Association and the Politics of Medicine* (Reno, Nev.: Greasewood Press, 2002), 65.

102. Shaun McKinnon, "Acupuncture Backer Arthur Steinberg Dies," *Las Vegas Review-Journal,* October 18, 1994, http://ccl.idm.oclc.org/login?url=http://search.proquest.com/docview/259939983?accountid=10141; Wu, *Traditional Chinese Medicine in the United States,* 31.

103. "Nevada to Allow Acupuncture," *Los Angeles Times,* April 21, 1973.

104. "Acupuncture in Nevada," *Time Magazine,* April 23, 1973, 16.

105. G. G. L., "The Two-Armed Bandit," *Journal of the American Medical Association* 225, no. 3 (1973): 297.

106. Nevada Assembly Concurrent Resolution no. 9, May 2, 2011, https://www.leg.state.nv.us/Session/76th2011/Bills/ACR/ACR9.pdf.

107. Eleanor Hoover, "When the Stars Tense Up, It's Acupuncturist Zion Yu Who Keeps Hollywood on Pins and Needles," *People Magazine,* November 14, 1983, http://people.com/archive/when-the-stars-tense-up-its-acupuncturist-zion-yu-who-keeps-hollywood-on-pins-and-needles-vol-20-no-20/.

108. Skurko, "Legalizing Acupuncture in California."

109. Pedro Chan, *Acupuncture, Electro-Acupuncture, Anaesthesia: A Small Needle Works Wonders* (Alhambra, Calif.: Borden, 1972), iv.

110. Pedro Chan, *Wonders of Chinese Acupuncture* (Alhambra, Calif.: Borden, 1973), ix–xi; Pedro Chan, *Finger Acupressure: Treatment for Many Common Ailments from Migraine to Insomnia by Using Finger Massage on Acupuncture Points* (Los Angeles: Price/Stern/Sloan, 1974).

111. Critically, the new legislation took a capacious approach to defining the practice it regulated. It focused on the needle therapy but also encompassed "Asian medicine," "Oriental medicine," and "Chinese medicine." "Brown Has Big Campaign Pot," *Desert Sun* (Palm Springs, Calif.), October 14, 1974; "The State: Brown Signs Bill Expanding Acupuncture," *Los Angeles Times,* July 15, 1975; National Policy Group, "Acupuncture State Law Summary," 2014, http://theacupunctureobserver.com/wp-content/uploads/2014/02/State+Law+Summary.pdf.

112. Baolin Wu, "National Healthcare Plan—From Aristocracy to Welfare—A Letter to President Obama," address, Tenth World Congress of Chinese Medicine, San Francisco, 2013, http://www.drbaolinwu.com/about_dr_wu.htm.

113. "Acupuncture Board History," California Department of Consumer Affairs, http://www.acupuncture.ca.gov/about_us/history.shtml.

114. McRae, "A Critical Overview of U.S. Acupuncture Regulation," 169.

115. As of 2014, nearly all states and the District of Columbia have recognized acupuncture and other traditional Chinese therapies as a practice of medicine and regulated them by statute. The exceptions are Alabama, where acupuncture is classified as an experimental procedure only, and Oklahoma, the Dakotas, and Wyoming, which do not regulate acupuncture or other traditional Chinese therapies by statute. National Policy Group, "Acupuncture State Law Summary."

116. In 1980, forty-six plaintiffs sued the Texas State Board of Medical Examiners for limiting their access to acupuncture. The board had broadly prohibited the practice of acupuncture by nonlicensed physicians since 1974, and the plaintiffs argued this policy violated their freedom to "obtain or reject medical treatment" encompassed by a privacy right. The court agreed. In *Andrews v. Ballard,* the U.S. District Court found that the board had overstepped its compelling interest in protecting public health when it restricted practitioners of Chinese medicine and made it effectively impossible for Texans to locate their services within the state. Testimony by desperate patients failed by Western-style biomedical science seemed to sway the sympathies of the court, and the defendants could offer no proof that they had consulted with experts in the field of traditional Chinese medicine before deeming it a merely "experimental" procedure. *Jack Andrews et. al., Plaintiffs, v. L. G. Ballard, D.O., et. al, Defendants,* United States District Court, S.D. Texas, Houston Division, July 9, 1980.

117. Advertisement, *Los Angeles Times,* April 18, 1978; *Los Angeles Times,* March 25, September 22, 1983.

118. Chan and Lee, *The Way Forward for Chinese Medicine,* 358.

119. National Policy Group, "Acupuncture State Law Summary."

120. Advertisement, *Los Angeles Times,* October 24, 1982.

121. Advertisement, *Los Angeles Times,* September 22, 1983.

122. Advertisement, *New York Times,* October 27, 1985.

123. Advertisement, *Los Angeles Times,* February 15, 1980.

124. Advertisement, *Los Angeles Times,* October 30, 1983.

125. Advertisement, *Los Angeles Times,* July 22, 1980.

126. Advertisement, *Call and Post* (Cleveland), September 13, 1984.

127. Advertisement, *Los Angeles Times,* June 21, 1979.

128. Morton W. Barke, interview with author, June 15, 2017.

129. Advertisement, *Los Angeles Times,* April 18, 1974.

130. Chan, *Acupuncture, Electro-Acupuncture, Anaesthesia,* iv.

131. Advertisement, *Los Angeles Times,* September 7, 1975.

Epilogue

1. Diploma, University of California, San Francisco, 1910, Ka-Kit Hui personal collection; Ka-Kit Hui, interviews with author, October 17, 2016; June 20, 2018.

2. Ibid.

3. Ka-Kit Hui, interview with author, October 17, 2016.

4. David M. Eisenberg et al., "Unconventional Medicine in the United States—Prevalence, Costs, and Patterns of Use," *New England Journal of Medicine* 328, no. 4 (1993): 246–252.

5. UCLA Center for East-West Medicine, https://cewm.med.ucla.edu/about/center-history/.

6. Ka-Kit Hui, interview with author, October 17, 2016; Ka-Kit Hui, "Integrative Medicine, a New Model for the World," *China Today* 54, no. 2 (2005): 34; Ka-Kit Hui, "The Potential for Incorporating Traditional Medicine into Clinical Practice," address, WHO International Symposium, Awaji Island, Hyogo Prefecture, Japan, September 11–13, 2000.

7. Reston, "Now, About My Operation in Peking."

8. Edgar Snow, "Report from China—III: Population Care and Control," *New Republic,* May 1, 1971, 20–21.

9. Dimond, *More Than Herbs and Acupuncture,* 9–13; E. G. Dimond, "Ward Rounds with an Acupuncturist," *New England Journal of Medicine* 272 (1965): 575–577.

10. Jennings Parrott, "Lon Nol Feels Much Better Now—Ouch!" *Los Angeles Times,* June 23, 1971.

11. The People's Republic also invited delegations from France, Italy, Germany, England, and Canada in the same period. Dimond, "Medical Education and Care in People's Republic of China," 1552–1557; Clyde Lanford Smith and Linnea Capps, "An Interview with Dr. Vic Sidel," *Social Medicine* 7, no. 3 (October 2013): 180–181.

12. "Nixon Doctor Says Acupuncture Is 'Very Superior' to Anesthesia," *Los Angeles Times,* April 12, 1972.

13. Dan Bensky, Andrew Gamble, and Ted J. Kaptchuk, *Chinese Herbal Medicine: Materia Medica* (Seattle: Eastland Press, 1986); Kaptchuk, *The Web That Has No Weaver.*

14. Dimond, "Medical Education and Care in People's Republic of China," 1552–1557.

15. Quoted in Wolpe, "The Maintenance of Professional Authority," 413.

16. John J. Bonica, "Acupuncture Anesthesia in the People's Republic of China," *Journal of the American Medical Association* 229, no. 10 (1974): 1549.

17. Wolpe, "The Maintenance of Professional Authority," 414.

18. Lawrence K. Altman, "A.M.A. Delegation Hails Chinese Medical Gains," *New York Times,* August 4, 1974, http://www.nytimes.com/1974/08/04/archives/ama -delegation-hais-chinese-medical-gains-surgeon-is-impressed.html?_r=0.

19. W. C. Liu, "Acupuncture Anesthesia: A Case Report," *Journal of the American Medical Association* 221, no. 1 (July 3, 1972): 87–88; Ronald Kotulak, "Acupuncture Used Here: May Have Been U.S. 1st," *Chicago Tribune,* June 3, 1972, http://archives.chi cagotribune.com/1972/06/03/page/4/article/acupuncture-used-here-may-have-been -u-s-1st.

20. Harry Schwartz, "The Needle Pain-Killer Comes to America," *New York Times,* June 4, 1972; James Y. P. Chen, *Acupuncture Anesthesia in the People's Republic of China* (Washington, D.C.: U.S. Department of Health, Education, and Welfare, Public Health Service, National Institutes of Health, 1973), 5–7.

21. Whorton, *Nature Cures,* 467; Lynda W. Freeman, *Mosby's Complementary and Alternative Medicine: A Research-Based Approach,* 3rd ed. (2000; St. Louis: Mosby Elsevier, 2009), 324–329; E. Ernst, "The Recent History of Acupuncture," *American Journal of Medicine* 121, no. 12 (2008): 1027–1028.

22. Bruce Lambert, "Frederick Kao, 73, Educator Who Led Acupuncture Effort," *New York Times,* July 31, 1992, http://www.nytimes.com/1992/07/31/nyregion/frederick -kao-73-educator-who-led-acupuncture-effort.html; *American Journal of Chinese Medicine* website, http://www.worldscientific.com/page/ajcm/aims-scope.

23. F. F. Kao, "Editorial," *American Journal of Chinese Medicine* 1 (1973): viii.

24. *American Journal of Chinese Medicine,* World Scientific (online database), http://www.worldscientific.com/toc/ajcm/01/02.

25. Devra Lee Davis, "The History and Sociology of the Scientific Study of Acupuncture," *American Journal of Chinese Medicine* 3, no. 1 (1975): 15.

26. K. K. Chen, "Half a Century of Ephedrine," *American Journal of Chinese Medicine* 2, no. 4 (1974): 359–365.

27. Paul Unschuld, "The Development of Medical-Pharmaceutical Thought in China," *American Journal of Chinese Medicine* 5, no. 2 (1977): 109–115; Unschuld, "The Development of Medical-Pharmaceutical Thought in China II," *American Journal of Chinese Medicine* 5, nos. 3–4 (1977): 211–231.

28. Chen would eventually publish case histories on the effects of acupuncture on smoking cessation and analgesia, and he used the research methods he had honed at the laboratory bench to consider the pharmacological action of ginseng. In the 1970s, he

became a licensed practitioner and ran an acupuncture clinic in Santa Monica up until his death in 2012. James Y. P. Chen, "Chinese Health Foods and Health Tonics," *American Journal of Chinese Medicine* 1, no. 2 (1973): 225–247; James Y. P. Chen, "Treatment of Cigarette-Smoking by Auricular Acupuncture—Report of 184 Cases," *American Journal of Acupuncture* 7, no. 3 (1979): 229–234; James Chen, obituary, *Los Angeles Times,* October 10, 2012.

29. James Chen, obituary, *Los Angeles Times,* October 10, 2012.

30. Chen, *Acupuncture Anesthesia in the People's Republic of China,* ix–x; Culliton, "Acupuncture," 592.

31. James Y. P. Chen, "Chinese Health Foods and Herb Tonics," *American Journal of Chinese Medicine* 1, no. 2 (January 1973): 225.

32. Bonica, "Acupuncture Anesthesia in the People's Republic of China," 1550; Lee Davis, "The History and Sociology of the Scientific Study of Acupuncture," 16.

33. Terri A. Winnick, "From Quackery to 'Complementary' Medicine: The American Medical Profession Confronts Alternative Therapies," *Social Problems* 52, no. 1 (February 2005): 53–54; Chan and Lee, *The Way Forward for Chinese Medicine,* 353–354.

34. For these records I searched using the topics "acupuncture" and "Chinese herb*" and limiting the years to 1970 to 2017. I then reviewed the results to determine whether the database returned duplicate or otherwise errant search results. This collection includes eighteen thousand peer-reviewed journals in science, social sciences, and humanities disciplines including the *Journal of the American Medical Association* and the *New England Journal of Medicine.* https://clarivate.libguides.com/webofscienceplatform/woscc.

35. B. Holmstedt, "Historical Perspective and Future of Ethnopharmacology," *Journal of Ethnopharmacology* 32, nos. 1–3 (1991): 7–24.

36. J. Gertsch, "How Scientific Is the Science in Ethnopharmacology? Historical Perspectives and Epistemological Problems," *Journal of Ethnopharmacology* 122, no. 2 (2009): 177.

37. Michael Heinrich and Anna K. Jäger, *Ethnopharmacology* (Chichester, West Sussex, U.K.: Wiley Blackwell, 2015), 7–8.

38. Carol Ferring Shepley, *Movers and Shakers, Scalawags and Suffragettes: Tales from Bellefontaine Cemetery* (St. Louis: Missouri History Museum Press, 2015), 255.

39. "Youyou Tu—Facts," Nobel Prize Committee, https://www.nobelprize.org/nobel_prizes/medicine/laureates/2015/tu-facts.html; P. Ram Manohar, "Nobel Prize, Traditional Chinese Medicine, and Lessons for Ayurveda?" *Ancient Science of Life* 35, no. 2 (October–December 2015): 67–69, https://www.ncbi.nlm.nih.gov/pmc/articles/PMC4728866/#ref1.

40. "Acupuncture," Mayo Clinic, http://www.mayoclinic.org/tests-procedures/acupuncture/basics/why-its-done/prc-20020778; "Acupuncture," Cleveland Clinic, http://my.clevelandclinic.org/services/wellness/integrative-medicine/treatments-services/acupuncture; "Acupuncture and Integrative Chinese Medicine: Find Balance for Well Being," Osher Center for Integrative Medicine, University of California, San

Francisco, http://www.osher.ucsf.edu/patient-care/treatments-services/acupuncture
-and-traditional-chinese-medicine/; "Complementary and Alternative Therapies,"
Mount Sinai Hospital, http://www.mountsinai.org/patient-care/service-areas/pain
-management/pain-management-services/integrative-medicine.

41. Victoria Maizes et al., "The Evolution of Integrative Medical Education and
the Influence of the University of Arizona Center for Integrative Medicine," *Journal of
Integrative Medicine* 13 (November 2015): 356–362.

42. Chiropractic Care and Acupuncture Rider Plan, Anthem Blue Cross, https://www
.cdrewu.edu/sites/default/files/documents/imported/2018%20-%20CDU%20-%20
Anthem%20-%20HMO%20-%20Chiropractic%20and%20Acupuncture%20Rider
.pdf; Combined Chiropractic and Acupuncture Services Amendment of the Kaiser
Foundation Health Plan, Evidence of Coverage for Sample Group Agreement, Kaiser
Permanente, http://info.kaiserpermanente.org/healthplans/plandocuments/california/
pdfs/2016/Small_Business_GF/NCR/2016%20Sample%20NCR%20Small%20
EOC%20Chiro-Acu%2015–20%20visits%20p4001.pdf; Acupuncture Policy, Aetna,
http://www.aetna.com/cpb/medical/data/100_199/0135.html.

43. Goldstein, "The Emerging Socioeconomic and Political Support for Alternative Medicine in the United States," 51.

44. Marks, *The Progress of Experiment,* 132–133.

45. Kaptchuk, *The Web That Has No Weaver,* 360.

46. Freeman, *Mosby's Complementary and Alternative Medicine,* 218–219.

47. Ke-Ji Chen et al., "Complementary/Alternative Medicine in Cardiovascular
Diseases 2014," *Evidence-Based Complementary and Alternative Medicine* 2015 (March
2015): 1–2.

48. Lu and Needham, *Celestial Lancets,* xlviii.

49. Rishma Walji and Heather Boon, "Redefining the Randomized Controlled
Trial in the Context of Acupuncture Research," *Complementary Therapies in Clinical
Practice* 12, no. 2 (2006): 91–96.

50. Florian Junne et al., "Key Issues in Clinical and Epidemiological Research
in Complementary and Alternative Medicine—A Systematic Literature Review,"
Forschende Komplementarmedizin 19, Suppl. no. 2 (2006): 51–60; Y. Veziari, M. J.
Leach, and S. Kumar, "Barriers to the Conduct and Application of Research in Comple-
mentary and Alternative Medicine: A Systematic Review," *BMC Complementary and
Alternative Medicine* 17, no. 1 (2017): 166.

51. Research Portfolio Online Reporting Tools, National Institutes of Health, U.S.
Department of Health and Human Services, https://projectreporter.nih.gov/reporter
_searchresults.cfm.

52. Chan and Lee, *The Way Forward for Chinese Medicine,* 351.

53. Hannah Flesch, "A Foot in Both Worlds: Education and the Transformation of
Chinese Medicine in the United States," *Medical Anthropology* 32, no. 1 (2013): 14.

54. Barnes, "The Acupuncture Wars," 261–301.

55. When Ginger McRae reviewed acupuncture regulation across the United
States in 1982, she argued that it was unlikely that acupuncture could survive in its

"authentic and rigorous form." McRae, "A Critical Overview of U.S. Acupuncture Regulation," 182.

56. Hannah Flesch reiterated that argument in her 2013 study of American schools of Oriental medicine, where she found that biomedicalization reinforces a hierarchy that places biomedicine above Chinese medicine. Wolpe, "The Maintenance of Professional Authority," 416–419; Flesch, "A Foot in Both Worlds," 17.

57. Zhan, *Other-Worldly,* 4.

58. D. P. Lu and G. P. Lu, "An Historical Review and Perspective on the Impact of Acupuncture on U.S. Medicine and Society," *Medical Acupuncture* 25, no. 5 (2013): 311–316; Shamly Austin et al., "Acupuncture Use in the United States: Who, Where, Why, and at What Price?" *Health Marketing Quarterly* 32, no. 2 (2015): 113–128; U.S.–China Trade Facts, Office of the U.S. Trade Representative, https://ustr.gov/countries-regions/china-mongolia-taiwan/peoples-republic-china; U.S. China Economic and Security Review Commission, Annual Report to Congress, 2015, https://www.uscc.gov/Annual_Reports/2015-annual-report.

59. Austin et al., "Acupuncture Use in the United States," 117–120.

60. P. M. Barnes, B. Bloom, and R. Nahin, "Complementary and Alternative Medicine Use among Adults and Children: United States 2007," *CDC National Health Statistics Report no. 12,* December 10, 2008, https://nccih.nih.gov/news/camstats/2007.

61. U.S.–China Trade Facts, Office of the U.S. Trade Representative; "Global Herbal Supplements and Remedies Market 2017—Demand, Insights, Analysis, Opportunities, Segmentation, and Forecast to 2022," MarketsNResearch, November 2017, http://www.marketsnresearch.com/global-herbal-supplements-and-remedies-market-2017-demand.html; "National Business Journal: The U.S. Supplements Industry Is $37 Billion, Not $12 Billion," Nutra Ingredients, June 1, 2015, https://www.nutraingredients-usa.com/Article/2015/06/01/NBJ-The-US-supplement-industry-is-37-billion-not-12-billion.

62. Chan and Lee, *The Way Forward for Chinese Medicine,* 355; Rowena K. Richter, *Herbal Medicine: Chaos in the Marketplace* (New York: Routledge, 2003), 14–29.

63. Goldstein, "The Emerging Socioeconomic and Political Support for Alternative Medicine in the United States," 58.

64. Analysis of Web of Science Core Collection search on the keyword "Chinese herb*" limited by the dates 1970–2017. Therapeutic exercise like qi gong and t'ai chi have also received some attention as interest in complementary and alternative medicine has grown. Guichen Li, Hua Yuan, and Wei Zhang, "Effects of Tai Chi on Health Related Quality of Life in Patients with Chronic Conditions: A Systematic Review of Randomized Controlled Trials," *Complementary Therapies in Medicine* 22, no. 4 (2014): 743–755; Kaptchuk, *The Web That Has No Weaver,* 369–379; Harrington, *The Cure Within,* 222–224.

65. Guo Chengqi, "Traditional Chinese Medicine? 100% Made in Japan," World-Crunch, March 30, 2017, https://www.worldcrunch.com/business-finance/traditional-chinese-medicine-100-made-in-japan.

66. Mary Esch, "Chinese Medicinal Herbs Provide Niche Market for U.S. Farmers," *San Diego Union-Tribune,* December 27, 2015, http://www.sandiegouniontribune .com/sdut-chinese-medicinal-herbs-provide-niche-market-for-2015dec27-story.html.

67. Goldstein, "The Emerging Socioeconomic and Political Support for Alternative Medicine in the United States," 53–54.

68. Taylor, *Ginseng, the Divine Root,* 144–145.

69. Johannsen, *Ginseng Dreams,* 8.

70. C. R. Roberts et al., *Proceedings of the First National Ginseng Conference* (Frankfort, Ky.: Governor's Council on Agriculture, 1979).

71. Johannsen, *Ginseng Dreams,* 149; Donna Leinwand, "States Seek Grip on Wild Ginseng Market," *USA Today,* December 4, 2007.

72. Daniel Wilcox, Nguyen D. T. Minh, and Lalita Gomez, "An Assessment of Trade in Bear Bile and Gall Bladder in Viet Nam," Animals Asia Report, November 2016, https://www.traffic.org/site/assets/files/2342/vn-bears-report.pdf; Uttam Babu Shrestha and Kamaljit S. Bawa, "Trade, Harvest, and Conservation of Caterpillar Fungus (Ophiocordyceps Sinensis) in the Himalayas," *Biological Conservation* 159 (2013): 514–520; Gertsch, "How Scientific Is the Science in Ethnopharmacology?" 177–183.

73. Richard Ellis, *Tiger Bone and Rhino Horn: The Destruction of Wildlife for Traditional Chinese Medicine* (Washington, D.C.: Island Press, 2005); "More Tigers Poached This Year So Far Than in 2015," *The Guardian* (London), April 29, 2016, http:// www.theguardian.com/environment/2016/apr/29/more-tigers-poached-india-so-far -this-year-than-2015; Javier C. Hernández, "China Reverses Ban on Rhino and Tiger Parts in Medicine, Worrying Activists," *New York Times,* October 29, 2018.

74. Jonathan Watts, "Fungus Gold Rush in Tibetan Plateau Rebuilding Lives after Earthquake," *The Guardian,* June 17, 2010, http://www.theguardian.com/environ ment/2010/jun/17/fungus-tibetan-plateau; Schultz, "Demand for Himalayan Viagra Fungus Heats Up, Maybe Too Much"; Yi Luo, "Chinese Medicine's Commercialization and Its Social and Environmental Impact" (2015), CMC Senior Theses, paper 1214, pp. 53–62, http://scholarship.claremont.edu/cmc_theses/1214.

75. Richter, *Herbal Medicine,* 5; Roxanne Nelson, "FDA Issues Alert on Ephedra Supplements in the USA," *The Lancet* 363 (January 10, 2004): 135.

76. David Cyranoski, "China to Roll Back Regulations for Traditional Medicine Despite Safety Concerns," *Nature,* November 29, 2017, https://www.nature .com/news/china-to-roll-back-regulations-for-traditional-medicine-despite-safety -concerns-1.23038.

77. Laura Landro, "Herbal Supplements Face New Scrutiny," *Wall Street Journal—Eastern Edition,* September 14, 2010.

78. W. Abebe, "Herbal Medication: Potential for Adverse Interactions with Analgesic Drugs," *Journal of Clinical Pharmacy and Therapeutics* 27, no. 6 (2002): 391–401; Ruth Kava, "More Bad News on Herbal Supplements," American Council on Science and Health, October 20, 2017, https://www.acsh.org/news/2017/10/20/more-bad -news-herbal-supplement-11995; Alex Berezow, "Sometimes Herbal Remedies Can Kill

You," American Council on Science and Health, May 9, 2016, https://www.acsh.org/news/2016/05/09/sometimes-herbal-remedies-can-kill-you.

79. Richter, *Herbal Medicine,* 42.

80. E. Ernst, "Adulteration of Chinese Herbal Medicines with Synthetic Drugs: A Systematic Review," *Journal of Internal Medicine* 252, no. 2 (2002): 107–113; W. F. Huang, K. C. Wen, and M. L. Hsiao, "Adulteration by Synthetic Therapeutic Substances of Traditional Chinese Medicines in Taiwan," *Journal of Clinical Pharmacology* 37, no. 4 (1997): 344–350; U.S. China Economic and Security Review Commission, Annual Report to Congress, 2015, 10, https://www.uscc.gov/Annual_Reports/2015-annual-report-congress.

81. "Measles Outbreak," Centers for Disease Control, 2018, https://www.cdc.gov/measles/cases-outbreaks.html; "Reported Cases of Pertussis," Centers for Disease Control, 2015, https://www.cdc.gov/pertussis/surv-reporting/cases-by-year.html; Julia Belluz, "I Was Skeptical That the Anti-Vaccine Movement Was Gaining Traction. Not Anymore," *Vox,* October 3, 2017, https://www.vox.com/science-and-health/2017/2/15/14231266/anti-vaccine-movement-trump.

82. Megan Thielking, "The FDA Has Proposed That Doctors Learn about Acupuncture as an Alternative Treatment for Pain," *Business Insider,* May 10, 2017, http://www.businessinsider.com/fda-doctors-acupuncture-pain-2017-5.

83. Josh Bloom, "All I Want for Christmas Is for People Not to Hurt," American Council on Science and Health, December 12, 2017, https://www.acsh.org/news/2017/12/12/all-i-want-christmas-people-not-hurt-12271.

84. Best Chinese Medicines, https://bestchinesemedicines.com/products/plum-flower-six-flavor-teapills-liu-wei-di-huang-wan.

85. Zhan, *Other-Worldly,* 94; Wu, *Traditional Chinese Medicine in the United States,* 148.

86. Zhan, *Other-Worldly,* 101.

Index

Italic page numbers indicate illustrations.